Soft Tissue Index: Essential Medical and Crash Studies

by Dr. Charles Davis, DC, QME
and
David N. Finley, Esq.

THOMSON
WEST

For Customer Assistance Call 1-800-328-4880

Mat #40591599

ISBN # 978-0-314-98102-8

ABOUT THE AUTHORS

Dr. Charles Davis, DC, QME

Dr. Charles G. Davis is a graduate of Los Angeles College of Chiropractic. He has been involved in sports medicine at the local and national levels and has additional training in traffic collision reconstruction and neurology. Dr. Davis is certified in industrial medicine as a State of California Qualified Medical Evaluator and is a Diplomate in the American Academy of Pain Management.

Dr. Davis is a published author and is recognized for his work on the effects of low speed impacts and on manipulation under anesthesia.

Dr. Davis was awarded *Educator-Researcher of the Year* by The International Chiropractors' Association of California in 2001.

David N. Finley, Esq.

David N. Finley, Esq., has nearly 20 years of combined experience in litigation and legal publishing. He has conducted extensive legal research in State and Federal courts, and has worked up a number of cases for trial and arbitration. He is the creator and co-author of Federal Motions in Limine and Federal Summary Judgment and Related Termination Motions as well as nearly two dozen additional state versions of the *in limine* motion line. He is the creator and former Editor-in-Chief of the national voir dire newsletter, The Jury Expert. He graduated from Hastings College of the Law, where he was a member of the Moot Court Honors Board and an award recipient for best written brief. He is also an adjunct Instructor of Legal Research and Writing at Chapman University School of Law.

HOW TO USE THIS BOOK

This manual is designed to provide quick access into the findings of essential medical and crash studies relevant to attorneys and medical professionals involved in injury litigation. The book is formatted and edited so that users can quickly find published literature to support injury claims or medical opinions.

The findings are organized by category in a logical outline format. Users can quickly locate their desired topic in the Table of Contents or Index. Each grouping contains brief summaries of studies relating to the category in information sought (e.g., whiplash symptoms, head restraint position, brain injury, etc.) and are cited to the source publication and date.

Note that the key finding in most studies will be formatted in bold-faced text to facilitate your research.

ADDITIONAL RESOURCES

Upon locating a relevant study, users can easily utilize online archives or traditional library resources to obtain abstracts or full-text copies of the source articles. Below is a list of popular Internet sites and journals that may be helpful. Fees to download full studies range from $0 to $35 each.

Archives

Pub Med/Medicine: www.ncbi.nlm.nih.gov/entrez/query.fcgi

Highwire Press: highwire.stanford.edu/

Journals

Journal of Bone and Joint Surgery, U.K. Edition: www.jbjs.org.uk/journal

Journal of Bone and Joint Surgery, U.S. Edition: www.efbjs.org

Spine: www.spinejournal.com

Lancet: www.thelancet.com

British Medical Journal: www.bmj.com

Journal of American Medical Association: www.jama.ama-assn.org

New England Journal of Medicine: www.content.nejm.org

Journal of Manipulative and Physiological Therapeutics: www.mosby.com/jmpt

Society of Automotive Engineers: www.sae.org

WESTLAW ELECTRONIC RESEARCH GUIDE

Westlaw—Expanding the Reach of Your Library

Westlaw is West's online legal research service. With Westlaw, you experience the same quality and integrity that you have come to expect from West books, plus quick, easy access to West's vast collection of statutes, case law materials, public records, and other legal resources, in addition to current news articles and business information. For the most current and comprehensive legal research, combine the strengths of West books and Westlaw.

When you research with westlaw.com you get the convenience of the Internet combined with comprehensive and accurate Westlaw content, including exclusive editorial enhancements, plus features found only in westlaw.com such as ResultsPlus™ or StatutesPlus™.

Accessing Databases Using the Westlaw Directory

The Westlaw Directory lists all databases on Westlaw and contains links to detailed information relating to the content of each database. Click Directory on the westlaw.com toolbar. There are several ways to access a database even when you don't know the database identifier. Browse a directory view. Scan the directory. Type all or part of a database name in the Search these Databases box. The Find a Database Wizard can help you select relevant databases for your search. You can access up to ten databases at one time for user-defined multibase searching.

Retrieving a Specific Document

To retrieve a specific document by citation or title on westlaw.com click **Find** on the toolbar to display the Find a Document page. If you are unsure of the correct citation format, type the publication abbreviation, e.g., **xx st** (where xx is a state's two-letter postal abbreviation), in the Enter Citation box and click **Go** to display a fill-in-the-blank template. To retrieve a specific case when you know one or more parties' names, click **Find by Title**.

KeyCite®

KeyCite, the citation research service on Westlaw, makes it easy to trace the history of your case, statute, administrative decision or regulation to determine if there are recent updates, and to find other documents that cite your document. KeyCite will also find pending legislation relating to federal or state statutes. Access the powerful features of KeyCite from the westlaw.com toolbar, the **Links** tab, or KeyCite flags in a document display. KeyCite's red and yellow warning flags tell you at a glance whether your document has negative history. Depth-of-treatment stars help you focus on the most important citing references. KeyCite Alert allows you to monitor the status of your case, statute or rule, and automatically sends you updates at the frequency you specify.

ResultsPlus™

ResultsPlus is a Westlaw technology that automatically suggests additional information related to your search. The suggested materials are accessible by a set of links that appear to the right of your westlaw.com search results:

- Go directly to relevant ALR® articles and Am Jur® annotations.
- Find on-point resources by key number.
- See information from related treatises and law reviews.

StatutesPlus™

When you access a statutes database in westlaw.com you are brought to a powerful Search Center which collects, on one toolbar, the tools that are most useful for fast, efficient retrieval of statutes documents:

- Have a few key terms? Click **Index**.
- Know the common name? Click **Popular Name Table**.
- Familiar with the subject matter? Click **Table of Contents**.
- Have a citation or section number? Click **Find by Citation**.

- Or, simply search with **Natural Language** or **Terms and Connectors**.

When you access a statutes section, click on the **Links** tab for all relevant links for the current document that will also include a KeyCite section with a description of the KeyCite status flag. Depending on your document, links may also include administrative, bill text, and other sources that were previously only available by accessing and searching other databases.

Additional Information

Westlaw is available on the Web at www.westlaw.com.

For search assistance, call the West Reference Attorneys at 1-800-REF-ATTY (1-800-733-2889).

For technical assistance, call West Customer Technical Support at 1-800-WESTLAW (1-800-937-8529).

Summary of Contents

Table of Contents

CHAPTER 1. OVERVIEW OF KEY ISSUES

CHAPTER 2. INJURY MECHANISM & CAUSATION

CHAPTER 3. CRASH STUDY COMPARISONS

CHAPTER 4. VEHICLE DAMAGE & OCCUPANT INJURY

CHAPTER 5. COMMON SYMPTOMS

CHAPTER 6. STRUCTURES INJURED

CHAPTER 7. TISSUE HEALING

CHAPTER 8. PAIN FROM WHIPLASH INJURIES

CHAPTER 9. WHIPLASH DIAGNOSIS

CHAPTER 10. SOFT TISSUE TREATMENT

CHAPTER 11. OUTCOME ASSESSMENTS

CHAPTER 12. PROGNOSIS

CHAPTER 13. GUIDELINES

CHAPTER 14. COMMONLY ENCOUNTERED DEFENSE STUDIES & METHODS

APPENDICES

Chapter 1

Overview of Key Issues

§ 1:1 Anatomy overview

The cervical spine is made up of 7 vertebrae. These are the bones of the spine. Their role is to support and protect the spinal cord. The facet joints provide a mobile link between each vertebra. Similar to other joints, they can wear down and become irritated. Intervertebral discs sit between each vertebra. The disc is made up of 2 parts: annulus (outer ring) and nucleus pulpous (center). The disc's main function is shock absorption. The spinal cord gives out nerve roots at each level of the spine. The nerve roots are responsible for carrying information between the brain and the upper extremity. The vertebral artery is a branch from the subclavian artery. It passes from C6 up to C1. The function of the vertebral artery is to supply the cervical segment of the spinal cord and approximately 2/5 of the brain. Its branches in the cervical spine supply the spinal cord, the vertebrae and the muscles.

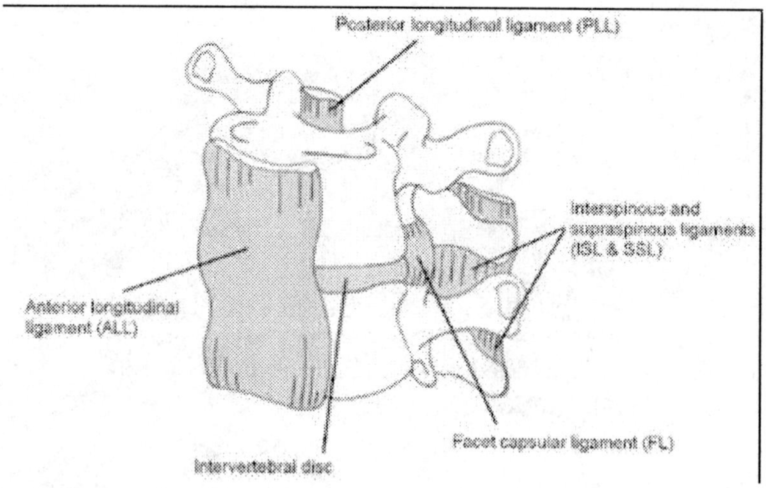

§ 1:2 Types of possible injuries

Whiplash is a general term indicating injury to the vertebral column from sudden acceleration/deceleration forces. A whiplash injury can involve various structures:

- Soft tissue: Strain or tear of tendons, muscles, fascia, discs, or joint capsule.
- Bone: Fracture(s) of the vertebrae.
- Ligament: The subluxation or dislocation of the facet joints due to unstable ligament.
- Spinal cord: Compression, stretching.
- Vertebral artery: Stretching, compression or tear.
- Headaches and TMJ injuries are also very common with whiplash injuries.

§ 1:3 Whiplash as defined by Quebec Task Force in 1995

"Acceleration/deceleration mechanism of energy transfer to the neck, which may result from a motor vehicle accident causing bony or soft tissue injuries, which in turn may lead to a variety of clinical manifestations."

These signs or symptoms could indicate damage beyond the usual injury: dizziness, drop attacks, difficulty with speech, difficulty swallowing and double vision.

§ 1:4 Imaging diagnosis—X-rays

- Show bones of the spine

- May show degenerative changes
- Do not show most soft tissue structures
- Usually the starting point for tests

§ 1:5 Imaging diagnosis—CAT scan (computer assisted tomography)

- X-ray slices or cuts taken at specific levels that are computer enhanced
- Allows one to view bones and some soft tissue
- Used to clearly define complicated bone injury

§ 1:6 Imaging diagnosis—MRI (Magnetic Resonance Imaging)

- Uses magnetic waves to obtain images of bone and soft tissue.
- Shows nerve roots and discs better than a CAT scan.

§ 1:7 Pain scales

Note:

See Chapter 8 for expanded discussion.

Below are several sources for rating pain levels.

- 0 being no pain and 10 the most severe pain.
- no pain.
- 1– 3 — annoying pain, able to perform all activities.
- 4– 7 — pain that slows the patient down; patient able to do activities with modifications, might be unable to do demanding activities.
- 8– 10 — pain level that prohibits some activities. A 9 or 10 would be incapacitating.

See Huskisson EC. Measurement of pain. Lancet. 1974 Nov 9;2(7889):1127–31.

In typical Workers' Compensation systems, there are 4 levels of pain:

- Minimal pain — would constitute an annoyance, no handicap in the performance of activity.
- Slight pain — could be tolerated, but would cause some handicap in the performance of the activity precipitating the pain.
- Moderate pain—could be tolerated, but would cause some marked handicap in performance of the activity precipitating pain.
- Severe pain—would preclude the activity precipitating the pain.

See Title 8. California Code of Regs. § 9727.

AMA Guidelines of Impairment 5th ed. classifies pain as follows:

- Class 1 Mild—Individual's pain is mildly aggravated by activities of daily living (ADL), is able to perform them with few modifications.
- Class 2 Moderate—Moderate difficulties in ADL, must make significant modifications to perform them.
- Class 3 Moderately Severe—Individual can perform ADL only with significant modifications. Unable to perform routine activities (driving a car).
- Class 4 Severe—Individual must get help from others for many ADL, or spend inordinate time in accomplishing them (2 hours to get out of bed and get dressed).

§ 1:8 Pain scales—Pathological pain conditions

- Allodynia is pain from non-painful sensations.
- Hyperalgesia is an increased pain response to a stimulus (a painful stimulus hurts more than it should).

"Acceleration/deceleration mechanism of energy transfer to the neck, which may result from a motor vehicle accident causing bony or soft tissue injuries, which in turn may lead to a variety of clinical manifestations."

These signs or symptoms could indicate damage beyond the usual injury: dizziness, drop attacks, difficulty with speech, difficulty swallowing and double vision.

§ 1:9 Abbreviated Injury Scale (AIS)

In 1971, the Association for the Advancement of Automotive Medicine AAAM (formerly the American Association for Automotive Medicine) and the Society of Automotive Engineers (SAE), under the sponsorship of the AMA, developed a scaling system for injuries sustained in vehicular trauma called the Abbreviated Injury Scale (AIS). By design, the scale is intended to consider the threat to life. Whiplash injuries by definition are Abbreviated Injury Scale (AIS) 1 level injuries. The AIS is a data collection scale for the chance of dying. An AIS 6 means a patient is virtually unsurvivable. The AIS does not take into count how long a patient will have pain and/or disability.

Below are the AIS categories:

Code	Category	
1	Minor	0% risk of death
2	Moderate	0.1% to 0.4%
3	Serious	0.8% to 2.3%
4	Severe	10%
5	Critical	(survival uncertain) 50%
6	Maximum	(virtually unsurvivable)

AIS 1 Includes most soft-tissue sprain strain injuries to the cervical, dorsal, and lumbar spine regions. Includes minor superficial lacerations, contusions, or abrasions. Includes disc bulging cases. No neurological deficits.

AIS 2 Includes disc herniations without nerve root damage, radiculopathy, or neurologic deficits. Incomplete brachial plexus or cauda equine injury with transient signs.

AIS 3 Includes disc herniations with nerve root damage, radiculopathy, and disc rupture.

AIS 4 Lacerations to major arteries or veins with neurologic deficit and strokes.

AIS 5 Complete cord syndrome C4 and below.

AIS 6 Complete cord syndrome C3 or above.

"Acceleration/deceleration mechanism of energy transfer to the neck, which may result from a motor vehicle accident causing bony or soft tissue injuries, which in turn may lead to a variety of clinical manifestations."

These signs or symptoms could indicate damage beyond the usual injury: dizziness, drop attacks, difficulty with speech, difficulty swallowing and double vision.

Chapter 2

Injury Mechanism & Causation

KeyCite®: Cases and other legal materials listed in KeyCite Scope can be researched through the KeyCite service on Westlaw®. Use KeyCite to check citations for form, parallel references, prior and later history, and comprehensive citator information, including citations to other decisions and secondary materials.

§ 2:1 Overview

In experimental studies and autopsy studies, soft tissue injuries have been found in a number of different structures and locations in the neck region. Neck injury may appear as a result of a whiplash trauma to muscles, ligaments, facet joints, discs, nerve tissue, etc. Several injury types may be present in the same patient at the same time.

There is a wide variation in human response and tolerance data. This is due to the large biological variations among humans and the effects of aging. Average values are useful in design but cannot be applied to individuals. See King et al. Fundamentals of impact biomechanics: Part I-Biomechanics of the head, neck, and thorax. Annu Rev Biomed Eng. 2000;2:55–81.

The following sections summarize the findings of many of the most important studies relating to typical trauma arising in low-speed cases.

§ 2:2 Intervertebral motion—The "S-shaped" curve—Description

Several studies have focused on the detailed motion of the cervical spinal segments during rear-end impact loading. These studies show that there is flexion in the upper cervical spine and extension in the lower cervical spine. The intervertebral motion appears to deviate from normal physiologic human neck motion.

The 1997 Grauer study showed that **whiplash produces**

an "S-shaped" curve of the neck with hyperextension at lower levels. This test used a head-neck model of cadavers with the following findings: In a rear-end impact, the neck forms an S-shaped configuration at 50 to 75 ms following accelerating motion. This time period shows cervical spine flexion at the upper levels and greater extension at the lower levels than in the later stages of maximum extension of the head. At 100–125 ms the cervical spine reverts to a C-shape curvature of the entire cervical spine. The physiological extension limits were exceeded at the intervetebral levels of C6–7 and C7–T1 at all four test levels (2.5g, 4.5g, 6.5g, and 8.5g forces). Physiological limits were also exceeded at C2–3 and C4–5 at 2.5g force, and C4–5 at 6.5g. Therefore, even as there is no gross hyperextension/hyperflexion with ranges of motion in whiplash experiments, segmental levels may exceed physiological limits. See Grauer JN, Panjabi MM, Cholewicki J, Nibu K, Dvorak J. Whiplash produces an S-shaped curvature of the neck with hyperextension at lower levels. Spine. 1997 Nov 1;22(21):2489–94.

In a study with human volunteers, the S-shaped curve was also found. The cervical spine showed an initial flexion and C6 rotated backward before the upper vertebrae in the early phase. After C6 reached its maximum rotation angle, C5 was induced to extend. As the upper segments went into flexion, and the lower segments into extension, the cervical spine took an S-shaped position. This showed an upward-shifted C5–C6 instantaneous axis of rotation. This motion differs from normal extension motion and is probably related to the injury mechanism. Instead of one vertebra gliding over another, the instantaneous axis of rotation raises, allowing for the posterior facets to slam together. *"This is a non-physiological motion of the vertebral segments."* On extension, the cervical facets collide, and there is opening of the anterior (front) of the vertebral segment. See Ono K, Kaneoka K, Wittek A, Kajzer J. Cervical injury mechanism based on the analysis of human cervical vertebral motion and head-neck-torso kinematics during low-speed rear impacts. 41st Annual Stapp Car Crash Conference, 1997, Florida, USA, SAE paper no. 973340 (Kaneoka K, Ono K, Inami S, Hayashi K. Motion analysis of cervical vertebrae during whiplash loading. Spine. 1999 Apr 15;24(8):763–9; Ono K, Kaneoka K, Wittk A, Kajzer J. 41st Cervical injury mechanism based on the analysis of human cervical vertebral motion and head-neck-torso kinematics during low-speed rear impact. Stapp Car Crash Conference, Lake Buena Vista, Fla 1997; Society for Automotive Engineers paper no. 973340:339–56.

Note that the pinching of the lower cervical facet joints may lead to local tissue injury and nociceptive pain. Cusick JF, Pintar FA, Yoganandan N. Whiplash syndrome: kinematic factors influencing pain patterns. Spine. 2001 Jun 1;26(11):1252–8.

Recent results obtained by Deng from cadavers and through the use of a bi-axial high-speed X-ray camera device, at a framing rate of 250 per second, demonstrated that **compression began early in the impact, even if the seat back was vertical, and that there were both relative translation and rotation between adjacent cervical vertebrae**. Deng B. 1999 Kinematics of human cadaver cervical spine during low-speed rear-end impacts. PhD. thesis. Detroit: Wayne State Univ.

See also Kaneoka K, Ono K, Inami S, Hayashi K. Motion analysis of cervical vertebrae during whiplash loading. Spine. 1999 Apr 15;24(8):763–9; Panjabi MM, Wang JL, Delson N. Neck injury criterion based on intervertebral motions and its evaluation using an instrumented neck dummy. 1999 International IRCOBI Conference on the Biomechanics of Impact, 1999, Barcelona, Spain, SAE paper no: 1999-13-0043; Winkelstein BA, Nightingale RW, Richardson WJ, Myers BS. Cervical facet joint mechanics: Its application to whiplash injury. 43rd Stapp Car Crash Conference, 1999, California, USA, SAE Paper no. 99SC15; Yoganandan, N; Pintar, F.A. Mechanics of Head Ache and Neck Pain in Whiplash. In: Eds. Yoganandan N, Pintar FA.: Frontiers in Whiplash Trauma. IOS Press, 2000. The Netherlands, ISBN 158603 012 4, pp. 173–185; Deng B, Begeman PC, Yang KH, Tashman S, King AI. Kinematics of Human Cadaver Cervical Spine During Low-Speed Rear-End Impacts. STAPP Car Crash Journal, 2000; 44:171–188.

§ 2:3 Intervertebral motion—The "S-shaped" curve—Crash studies relating to S-shaped curve

Muscular measurement of the deep cervical muscle, semispinalis capitis, had its maximum contraction during the rebound phase. (Phases: extension, head-impact, rebound). Additional findings that Injury does not relate to Delta-V. See Hell W, Schick S, Langwieder K, Zellmer H. Biomechanics of cervical spine injuries in rear-end car impacts: influence of car seats and possible evaluation criteria. Traffic Injury Prevention 2002;3:127–40.

During the rebound movement of the head, there is eccentric contraction of the deep muscles. One of the deep muscles is the multifidus, and it covers part of the facet joint. Research has indicated that there is enough force to cause a sub-catastrophic injury to the facet joint. See Winkelstein BA, McLendon RE, Barbir A, Myers BS. An anatomical investigation of the human cervical facet capsule, quantifying muscle insertion area. J Anat. 2001 Apr;198 (Pt 4):455–61.

The S-shaped configuration occurs in the lateral axis following a side impact. See Harrison DE, Harrison DD, Cailliet R, Janik TJ, Troyanovich SJ. Cervical coupling during lateral head translations creates an S-configuration. Clin Biomech (Bristol, Avon). 2000 Jul; 15(6):436–40.

Using X-ray movies of volunteer neck motion at 90 frames per second, Matsushita et al found that **the neck was in compression due to the upward ramping of the torso on an inclined seat back, and that there was more relative rotation in the lower cervical vertebrae (C5–6), leading to the hypothesis that the injury could be in the facet capsules in low-speed rear-end collisions**. See Matsushita T, Sato TB, Hirabyashi K, Fujimura S, Asazuma T, Takatori T. X-ray study of the human neck motion due to head inertia loading. Proceedings Stapp Conf. 38th, 1994, Fort Lauderdale, Florida. # 942208 Warrendale, PA: Society Automotive Engineers.

§ 2:4 Intervertebral motion—The "S-shaped" curve—Testing on whole body cadavers

In testing with whole body cadavers, complex motion of the spine was also found. Compression, tension, shear force, flexion and extension all contribute to stretch the facet capsular ligaments. Shear force dominated the capsular deformation at the lower cervical levels, while flexion-tension was the predominant factor in determining the capsular stretch at higher cervical levels. See Luan F, Yang KH, Deng B, Begeman PC, Tashman S, King AI. Qualitative analysis of neck kinematics during low-speed rear-end impact. Clin Biomech (Bristol, Avon). 2000 Nov; 15(9):649–57.

During a rear-end impact, the neck kinematics are quite complicated and can be roughly divided into three stages, as adapted from the Luan study, referenced above:

1) **The first 100 ms after the impact (0.00 sec – 0.100 sec), flexural deformity of the neck is observed along with a loss of lordosis. The lordotic neck becomes straight due to flexion.** Only minimal relative rotations (flexion/extension) are observed for the first 50 ms. After 50

ms, both upper and lower parts of the cervical spine are subjected to a flexion movement. The shear force is transmitted initially though the lower levels and eventually through the upper levels, but does not reach the superior end of the cervical spine. The shear formation also contributes to the straightening of the neck. The axial force then changes from compressive to tensile at about 60 ms (0.060 sec).

2) **In the next 30 ms, the cervical spine assumes an S-shaped curve as the lower cervical spine begins to extend and gradually cause the upper spine to extend.** Eventually, the straightened neck once becomes lordotic. An extension moment acts at the lower levels, while a flexion moment acts at the upper levels. Shear forces also act at all levels of the cervical spine along with a tensile force.

3) **During the final stage, the entire neck is in extension due to moments at both ends.** Shear forces and tensile axial forces continue to act at all levels. At 180 ms (0.180 sec) after the onset of impact, the head reaches its maximum extension and begins to rebound. Subsequently, the extension moment at the upper neck is reduced.

Compression of the neck is due to the straightening of the thoracic spine and possible upward ramping of the torso on the seat back during the initial stage of the impact. Tension occurs immediately after compression ends. Tension occurs in the neck because of the relatively faster upward motion of the head with respect to the neck. The torso moves faster than the head in the horizontal direction as it drags the head forward by stretching the neck, causing the 'head lag' phenomenon. Shear forces are generated in the neck when the torso moves forward due to an impact from behind. The shear force is transmitted from the lower cervical vertebrae to the upper ones one level at a time. This shearing motion contributes to the straightening of the lordotic curve of the neck and to the stretching of the fact capsular ligaments.

The shear moment is greater at higher cervical levels due to a longer movement arm. It compresses the anterior portion of the discs and stretches the posterior portion. It takes approximately 130 ms to transit from full flexion to full extension.

Neck forces at the occipital condyle approximate 250 newtons (56 lbs.) with peak sled acceleration of 5.18 g, simulating a 1.98 m/s (4.46 mph) rear-end impact.

Compression, **tension**, **shear force**, **flexion** and **extension** all contribute to stretch the facet capsular ligaments. Shear force dominated the capsular deformation at the lower cervical levels, while flexion-tension was the predominant factor in determining the capsular stretch at higher cervical levels. Neck kinematics during whiplash are complicated and greatly influenced by the rotation of the thoracic spine.

See Luan F, Yang KH, Deng B, Begeman PC, Tashman S, King AI. Qualitative analysis of neck kinematics during low-speed rear-end impact. Clin Biomech (Bristol, Avon). 2000 Nov; 15(9):649–57.

§ 2:5 Tissue injuries

In a low-velocity impact, the soft tissue is seldom torn completely. It is most likely stretched beyond its elastic limit, resulting in an incomplete injury. Panjabi MM, Cholewicki J, Nibu K, Babat LB, Dvorak J. Simulation of whiplash trauma using whole cervical spine specimens. Spine. 1998 Jan 1;23(1):17–24. A subfailure injury to a ligament significantly alters its mechanical properties. Panjabi MM, Yoldas E, Oxland TR, Crisco JJ 3rd. Subfailure injury of the rabbit anterior cruciate ligament. J Orthop Res. 1996 Mar;14(2):216–22. Many subfailure injuries have potential injury consequence. Herkowitz HN, Rothman RH. Subacute instability of the cervical spine. Spine. 1984 May–Jun;9(4):348–57.

Incomplete injuries of the ligaments are more prevalent than complete injuries. The incomplete injury is a subfailure stretch delivered at high speed. Panjabi MM, Courtney TW. High-speed subfailure stretch of rabbit anterior cruciate ligament: changes in elastic, failure and viscoelastic characteristics. Clin Biomech (Bristol, Avon). 2001 May;16(4):334–40; Panjabi MM, Crisco JJ 3rd, Lydon C, Dvorak J. The mechanical properties of human alar and transverse ligaments at slow and fast extension rates. Clin Biomech (Bristol, Avon). 1998 Mar;13(2):112–120.

A single application of whiplash acceleration pulse can induce soft tissue-related and ligament-related alterations to cervical spine structures. Structural alterations in the lower cervical spine included stretch and tear of the ligamentum flavum, anulus disruption, anterior longitudinal ligament rupture, and zygopophysial joint compromise with tear of the capsular ligaments. Yoganandan N, Cusick JF, Pintar FA, Rao RD. Whiplash injury determination with conventional spine imaging and cryomicrotomy. Spine. 2001 Nov 15;26(22):2443–8.

According to medical literature, automobile collisions can cause injury to facets, discs, muscles, nerves, liga-

ments, vertebrae, vertebral artery and even the brain. *See* Malanga GA. Cervical flexion-extension/whiplash injuries. Spine State of the Art Reviews. Hanley & Belfus, Philadelphia, 1998, Vol 12, No 2; Barnsley L, Lord S, Bogduk N. Whiplash injury. Pain. 1994 Sep;58(3):283–307; Foreman SM, Croft AC eds. Whiplash injuries: The Cervical Acceleration/Deceleration Syndrome. 3 ed. Philadelphia: Lippincott Williams & Wilkins; 2002.

The S-shaped phase shift of the spine may also have effects in vertebral artery. See Nibu K, Cholewicki J, Panjabi MM, Babat LB, Grauer JN, Kothe R, Dvorak J. Dynamic elongation of the vertebral artery during an in vitro whiplash simulation; Eur Spine J. 1997;6(4):286–9; Seric V, Blazic-Cop N, Demarin V. Haemodynamic changes in patients with whiplash injury measured by transcranial Doppler sonography (TCD). Coll Antropol. 2000 Jun;24(1):197–204; Chung YS, Han DH. Vertebrobasilar dissection: a possible role of whiplash injury in its pathogenesis. Neurol Res. 2002 Mar;24(2):129–38.

The anatomical basis of spinal pain arises primarily in the discs, zygapophyseal joints and spinal muscles. There are no scientific data, however, that sustain the belief that muscles may be a source of chronic pain. On the other hand, controlled studies have shown how common discogenic pain and zygapophyseal joint pain are. Cervical zygapophyseal joint pain accounts for more than 50% of chronic neck pain after whiplash. Collectively, lumbar zygapophyseal joint pain, internal disk disruption and sacroiliac joint pain account for nearly 70% of chronic low-back pain. Bogduk N. The anatomical basis for spinal pain syndromes. J Manipulative Physiol Ther. 1995 Nov–Dec;18(9):603–5.

Injuries have been reported in several ligaments, the intervertebral discs and the facet joint structures. Yoganandan N, Pintar FA, Stemper BD. Schlick MB, Philippens M, Wismans J. Biomechanics of Human Occupants in Simulated Rear Crashes: Documentation of Neck injuries and Comparison of Injury Criteria. Stapp Car Crash Journal 2000; 44: 189–204.

Indications of muscle injury due to eccentric muscle loading in the early phase of the neck motion in rear impacts have been found. Siegmund GP. Brault, JR. Role of Cervical Muscles During Whiplash. In: Eds. Yoganandan, N; Pintar, F.A.: Frontiers in Whiplash Trauma. 2000, IOS Press, The Netherlands, ISBN 1 58603 012 4; Brault JR, Siegmund

GP, Wheeler JB. Cervical muscle response during whiplash: evidence of a lengthening muscle contraction. Clin Biomech (Bristol, Avon). 2000 Jul;15(6):426–35.

Eccentric muscle contraction of the multifidus muscle may cause damage to the facet capsule. Winkelstein BA, McLendon RE, Barbir A, Myers BS. An anatomical investigation of the human cervical facet capsule, quantifying muscle insertion area. J Anat. 2001 Apr;198(Pt 4):455–61.

Interstitial hemorrhage in cervical dorsal root ganglia was reported in an autopsy study of victims who had sustained severe inertial neck loading during impacts to the torso or to the head. The structures around the ganglia were mostly uninjured. These findings correlate to experimental findings in pigs of nerve cell membrane dysfunction in cervical spinal root ganglia. Taylor JR, Twomey LT, Kakulas BA. Dorsal root ganglion injuries in 109 blunt trauma fatalities. Injury. 1998 Jun;29(5):335–9; Ortengren T, Hansson HA, Lovsund P, Svensson MY, Suneson A, Saljo A. Membrane leakage in spinal ganglion nerve cells induced by experimental whiplash extension motion: a study in pigs. J Neurotrauma. 1996 Mar;13(3):171–80; Svensson MY, Bostrom O, Davidsson J, Hansson HA, Haland Y, Lovsund P, Suneson A, Saljo A. Neck injuries in car collisions—a review covering a possible injury mechanism and the development of a new rear-impact dummy. Accid Anal Prev. 2000 Mar;32(2):167–75.

Soft tissue injury was defined as a significant increase ($P < 0.05$) in the intervertebral flexibility parameters of neutral zone or range of motion resulting from simulated whiplash. The injury threshold, based on the peak T1 horizontal acceleration, was **5 g** and the mode of injury was extension as evidenced by a 39.8% increase in the C5–C6 extension neutral zone. At higher accelerations, the injuries spread among the lower cervical spine. The neutral zone was a more sensitive parameter than the range of motion for determining the injury threshold. **A rear-end collision is most likely to injure the lower cervical spine by intervertebral hyperextension.** Ito S, Ivancic PC, Panjabi MM, Cunningham BW. Soft Tissue Injury Threshold During Simulated Whiplash: A Biomechanical Investigation. Spine 2004;29:979–987.

§ 2:6 Facet joint injury

Since about 1995, the facet joint of the cervical spine has been the center of attention in the study of whiplash injuries. It has been stated that as many as 60% of chronic whiplash patients' pain could be attributed to the facets. A number of many respected engineers from around the world have demonstrated that the cervical spine undergoes abnormal motion during low speed crashes, and this abnormal motion may be responsible for chronic whiplash symptoms.

A head turned posture increases facet capsular ligament neck strain compared to a neutral head posture — a finding consistent with the greater symptom severity and duration observed in whiplash neck injury patients who have their head turned at impact.

A review of whiplash-type injuries indicates most minor injuries will heal in 2–3 months and 25% will become chronic. Injuries involving the disc, zygapophysial (facet) joints or alar ligaments will not resolve spontaneously and will become chronic. These patients may improve over a period of 2 years and are unlikely to improve after 2 years. Barnsley L, Lord S, Bogduk N. Whiplash injury. Pain. 1994 Sep;58(3):283–307.

In rear-end impacts, axial compression together with shear force may be responsible for injuries to the cervical facet joints. The geometry of the cervical spine zygapophysial (facet) joints plays an important role. Cervical zygapophysial (facet) joint pain is common among patients with chronic neck pain after whiplash. Lord SM, Barnsley L, Wallis BJ, Bogduk N. Chronic cervical zygapophysial joint pain after whiplash. A placebo-controlled prevalence study. Spine. 1996 Aug 1;21(15):1737–44.

The pinching of the lower cervical facet joints may lead to local tissue injury and nociceptive pain. Cusick JF, Pintar FA, Yoganandan N. Whiplash syndrome: kinematic factors influencing pain patterns. Spine. 2001 Jun 1;26(11):1252–8.

The forces acting on the facet capsular ligament, due to vertebral motions and eccentric muscle contractions, can be as high as 66 N. (N = Newton, which is equal to about 0.225 pounds.)

The multifidus muscle insertion was found to cover 22.4 ± 9.6% of the capsule area. These anatomical data provide quantitative evidence of substantial muscle insertions into the cervical facet capsular ligament and provide a possible mechanism for injury to this ligament and the facet joint as a whole. Winkelstein BA, McLendon RE, Barbir A, Myers BS. An anatomical investigation of the human cervical facet capsule, quantifying muscle insertion area. J Anat. 2001 Apr;198(Pt 4):455–61.

Cervical facet capsular ligaments may be injured under loading conditions similar to those generated during whiplash (rear-end 8km/h [5mph] rear-end collision). Siegmund GP, Myers BS, Davis MB, Bohnet HF, Winkelstein BA. Human cervical motion segmental flexibility and facet capsular ligament strain under combined posterior shear, extension and axial compression. Stapp Car Crash Journal 2000; 44:159–170.

§ 2:7 Facet joint injury—Facet joint mechanics

The Siegmund study showed that unembalmed human cadaveric cervical spines were free from other obvious spinal disorders or diseases that could have adversely affected their structural properties. The cervical facet capsular ligaments may be injured under whiplash-like loads of combined shear, bending, and compression. The results provide a mechanical basis for injury caused by whiplash loading. *See* Siegmund GP, Myers BS, Davis MB, Bohnet HF, Winkelstein BA. Mechanical evidence of cervical facet capsule injury during whiplash: a cadaveric study using combined shear, compression, and extension loading. Spine. 2001 Oct 1;26(19):2095–101.

Specific findings from this study include the following:

"Cervical motion segments were quasi-statically tested using combined loads similar to those measured during whiplash loading to quantify intervertebral flexibility and maximum principal strain in the facet capsule." The range of axial compressive preloads used in this study were comparable to those used during staged rear-end collisions with human volunteers. **"The applied forces and moments used in the current study were similar to, and did not exceed, those that might be expected in vivo under whiplash loading at a speed change of 8 km/h." [8 km/h X .62 = 5 mph].** On average, the facet capsule is not injured by the intervertebral loads and motions that have been observed in human subjects exposed to staged rear-end collisions. But, **"of considerable interest, however, were the two specimens that exceeded their subcatastrophic failure strains under the whiplash-like loads of the flexibility tests."** "These findings suggest that capsular ligament fibers within these two specimens experienced subcatastrophic failures under the whiplash-like loading of the flexibility test." "Given the presence of nociceptive nerve endings in the cervical facet capsule ligament, **such subcatastrophic failures suggest a mechanical hypothesis for the development of pain observed in some clinical populations**."

"Assuming the ratio of flexibility strains to initial failure strains is normally distributed, then approximately **7.3% of specimens exposed to these spinal loads will undergo subcatastrophic failure of a facet capsular ligament.**" "In the current sample, 2 of 13 (15%) specimens and 2 of 7 donors (28%) reached this level." "Therefore, based on the data presented here, the risk of facet capsular ligament injury may be related more to individual differences in subcatastrophic failure thresholds than to the magnitude of the loads to which an individual is exposed."

The Siegmund study was done without the effects of the full spine. Luan et al. found that neck kinematic during whiplash is complicated and greatly influenced by the rotation of the thoracic spine, which would add more variables and more complex motions. **The Siegumd study was also done at a speed less than what would have occurred during a whiplash injury.**

Peak facet joint compression and facet joint sliding exceeded the physiologic limits at 3.5 and 5 g, respectively. Capsular ligament strains exceeded the physiologic strains at 6.5 g and were largest in the lower cervical spine. Peak facet joint compression occurred at maximum intervertebral extension, whereas peak capsular ligament strain occurred after the maximum intervertebral extension had been reached as the facet joint was returning to its neutral position. **Facet joint components are at risk for injury during whiplash due to facet joint compression and excessive capsular ligament strain.** Pearson AM, Ivancic PC, Ito S. Panjabi MM. Facet Joint Kinematics and Injury Mechanisms During Simulated Whiplash. Spine 2004;29:390–397.

§ 2:8 Neck injury risk—Foreman and Croft study

Foreman and Croft list the following injury risks in automobile accidents:

§ 2:9 Neck injury risk—Foreman and Croft study—Risk for acute injury

1) Female gender
2) History of neck injury
3) Poor head restraint geometry/tall occupant
4) Rear impact
5) Use of seat belts/shoulder harness
6) Body mass index/head neck index (decreased risk with increasing mass and neck size)

7) Out-of-position occupant (leaning forward/slumped)
8) Non-failure of seat back
9) Having the head turned at impact
10) Non-awareness of impending impact
11) Increasing age (middle age and beyond)
12) Front vs. rear seat position
13) Impact by vehicle of greater mass (25% greater)
14) Crash speed under 10 mph.

§ 2:10 Neck injury risk—Foreman and Croft study—Risk for chronic whiplash

1) Female gender
2) Body mass index in females only
3) Immediate/early onset of symptoms (within 12 hours) and/or severe initial symptoms
4) Ligamentous instability
5) Initial back pain
6) Greater subjective cognitive impairment
7) Greater number of initial symptoms
8) Use of seatbelt shoulder harness
9) Initial physical findings of limited range of motion
10) Initial loss of ROM
11) Initial neurological symptoms
12) Past history of neck pain or headache
13) Initial degenerative changes seen on radiographs
14) Loss or reversal of cervical lordosis
15) Increasing age (middle age and beyond)
16) Front seat position

See Foreman SM, Croft AC eds. Whiplash Injuries: The Cervical Acceleration/Deceleration Syndrome. 3 ed. Philadelphia: Lippincott, Williams & Wilkins; 2002.

§ 2:11 Neck injury risk—Other studies

The neck injury risk differs significantly between different car models of similar size in rear impacts. Krafft M. (2000): Influence of velocity change and car acceleration on short- and long-term disability risk in rear impact. In: Eds. Yoganandan, N; Pintar, F.A.: Frontiers in Whiplash Trauma. IOS Press, The Netherlands, ISBN 1 58603 012 4, pp.99–117.

Taller drivers have an increased injury risk in rear impacts. Jakobsson, L.; Norin, H.; Isaksson-Hellman, I. (2000) Parameters Influencing the Risk of AIS1 Neck Injuries in

Frontal and Side Impacts. Proc. IRCOBI Conf. Montpellier, France, September 20–22, pp. 235–247.

Phase 1, flexion and compression injuries over pretensioned lap and shoulder belts resulted in severe thoracoabdominal and spine injuries in restrained occupants, with a high associated mortality. Increased lower extremity injuries from additional force loads into bolsters and panels were also noted. Phase 2, the majority (>50%) of front-seat occupants was partially reclined. Fully reclined occupants were younger (30 vs. 39 years, $p < 0.0001$), more likely to be male (70% vs. 49%, $p < 0.0001$) and less likely to wear a seat belt (58% vs. 78%, $p < 0.0001$) than upright or partially reclined occupants. Mortality was increased in both partially (adjusted odds ratio 1.15, 95% confidence interval 1.05–1.26) and fully reclined occupants (adjusted odds ratio 1.77, 95% confidence interval 1.09–2.88).

The reclined position is associated with increased occupant mortality in motor vehicle collisions.

Dissanaike S, Kaufman R, Mack CD, Mock C, Bulger E. The effect of reclined seats on mortality in motor vehicle collisions. J Trauma. 2008 Mar;64(3):614–9.

§ 2:12 Muscle activation

The joints of the cervical spine undergo maximum deformation during the early part of the whiplash acceleration when the muscle tone activations are minimal or absent; Deng B, Begeman P, Yang K, et al. Kinematics of human cadaver cervical spine during low-speed rear-end impacts. Stapp Car Crash J. 2000;171–88.

Because the spine cannot support itself, and depending on the sample tested, the amount of force to produce failure of the ligaments can be low. Muscles are needed for protection, and the deep extensor muscles may have a different response than superficial muscles. Kunita K, Fujiwara K. Relationship between reaction time of eye movement and activity of the neck extensors. Eur J Appl Physiol Occup Physiol. 1996;74(6):553–7.

The deep, segmental muscles are under non-voluntary control. The bigger muscles that cross over multiple segments are under voluntary control. In sled acceleration testing, the average muscle response was first in the levator scapulae (73.2 ms, 15.2 SD) followed by the sternocleidomastoid (73.3 ms, 14.7 SD). Magnusson ML, Pope MH, Hasselquist L, Bolte KM, Ross M, Goel VK, Lee JS, Spratt K, Clark CR, Wilder DG. Cervical electromyographic activity during low-speed rear impact. Eur Spine J. 1999;8(2):118–25.

Testing has indicated it takes approximately 200 ms to develop sufficient muscle force to limit motion. Tennyson SA, Mital NK, King AI. Electromyographic signals of the spinal musculature during +Gz impact acceleration. Orthop Clin North Am. 1977 Jan;8(1):97–119. It appears that the muscle reflex contraction would be too little and too late to restrict motion. Foust DR, Chaffin DB, Snyder RG, Baum JK. Cervical range of motion and dynamic response and strength of cervical muscles. 17th Stapp car crash conference. Oklahoma City (OK): Society of Automotive Engineers; 1973.

It takes time for protective muscle to contract. Laboratory studies using animals have demonstrated the time to develop muscle forces to be approximately 200 msec. The reaction time of the experimental animal is shorter than that of the human. Tennyson SA, Mital NK, King AI. Electromyographic signals of the spinal musculature during +Gz impact acceleration. Orthop Clin North Am. 1977 Jan;8(1):97–119.

The rate of change of accelerations, and not the amplitude of the body or head, might be a critical factor in why sensorimotor control sometimes fails to protect the neck. 1/3 of the subjects displayed either a fully passive behavior or inappropriate muscle activity. Vibert N, MacDougall HG, de Waele C, Gilchrist DP, Burgess AM, Sidis A, Migliaccio A, Curthoys IS, Vidal PP. Variability in the control of head movements in seated humans: a link with whiplash injuries? J Physiol. 2001 May 1;532(Pt 3):851–68.

§ 2:13 Variables affecting injury—Turned or rotated head

The effects of pretorque direction, compression, and posterior shear on motion segment motion and maximum principal strain in the capsule were examined using repeated-measures analyses of variance. Axial pretorque affected peak capsule strains more than axial compression or posterior shear. Peak strains reached 34% +/- 18% and were higher for pretorques toward rather than away from the facet capsule (i.e.-, head rotation to the right caused higher strain in the right facet capsule).

Compared to previously-reported data for these specimens, peak capsule strains with a pretorque were double those without a pretorque (17% +/- 6%) and not significantly different from those at partial failure of the ligament (35% +/- 21%). **Axial rotation doubles the maximum principal strain (MPS) in the capsular ligament compared to the neutral posture. A head-turned posture increases facet capsular**

ligament strain compared to a neutral head posture-a finding consistent with the greater symptom severity and duration observed in whiplash patients who have their head turned at impact.

Siegmund GP, Davis MB, Quinn KP, Hines E, Myers BS, Ejima S, Ono K, Kamiji K, Yasuki T, Winkelstein BA. Head-turned postures increase the risk of cervical facet capsule injury during whiplash. Spine. 2008 Jul 1;33(15):1643–9.

This study documents intervertebral foramen width, height, and area narrowing during simulated head-turned rear impact in a whole-cervical spine model with muscle force replication and a surrogate head. "The cervical nerve root and ganglion complex are anatomically localized within the medial zone of the intervertebral foramen and thus, are at risk for compression injury." "Foraminal width narrowing due to head-turned rear impact can potentially compress the cervical ganglia and nerve roots causing injury and leading to chronic radicular symptoms, especially in individuals with stenotic spines." The mean age of the study's specimens was 80.2 years and therefore, typically stiffer than those of the younger population most likely to suffer whiplash trauma. Thus, "the peak dynamic foraminal narrowing data acquired in the present study are conservative, relative to those that might be obtained in a younger population."

In a stenotic foramen, the injury risk greatly increases and extends to include the C3–4 through C6–7 foramina and nerve roots. The potential "increased severity of C3–4 through C6–7 injury resulting from head-turned compared with head-forward rear impact may result in more severe acute symptoms of radicular irritation, including increased dermatomal pain, paresthesias, numbness, and weakness." This "increase in nerve injury and symptom severity may also lead to a worse clinical prognosis, including increased chronic radicular symptoms." Head-turned rear impact causes ganglion compression in nonstenotic C5–6 and C6–7 foramina, and the injury risk greatly increases and extends to the C3–7 foramina and nerve roots, in cases involving a stenotic foramen. "The greater potential severity of ganglion injury observed as a result of head-turned compared with head-forward rear impact is supported by clinical and epidemiological observations." **"Chronic radicular symptoms reported by whiplash-injured patients may be caused by dynamic cervical ganglion or nerve root compressive injury or repeated and less severe compression due to cervical instability."** Tominaga Y, Maak TG, Ivancic PC, Panjabi MM, Cunningham BW.

Head-turned rear impact causing dynamic cervical intervertebral foramen narrowing: implications for ganglion and nerve root injury. J Neurosurg Spine. 2006 May;4(5):380–7.

A rotated head posture at the time of vehicular rear impact has been correlated with a **higher incidence and greater severity of chronic radicular symptoms** than accidents occurring with the occupant facing forward. No studies have been conducted to quantify the dynamic changes in foramen dimensions during head-turned rear-impact collisions. The objectives of this study were to quantify the changes in foraminal width, height, and area during head-turned rear-impact collisions and to determine if dynamic narrowing causes potential cervical nerve root or ganglion impingement. The authors subjected a whole cervical spine model with muscle force replication and a surrogate head to simulated head-turned rear impacts of 3.5, 5, 6.5, and 8 g following a noninjurious 2 g baseline acceleration. Continuous dynamic foraminal width, height, and area narrowing were recorded, and peaks were determined during each impact; these data were then statistically compared with those obtained at baseline. The authors observed significant increases ($p < 0.05$) in mean peak foraminal width narrowing values, greater than baseline values, of up to 1.8 mm in the left C5–6 foramen at 8 g. At the right C2–3 foramen, the mean peak dynamic foraminal height was significantly narrower than baseline when subjected to rear impacts of 5 and 6.5 g, but no significant increases in foraminal area were observed. Analysis of the results indicated that the greatest potential for cervical ganglion compression injury existed at C5–6 and C6–7. Greater potential for ganglion compression injury existed at C3–4 and C4–5 during head-turned rear impact than during head-forward rear impact. Extrapolation of present results indicated potential ganglion compression in patients with a non-stenotic foramen at C5–6 and C6–7; in patients with a stenotic foramen the injury risk greatly increases and spreads to include the C3–4 through C6–7 as well as C4–5 through C6–7 nerve roots. Ivancic PC, Ito S, Tominaga Y, Carlson EJ, Rubin W, Panjabi MM. Effect of rotated head posture on dynamic vertebral artery elongation during simulated rear impact. Clin Biomech (Bristol, Avon). 2006 Mar;21(3):213–20.

Head-turned whole cervical spine model was stabilized with muscle force replication and subjected to simulated rear impacts of increasing severity. Multiplanar flexibility testing evaluated any resulting injury to identify and quantify cervical spine soft tissue injury and injury threshold acceleration for head-turned rear impact, and to compare these data with previously published head-forward rear and frontal impact results. Epidemiologically and clinically, head-turned rear impact is associated with increased injury severity and symptom duration, as compared to forward facing. It appears that no biomechanical data exist to explain this finding. Six human cervical spine specimens (C0–T1) with head-turned and muscle force replication were rear impacted at 3.5, 5, 6.5, and 8 g, and flexibility tests were performed before and after each impact. Soft tissue injury was defined as a significant increase ($P < 0.05$) in intervertebral flexibility above baseline. Injury threshold was the lowest T1 horizontal peak acceleration that caused the injury. The injury threshold acceleration was 5 g with injury occurring in extension or axial rotation at C3–C4 through C7–T1, excluding C6–C7. Following 8 g, 3-plane injury occurred in extension and axial rotation at C5–C6, while 2-plane injury occurred at C7–T1. **Head-turned rear impact** caused significantly greater injury at C0–C1 and C5–C6, as compared to head-forward rear and frontal impacts, and resulted in multiplanar injuries at C5–C6 and C7–T1. Panjabi MM, Ivancic PC, Maak TG, Tominaga Y, Rubin W. Multiplanar cervical spine injury due to head-turned rear impact. Spine. 2006 Feb 15;31(4):420–9.

Determination of alar, transverse, and apical ligament strains during simulated head-turned rear impact. The objectives were to quantify the alar, transverse, and apical ligament strains during head-turned rear impacts of increasing severity, to compare peak strains with baseline values, and to investigate injury mechanisms. Clinical and epidemiologic studies have documented upper cervical spine ligament injury due to severe whiplash trauma. There are no previous biomechanical studies investigating injury mechanisms during head-turned rear impacts. Whole cervical spine specimens (C0–T1) with surrogate head and muscle force replication were used to simulate head-turned rear impacts of 3.5, 5, 6.5, and 8 g horizontal accelerations of the T1 vertebra. The peak ligament strains during impact were compared ($P < 0.05$) to baseline values, obtained during a noninjurious 2 g acceleration. The highest right and left alar ligament average peak strains were 41.1% and 40.8%, respectively. The highest transverse and apical ligament average strain peaks were 17% and 21.3%, respectively. There were no significant increases in the average peak ligament strains at any impact acceleration compared with baseline. The alar, transverse, and apical ligaments are not at risk for injury due to head-turned rear impacts up to 8

g. **The upper cervical spine symptomatology reported by whiplash patients may, therefore, be explained by other factors, including severe whiplash trauma in excess of 8 g peak acceleration and/or other impact types, e.g., offset, rollover, and multiple collisions.** Maak TG, Tominaga Y, Panjabi MM, Ivancic PC. Alar, transverse, and apical ligament strain due to head-turned rear impact. Spine. 2006 Mar 15;31(6):632–8.

A turned or rotated head pre-tightens some of the cervical muscles, facets, ligaments, the annulus of the discs. Ligaments could be irreversibly overstretched or even ruptured when the head is rotated and, in addition, flexed by impact trauma, especially in unexpected rear-end collisions. Saldinger P, Dvorak J, Rahn BA, Perren SM. Histology of the alar and transverse ligaments. Spine. 1990 Apr; 15(4):257–61; Sturzenegger M, DiStefano G, Radanov BP, Schnidrig A. Presenting symptoms and signs after whiplash injury: the influence of accident mechanisms. Neurology. 1994 Apr; 44(4):688–93.

Pre-tightening of the head and neck increases facet capsular strains, increasing its role in the whiplash mechanism. Although the facet capsule does not appear to be at risk for gross injury during normal bending motions, a portion of the population may be at risk for subcatastrophic injury. Axial pretorque of the head and neck increases facet capsular strains, supporting the role of head pretorque in the whiplash mechanism. Winkelstein BA, Nightingale RW, Richardson WJ, Myers BS. The cervical facet capsule and its role in whiplash injury: a biomechanical investigation. Spine. 2000 May 15;25(10):1238–46.

§ 2:14 Variables affecting injury—Turned or rotated head—Compare: EMG studies on head rotation:

Note that the authors of the following studies have been criticized in published commentary. See 14:23, infra.

Compared to a lateral impact with the volunteer's head in the neutral position, a lateral impact with head rotation to either right or left may reduce the muscle response. **Further studies are needed to determine whether or not head rotation at the time of lateral impact reduces overall injury risk.** Kumar S, Ferrari R, Narayan Y. Cervical muscle response to head rotation in whiplash-type left lateral impacts. Spine. 2005 Mar 1;30(5):536–41.

If the head is rotated out of neutral posture at the time of rear impact, the injury risk tends to be greater for the sternocleidomastoid muscle contralateral to the side of rotation. **Measures to prevent whiplash injury may have to account for the asymmetric response because many victims of whiplash are expected to be looking to the left or right at the time of collision.** Kumar S, Ferrari R, Narayan Y. Looking away from whiplash: effect of head rotation in rear impacts. Spine. 2005 Apr 1;30(7):760–8.

Direction of impact is a factor in determining the muscle response to whiplash, but head rotation at the time of impact is also important in this regard. More specifically, when a rear impact is left posterolateral, it results in increased EMG generation mainly in the contralateral sternocleidomastoid, as expected, but head rotation at the same time in this type of impact reduces the EMG response of the cervical muscles. Muscle injury seems less likely under these conditions in low-velocity impacts. Kumar S, Ferrari R, Narayan Y. Effect of head rotation in whiplash-type rear impacts. Spine J. 2005 Mar–Apr;5(2):130–9.

Compared to a lateral impact with the volunteer's head in the neutral position, a lateral impact with head rotation to either right or left may reduce the muscle response. Further studies are needed to determine whether or not head rotation at the time of lateral impact reduces overall injury risk. Kumar S, Ferrari R, Narayan Y. Cervical muscle response to head rotation in whiplash-type left lateral impacts. Spine. 2005 Mar 1;30(5):536–41.

§ 2:15 Variables affecting injury—Effect of sitting posture

As the head and neck are tilted together forward from 0 to 15 degrees, the peak G' s for the occupant's head vary from 5.35 Gs to 16.72 Gs. *See* Ojalvo IU, Yanowitz, H. Vehicle and occupant responses to low-speed impact: comparison of analysis with test and parametric study. Society of Automotive Engineers 1998: 980300.

§ 2:16 Variables affecting injury—Awareness of collision

Startle Response to Collision. This study seeks **neurophysiological evidence of startle responses in the neck muscles** of 120 healthy subjects exposed to between 1 and 16 rear-end impacts or forward perturbations of different speeds. Startle responses were quantified by the synchronous electromyographic (EMG) activity between 10 and 20 Hz in bilaterally-homologous sternocleidomastoid, scalene, and cervical paraspinal neck muscles. Coherence analyses of EMG from the left and right muscles were used to estimate synchrony for: i) the first unexpected trial; ii) subsequent habituated trials; and iii) the superposition of habituated trials and a loud acoustic stimulus (40 ms, 124dB sound). The peak in coherent EMG activity between contralateral muscle pairs in the 10 to 20 Hz bandwidth was related to startle. Synchrony in this bandwidth was observed between the left and right muscles during the first impact or whiplash-like perturbation. This synchrony decreased significantly in the habituated trials but reappeared when the loud acoustic stimulus was introduced. Its presence in the first trial indicates that **startle is part of the neuromuscular response to an unexpected rear-end impact**. This startle component of the neuromuscular response could play a role in the aetiology of whiplash injuries. Blouin JS, Inglis JT, Siegmund GP. Startle responses elicited by whiplash perturbations. J Physiol. 2006 Jun 15;573(Pt 3):857–67.

Stabilizing effect of precontracted neck musculature in whiplash. This study investigated the effect of neck muscle precontraction in aware occupants in whiplash. Head angulation relative to T1 and facet joint capsular ligament distractions were compared between aware and unaware occupants to quantify changes in facet joint capsular ligament distractions between aware occupants with precontracted neck muscles and unaware occupants with reflex muscle contraction. While clinical studies have reported that patients aware of the impending impact had decreased symptom intensity and faster recovery after whiplash, to date, no study has investigated the effects of precontracted neck musculature on localized spinal soft tissue distortions in whiplash. In this study aware occupants with precontracted neck muscles and unaware occupants with reflex muscle contraction in whiplash were simulated using a validated computational model. Muscle contraction attained maximum levels before impact in the aware occupant and implemented reflex delay, electromechanical delay, and finite muscle rise time in the unaware occupant. Results showed that precontraction of neck muscles in aware occupants resulted in 63% decreased maximum head angles, elimination of cervical S-curvature, and up to 75% decrease in maximum facet joint capsular ligament distractions. **Occupants aware of an impending whiplash impact with precontracted neck muscles can markedly reduce overall head-neck and spinal motions. It is our theory that this would**

reduce whiplash injury likelihood. Stemper BD, Yoganandan N, Cusick JF, Pintar FA. Stabilizing effect of precontracted neck musculature in whiplash. Spine. 2006 Sep 15;31(20):E733–8.

Reflex muscle contraction in the unaware occupant in whiplash injury. Computer modeling and parametric analysis were used to determine the effect of reflex contraction of the neck muscles in the unaware occupant in whiplash and to delineate effects of reflex contraction on spinal segmental kinematics during the retraction phase. **The ability of reflex neck muscle contraction to mitigate whiplash injury in the unaware occupant remains unclear.** Analyzing relative timing between electromyographic and head-neck kinematics, previous investigators theorized that muscle contraction alters spinal kinematics, decreasing injury likelihood. Other investigators suggested that injury occurs during the initial (retraction) phase of head-neck kinematics, before significant muscle force generation. Computer modeling was used to determine reflex contraction effects on segmental angulations, implementing parametric analysis techniques to vary reflex delay and impact severity. Shorter reflex delays had a greater effect on segmental angulations later in the event and at lower impact severities. However, the magnitude of this effect, particularly at higher impact severities and during maximum cervical S-curvature (factors implicated in the whiplash injury mechanism) was minimal, altering segmental angulations by a maximum of 19%. **Because reflex contraction did not substantially alter spinal kinematics, muscle contraction likely does not initiate in sufficient time to mitigate whiplash injuries that may occur during the retraction phase.** Stemper BD, Yoganandan N, Rao RD, Pintar FA. Reflex muscle contraction in the unaware occupant in whiplash injury. Spine. 2005 Dec 15;30(24):2794–8; 2799 (discussion).

The larger retractions observed in surprised females likely produce larger tissue strains and may increase injury potential. **Aware human subjects may not replicate the muscle response, kinematic response, or whiplash injury potential of unprepared occupants in real collisions.** Siegmund GP, Sanderson DJ, Myers BS, Inglis JT. Awareness affects the response of human subjects exposed to a single whiplash-like perturbation. Spine. 2003 Apr 1;28(7):671–9.

Results of the unaware occupant model were compared to the model exercised without muscle contraction. Reflexive muscle contraction altered segmental angulations by less than 10% and facet joint capsular ligament distractions by less than

16% during the time of maximum S-curvature. At the C5–C6 and C6–C7 levels, muscle contraction increased capsular ligament distractions. Due to the nominal affect of reflexive muscle contraction on segmental angulations and facet joint capsular ligament distractions during S-curvature, it is **unlikely that this contraction can alter the cervical kinematics responsible for whiplash injury**. Stemper BD, Yoganandan N, Pintar FA. Influence of muscle contraction on whiplash kinematics. Biomed Sci Instrum. 2004;40:24–9.

In response to right anterolateral impacts, muscle responses were greater with higher levels of acceleration, and more specifically, when a frontal impact is offset to the subject's right, it results in not only increased EMG generation in the contralateral trapezius, but the splenius capitis contralateral to the direction of impact also bears part of the force of the neck perturbation. **Expecting or being aware of imminent impact plays a role in reducing muscle responses in low-velocity anterolateral impacts.** Kumar S, Ferrari R, Narayan Y. Cervical muscle response to whiplash-type right anterolateral impacts. Eur Spine J. 2004 Aug;13(5):398–407.

Because the muscular component of the head-neck complex plays a central role in the abatement of higher acceleration levels, it may be a primary site of injury in the whiplash phenomenon in lateral collisions. Expecting or being aware of imminent impact may play a role in reducing muscle responses in low-velocity impacts. Kumar S, Ferrari R, Narayan Y. Electromyographic and kinematic exploration of whiplash-type neck perturbations in left lateral collisions. Spine. 2004 Mar 11;29(6):650–9.

It would be inappropriate to extrapolate controlled testing injury data and apply them to real-world injury occurances. Aware human subjects may not replicate the muscle response, kinematic response, or whiplash injury potential of unprepared occupants in real collisions. Siegmund GP, Sanderson DJ, Myers BS, Inglis JT. Awareness affects the response of human subjects exposed to a single whiplash-like perturbation. Spine. 2003 Apr 1;28(7):671–9.

Awareness of the impending impact serves to significantly reduce the level of accelerations of the head and neck. Kumar S, Narayan Y, Amell T. Role of awareness in head-neck acceleration in low-velocity rear-end impacts. Accid Anal Prev. 2000 Mar;32(2):233–41.

Sturzenegger et al. found **awareness** to be a significant

outcome variable. **The 28% of their group who were aware reported significantly fewer symptoms and a lower intensity of headache.** Ryan et al. followed a small group (n=29) of CAD patients for 6 months and found awareness to be a strong prognostic indicator, with unaware patients 15 times more likely to have long-term pain. Sturzenegger M, DiStefano G, Radanov BP, Schnidrig A. Presenting symptoms and signs after whiplash injury: the influence of accident mechanisms. Neurology. 1994 Apr;44(4):688–93; Ryan GA, Taylor GW, Moore VM, Dolinis J. Neck strain in car occupants: injury status after 6 months and crash-related factors. Injury. 1994 Oct;25(8):533–7.

Kinematics of head movement in simulated low velocity rear-end impacts. Thirty individuals were subjected in random order to three rear-end impacts: two unexpected impacts causing chair acceleration of 4.5m/s2 (slow) and 10.0m/s2 (fast), and one 10.0m/s2 expected impact. Rearward head displacement, and linear and angular head accelerations were recorded. Angular head displacement was almost two times higher for the fast than the slow unexpected impacts (P=0.04). Rearward and forward angular head accelerations increased two to three times with increased impact magnitude (P<0.05). Rearward and forward linear head accelerations were two and a half to three and a half times higher for the fast than for the slow unexpected impacts (P<0.05). Males presented two times higher upward linear head acceleration than females in the unexpected fast impact. No significant magnitude differences were identified for impact awareness in kinematics of head movement (p>0.05). Rearward angular head acceleration reached the peak between 62 and 84 ms later than the rearward linear head acceleration (P<0.05) in all impacts. No significant differences were identified for timing of kinematics of head movement (p>0.05) with increased impact magnitude; however, statistical powers were low. **Kinematics of head movement increases with increased impact magnitude. Gender differences exist for vertical linear head acceleration only.** Temporal and amplitude awareness do not change the magnitude in kinematics of head movement. There are temporal differences between angular and linear head accelerations. Hernandez IA, Fyfe KR, Heo G, Major PW. Kinematics of head movement in simulated low velocity rear-end impacts. Clin Biomech (Bristol, Avon). 2005 Dec;20(10):1011–8.

Effect of head restraint backset on head-neck kinematics in whiplash. Head retraction values increased with increasing backset, reaching a maximum value of 53.5mm for backsets greater than 60mm. Segmental angulation magnitudes, greatest at levels C5–C6 and C6–C7, reached maximum values during the retraction phase and increased with increasing backset. Results were compared to a previously published head restraint rating system, in which lower cervical extension magnitudes from this study exceeded mean physiologic limits for restraint positions rated good, acceptable, marginal, and poor. As head restraint contact was the limiting factor in head retraction and segmental angulations, the present study indicates that minimizing whiplash injury may be accomplished by **limiting head restraint backset to less than 60mm** either passively or actively after impact. Stemper BD, Yoganandan N, Pintar FA. Effect of head restraint backset on head-neck kinematics in whiplash. Accid Anal Prev. 2006 Mar;38(2):317–23.

Vehicle stiffness has a strong influence on the retraction (70%), rebound (43%), and protraction (47%) phases. Headrest backset demonstrates a strong influence on the extension (49%) and rebound (39%) phases. For **WAD protection rating, the vehicle should be viewed as a system whereby the complex interactions among the vehicle, seat, and occupant characteristics all contribute to the WAD potential**. Sendur P, Thibodeau R, Burge J, Tencer A. Parametric analysis of vehicle design influence on the four phases of whiplash motion. Traffic Inj Prev. 2005 Sep;6(3):258–66.

§ 2:17 Variables affecting injury—Head restraints and occupant position

Distance from the head restraint and height of the head restraint are key factors. Two important distances are "topset" and "backset." The topset is how high the head restraint is; whereas, backset is how far the head is from the head restraint. **The optimal topset and backset is zero inches.** Rarely are these optimal positions achieved.

The Insurance Institute for Highway Safety found that only 5% of the model year 1995 automobiles had head restraints that allowed positioning above the ear level and closer than about 7.6 cm (2 inches) to the back of the head.

The seat-back and the head restraint influence the head-neck kinematics. Svensson MY, Lousund P, Haland Y, Larsson S. The influence of seat-back and head-restraint properties on the head-neck motion during rest-impact.

IROCBI 1994; Biomechanics of impacts Seeptember 21–23, 1994, Lyon, France. Pp 395–406.

The horizontal head-to-head restraint gap proved to have the largest influence on the head-neck motion during rear-impact speeds of 3–8 mph. Svensson MY, Lovsund P, Haland Y, Larsson S. The influence of seat-back and head-restraint properties on the head-neck motion during rear-impact. Accid Anal Prev. 1996 Mar; 28(2):221–7.

§ 2:18 Variables affecting injury—Relationship between head restraint positions and neck injury (Farmer study)

A study by Farmer, Wells & Werner evaluated 5083 State Farm files with respect to information on crash circumstances, vehicle damage, driver demographics, injury diagnosis and treatment. See Farmer CM, Wells JK, Werner JV. Relationship of head restraint positioning to driver neck injury in rear-end crashes. Accid Anal Prev. 1999 Nov;31(6):719–28. (Note that these authors are from the Insurance Institute for Highway Safety and State Farm Mutual Automobile Insurance Company.)

The following paragraphs highlight key findings from this study:

§ 2:19 Variables affecting injury—Relationship between head restraint positions and neck injury (Farmer study)—Study overview

The study showed that approximately 35% of the cases involve bodily injuries among the police reported rear-end crashes. "It is not unusual for injuries from rear-end crashes, especially soft-tissue neck injuries, to go unnoticed until several hours or days after the crash," and these crashes are often not reported to police. "Neck injuries were more likely among drivers involved in impacts to the rear center rather than a rear corner, crashes occurring on the road rather than in a parking lot, and crashes involving more severe damage. All of these variables may be related to the change in velocity of the struck vehicle, which could not be determined directly."

Crash circumstances from the claim folders included the location of the crash (intersection, mid-block, parking lot), and speed limit of the roadway where the crash occurred. Vehicle information included the make, model, year, impact point and damaged to both the struck and striking vehicles, and whether or not the struck vehicle was moving at the time of impact.

Information on the driver of the struck vehicle included gender, age, diagnosis (ICD-9) and treatment codes (CPT) for any sustained injury. "Drivers were coded as having sustained a neck injury if there was an explicit reference to neck injury in the claim folder, or if any of the diagnostic codes listed in the medical forms referred to neck injuries. For example, an ICD-9 code of 847.0 (whiplash) was taken as evidence of neck injury, even if no such injury was explicitly mentioned."

Damage to the struck vehicle was coded as minor if only the bumper, bumper cover, rear body panel, or tail lamp were repaired; moderate damage if there were repairs to the bumper reinforcement, bumper energy absorber, deck lid, or quarter panels; and severe if either the trunk floorpan or frame were repaired, or if the car was declared a total loss. These categories of vehicle damage grading may differ depending on who is making the classification. The authors note that there is a difference between "repair costs" and "damage severity."

Female drivers were significantly more likely to claim neck injuries than male drivers in this study by approximately two times the injury rate. Drivers age 65 or older were significantly less likely to claim neck injuries than drivers younger than age 65.

"In the tort and add-on states, 30% of female drivers and 23% of male drivers reported neck injuries. Thus female drivers in the study were approximately 30% more likely than male drivers to claim neck injuries in rear-end crashes. This gender differential is similar to that seen in previous studies." Elderly drivers, both male and female, reported neck injuries at a much lower rate than younger drivers. "There is no obvious explanation for this result. One could speculate that as drivers age, they are less likely to notice or complain of minor aches and pains than drivers who are accustomed to being pain-free."

Women are more likely than men to suffer neck injuries in rear impacts, and they are more affected by changes in head restraint positioning. "Drivers of cars with good-rated head restraints are 24% less likely than drivers of cars with poor-rated head restraints to suffer neck injuries in rear-end crashes." "For women drivers, even acceptable-rated head restraints are a major improvement over poor-rated ones. This is probably due to the fact that women tend to be shorter on average than men, and a head restraint positioned slightly too low for the average man may be sufficiently high for the average woman."

Among male drivers, the injury rate was lowest in the good head restraint group, highest in the acceptable head restraint group, and intermediate for the cars with head restraints rated marginal or poor. 1990 research reported that proper head restraint positioning was most effective in preventing long-term neck injuries. "Duration of treatment was determined from medical bills submitted with each claim. Long-term neck injury rates were lowest among drivers of cars with head restraints rated as good and highest among drivers of cars with head restraints rated poor." **Among female drivers, neck injury rates rose consistently with poorer head restraint ratings.**

"For both male and female drivers, head restraints rated good were associated with less likelihood of neck injury than head restraints rated poor."

§ 2:20 Variables affecting injury—Relationship between head restraint positions and neck injury (Farmer study)—Historical overview of head restraints

In the 1950s, head restraints were proposed as countermeasures to the hyperextension phase of whiplash. Federal Motor Vehicle Safety Standard (FMVSS) 202 requires that all passenger cars manufactured for sale in the United States after December 31, 1968 include head restraints in the front positions. These head restraints must extend at least 27.5 inches above the seating reference point in their highest position (measured parallel to the plane of the torso) and not deflect more than 4 inches under a 120-pound load.

The effectiveness of head restraints subsequent to FMVSS 202 has ranged from between a 13%–18% reduction in injuries; 17% for fixed head restraints and 10% for adjustable head restraints. In 1959, 8% of all occupants exposed in rural highway rear-end collisions sustained whiplash injuries. In 1969, the risk of flexion-torsion neck injury was significantly higher among front-seat passengers than among rear-seat passengers, and twice as high among women as men.

The 27.5 inch height required by FMVSS 202 is based on the conclusion of Severy et al. in 1968 that front-seat occupants are adequately protected from rear-end collision injuries for striking car speeds through 30 mph if they have a properly structured 28-inch seat-back. Severy DM, Mathewson JH, Bechtol CO. Controlled Automobile Rear-End Collisions, An Investigation of Related Engineering and Medical Phenomena. Canadian Medical Journal 1955;11:152–184.

Adjustable head restraints in the lowest position may be several inches below this optimal height. Studies have shown that more than 70% of drivers leave their adjustable head restraints in the down position. Head restraint regulations in Europe are more stringent, where head restraints must extend at least 29.5 inches above the seating reference point in their lowest position and at least 31.5 inches above the seating reference point in their highest position. These requirements are consistent with the conclusions of an international group of neck injury experts that met in 1994 in France: head restraints should be as high as the top of the head of an average-size male.

§ 2:21 Variables affecting injury—Relationship between head restraint positions and neck injury (Farmer study)—Importance of vertical and horizontal distance of head restraint

The study by Farmer, et al, supra, stated, **"Even a head restraint that is sufficiently high may not prevent whiplash injuries, if the horizontal distance between the head and the head restraint is too great."** A 1990 study in Sweden on rear-struck Volvos reported more serious neck injuries among those whose heads were more than 4 inches in front of the head restraint. Consistent with this finding, experts meeting in France (1994) also recommended that head restraints should be as close to the back of the head as possible, and a number of studies have reported that adjustable head restraints are often improperly positioned by drivers.

There were relatively few claims for cars with head restraints rated good or acceptable.

Previous studies have reported that both vertical and horizontal distances between the head restraint and the head are important in preventing neck injuries. Ninety-eight percent of the claims in this study involved cars for which the top of the unadjusted head restraint was more than 9 cm below the top of the head form, i.e. the head restraint was below the center of gravity of the average-size male's head.

Farmer, et al concluded: "When the head restraint is this low, it no longer stops rearward motion of the head, but instead can act as a fulcrum for the head. Therefore, reducing the horizontal distance between the head restraint and the head can be advantageous only if the head restraint is sufficiently high." Further, "[r]ecent advances have been made in head restraint design. In the 1997 model year, Mercedes and BMW introduced head restraints that position themselves automatically whenever the seats are adjusted."

Saab debuted the "active head restraint" in 1998. When an occupant's body presses into the seat-back during a rear-end collision, the active head restraint is mechanically pushed upward and forward to meet the head and reduce the possibility of whiplash injury.

"Improving the designs of head restraints to reduce neck injury is a focus of both car makers and US and European regulators as they work toward international harmonization of vehicle standards." **"This study provides convincing evidence that head restraints with good geometric characteristics reduce the incidence of whiplash injuries, especially for females who are more vulnerable to this injury than males."**

See Farmer CM, Wells JK, Werner JV. Relationship of head restraint positioning to driver neck injury in rear-end crashes. Accid Anal Prev. 1999 Nov;31(6):719–28.

§ 2:22 Variables affecting injury—Relationship between head restraint positions and neck injury (Farmer study)—Other findings

Note, too, that even after headrest contact, continuing head reclination was recorded in several experiments. This suggests a portion of the force exerted to the head acceleration is still transmitted by the neck, even during full headrest contact, resulting in a prolonged period of loading. **This finding suggests that the normally insignificant acceleration peaks are beyond the threshold for injury.** Muhlbauer M, Eichberger A, Geigl BC, Steffan H. Analysis of kinematics and acceleration behaviour of the head and neck in experimental rear-impact collisions. Neuro-Orthopedics 1999; 25: 1–17.

With vehicle acceleration at 8–10 km/h (about 5 mph), the head acceleration ranged from 5.0 to 16.6 g. That is a variation in acceleration factors greater than three in controlled testing conditions. Siegmund GP, King DJ, Lawrence JM, Wheeler JB, Brault JR, Smith TA. Head/neck kinematic response of human subjects in low-speed rear-end collisions. Society of Automotive Engineers 1997; 973341.

§ 2:23 Variables affecting injury—Seatbelts

Motor Vehicle Restraint System Use and Risk of Spine Injury. Motor vehicle collision (MVC)-related spinal injury is a severe and often permanently disabling injury. In addition, strain injuries have been reported as a common outcome of MVCs. Although advances in automobile crashworthiness have reduced both fatalities and severe injuries, the impact of varying occupant restraint systems (seatbelts and airbags) on thoracolumbar spine injuries is unknown. **This study examined the relationship between the occurrence of mild to severe cervical and thoracolumbar spine injury and occupant restraint systems among front seat occupants involved in frontal MVCs.** A retrospective cohort study was conducted among subjects obtained from the 1995–2004 National Automotive Sampling System. Cases were identified based on having sustained a spine injury of >/=1 on the Abbreviated Injury Scale (AIS), 1990 Revision. Risk risks (RRs) and 95% confidence intervals (CIs) were computed comparing occupant restraint systems with unrestrained occupants, and an overall incidence of AIS1 cervical (11.8%) and thoracolumbar (3.7%) spinal injury was found. Seatbelt-only restraints were associated with increased cervical AIS1 injury (RR = 1.40, 95% CI 1.04–1.88). However, seatbelt-only restraints showed the greatest risk reduction for AIS2 spinal injuries. Airbag-only restraints reduced thoracolumbar AIS1 injuries (RR = 0.29, 95% CI 0.08–1.04). Seatbelt restraints combined with airbag use was protective for cervical AIS3+ injury overall (RR = 0.29, 95% CI 0.14–0.58), cervical neurological injury (RR = 0.19, 95% CI 0.05–0.81), and thoracolumbar AIS3+ injury overall (RR = 0.20, 95% CI 0.05–0.70). The results of this study suggest that **seatbelts alone or in combination with an airbag increased the incidence of AIS1 spinal injuries**, but provide protection against more severe injury to all regions of the spine. Airbag deployment without seatbelt use did not show increased protection relative to unrestrained occupants. Reed MA, Naftel RP, Carter S, MacLennan PA, McGwin G Jr, Rue LW 3rd. Motor vehicle restraint system use and risk of spine injury. Traffic Inj Prev. 2006 Sep;7(3):256–63.

Vertebral column injuries and lap-shoulder belts. To present cases of vertebral column fractures or fracture dislocations that occur to restrained front-seat occupants where there is no evidence of body contact with interior car components based on both medical records and car inspection. Car crash injury cases investigated at the University of Michigan Transportation Research Institute and at the University of Birmingham (England) were reviewed, as well as the National Accident Severity Study files of the National Highway Traffic Safety Administration. Medical records and car inspections in the cases presented did not indicate any evidence of body contact with interior car structures. Vertebral fractures or fracture dislocations sustained by front-seat occupants who were wearing lap-shoulder belts are rare, as evidenced by the relatively few cases identified in the literature and in the crash injury files reviewed. Infrequently, in frontal crashes, vertebral fractures or fracture dislocations can occur to lap-shoulder belted front-seat car occupants without head or torso impacts with interior car structures. Cervical spine injuries are due to neck flexion over the shoulder portion of the restraint. Thoracolumbar fractures can occur in the frontal crash even at low crash velocity. Huelke DF, Mackay GM, Morris A. Vertebral column injuries and lap-shoulder belts. J Trauma. 1995 Apr;38(4):547–56.

Some studies have shown that seatbelts increase the risk for neck injury. See Morris AP, Thomas P. A study of soft tissue neck injuries in the UK. Paper No. 96-S9-O-08, Proc of 15th ESV Conference, Melbourne, Australia, May 1996:1412–24; Koch M, Kullgren A, Lie A, Nygren A, Tingvall C. Soft tissue injury of the cervical spine in rear-end and frontal car collisions, Proc. of IRCOBI Conference on Biomechanics of Impacts, Brunnen, Switzerland, 1995; Kraft M, Thomas A, Nygren A, Lie A, Tingvall C. Whiplash associated disorder — factors influencing the incidence in rear-end collisions. Paper No. 96-S9-O-09; Proc. of 15th ESC Conference, Melbourne, Australia; May 1996:1426–32.

Shoulder and lap belts should always be worn. This protects against major injury, including ejection during motor vehicle crashes. **"Using a shoulder belt without a lap belt is not as effective as the use of a shoulder and lap belt together, or only a lap belt in reducing motor vehicle crash ejection and fatal or hospitalizing injuries."** "These results stress the need for lap-shoulder restraint use to decrease the morbidity and mortality associated with motor vehicle crashes." Knight S, Cook LJ, Nechodom PJ, Olson LM, Reading JC, Dean JM. Shoulder belts in motor vehicle crashes: a statewide analysis of restraint efficacy. Accid Anal Prev. 2001 Jan;33(1):65–71.

§ 2:24 Variables affecting injury—Seatbelts—Neck and chest injuries from seatbelts

The literature is quite clear that seatbelts lower serious injuries and fatalities. It is also clear that **seatbelts increase the frequency of soft-tissue injuries.** In addition to the backward-forward movement of the head in a typical rear-end collision, seatbelts add rotational forces to the head, making the injury more complex. Huston BL, King TP. An analytical assessment of three-point restraints in several accident configurations. Paper presented to Automatic Occupant Protection Systems, International Congress and Exposition, Detroit, Michigan, February 29–March 4, 1988, pp. 55–59.

Bourbeau et al found that, in a survey of 3,927 accident victims, belted patients were 1.58 times more likely to suffer cervical strain than unbelted patients. Bourbeau R, Desjardins D, Maag U, Laberge-Nadeau C. Neck injuries among belted and unbelted occupants of the front seat of cars. J Trauma. 1993 Nov;35(5):794–9.

§ 2:25 Variables affecting injury—Seatbelts—Other potential seatbelt related injuries

Breast injuries. DiPiro PJ, Meyer JE, Frenna TH, Denison CM. Seatbelt injuries of the breast: findings on mammography and sonography. AJR Am J Roentgenol. 1995 Feb;164(2):317–20.

Heart and Sternal Injuries. (Steve Allen's injury). Restifo KM, Kelen GD. Case report: sternal fracture from a seatbelt. J Emerg Med. 1994 May–Jun;12(3):321–3; Bu'Lock FA, Prothero A, Shaw C, Parry A, Dodds CA, Keenan J, Forfar JC. Cardiac involvement in seatbelt-related and direct sternal trauma: a prospective study and management implications. Eur Heart J. 1994 Dec;15(12):1621–7.

Thyroid Injury and Laryngeal Trauma. Leckie RG, Buckner AB, Bornemann M. Seatbelt-related thyroiditis documented with thyroid Tc-99m pertechnetate scans. Clin Nucl Med. 1992 Nov;17(11):859–60; Rupprecht H, Rumenapf G, Braig H, Flesch R. Acute bleeding caused by rupture of the thyroid gland following blunt neck trauma: case report. J Trauma. 1994 Mar;36(3):408–9; Steuart RD, Morrison RT. Fracture of the laryngeal cartilage. An incidental finding on bone scintigraphy. Clin Nucl Med. 1992 Oct;17(10):815–7; Guertler AT. Blunt laryngeal trauma associated with shoulder harness use. Ann Emerg Med. 1988 Aug;17(8):838–9; Hartmann PK, Mintz G, Verne D, Timen S. Diagnosis and primary management of laryngeal trauma. Oral Surg Oral Med Oral Pathol. 1985 Sep;60(3):252–7.

§ 2:26 Variables affecting injury—Predicting injury

In a whiplash-type collision, the dynamic loads generated in the cervical spine are more complex than previ-

ously thought. Within the physiological range of cervical motion, considerable shear load was partially produced in the cervical spine, and was able to create micro-injury of soft tissues. This mechanical model cannot predict the tolerances of the neck structures and injury criteria. Matsushita T, Yamazaki N, Sato T, Hirabayashi K. Biomechanical and medical investigations of human neck injury in low-velocity collisions. Neuro-Orthopedics 1997; 21:27–45.

The model did not discriminate between the presence and absence of symptoms in all tests, and indicated that factors other than the selected peak kinematic responses influenced production. Siegmund GP, Brault JR, Wheeler JB. The relationship between clinical and kinematic responses from human subject testing in rear-end automobile collisions. Accid Anal Prev. 2000 Mar;32(2):207–17.

Studies have shown that one cannot depend on one variable to determine if an injury will occur. **Injury cannot be reliably predicted by knowing the Delta-V.** Krafft M, Kullgren A, Tingvall C, Bostrom O, Fredriksson R. How crash severity in rear impacts influences short- and long-term consequences to the neck. Accid Anal Prev. 2000 Mar;32(2):187–95.

So even under controlled test conditions, no one parameter can predict injury. Yet, the defense will state with certainty they can predict injury in real world, uncontrolled conditions.

An injury or noninjury cannot be deduced from the vehicle alone. Injury has been produced with in vitro ligament tensile tests with the force of less than the weight of the average head in volunteers with a speed change of 4 km/hour (2.5 mph), torso acceleration of 4.5g; a person in 5g acceleration may have a 50% chance of a concussion. For detailed references, see Davis CG. Injury threshold: whiplash-associated disorders. J Manipulative Physiol Ther. 2000 Jul–Aug;23(6):420–7.

With the possibility of more than 130 million human postures, variability of tensile strength of the ligaments among individuals, body positions in the vehicle, the differences of collagen fibers in the same specimen segment, the amount of muscle activation and inhibition of muscles, the size of the spinal canals, and the excitability of the nervous system, one specific threshold is not possible. How individuals react to a stimulus varies widely, and it is clearly evident that peripheral stimulation has effects on the central nervous system. Evaluation of the individual patient should include more than a traditional orthopedic examination geared to find ablative lesions. Dysfunction may be apparent in muscles, joints, and motor, sensory, vestibular, and eye function. The forces applied may be harmless to one person, may cause an injury in another, and may create a chronic condition in some. Individual evaluation is required. *See* Davis CG. Injury threshold: whiplash-associated disorders. J Manipulative Physiol Ther. 2000 Jul–Aug;23(6):420–7.

§ 2:27 Variables affecting injury—Gender variability in whiplash injuries—Gender dependent cervical spine kinematics

Although catastrophic tissue failure was not detected during experimentation or in the motion analysis phase, **it has been shown that subcatastrophic failure may lead to injury in cervical spine soft tissues**. Subcatastophic failure can occur without discernible changes in physical structure or cervical motion. Peripheral sensitization is a possible result of subcatastrophic failure, leading to allodynia in nociceptive nerve endings (lowered mechanical thresholds). In turn, lower thresholds result in nociceptive firing with decreased mechanical stimuli. Innervated structures of the cervical spine that can experience peripheral sensitization are the intervertebral ligaments, intervertebral discs, and facet joints. Stemper BD, Narayan Yoganandana N, Pintar FA. Gender dependent cervical spine segmental kinematics during whiplash. Journal of Biomechanics 2003;36: 1281–89.

Joint injury is of particular interest in whiplash, due to the findings by Barnsley et al. (1994) and the high concentration of pain facilitating neuropeptides such as substance P and calcitonin gene related peptide, which play a role in the inflammation of injured tissue, and Barnsley et al. (1994) mapped the distribution of pain as a function of spinal level. Studies have reported that injuries at the lower cervical spine (C4–C7) are responsible for posterior neck and shoulder pain and injuries at the upper levels for occipital headaches. Posterior neck pain and occipital headaches are the most common symptoms reported by whiplash patients. Results of the current study, i.e., **segmental motions are statistically greater (p<0:05) for females** than males at C2–C3, C4–C5, C5–C6, and C6–C7 levels, indicate that female soft tissues sustain greater magnitudes of stretch in rear impact. Stemper BD, Narayan Yoganandana N, Pintar FA. Gender dependent cervical spine segmental kinematics during whiplash. Journal of Biomechanics 2003;36: 1281–89.

Intervertebral kinematics were analyzed as a function of

spinal level at the time of maximum cervical S-curve, which occurred during the loading phase. Segmental angles were significantly greater (p<0:05) in female specimens at C2–C3, C4–C5, C5–C6, and C6–C7 levels. Because greater angulations are associated with stretch in the innervated components of the cervical spinal column, **these findings may offer a biomechanical explanation for the higher incidence of whiplash-related complaints in female patients secondary to rear impact acceleration.** Stemper BD, Narayan Yoganandana N, Pintar FA. Gender dependent cervical spine segmental kinematics during whiplash. Journal of Biomechanics 2003;36: 1281–89.

Seat stiffness is not sufficiently low in proportion to the female mass in comparison to males. The ***j*** and ***k*** seat properties influence neck biomechanics and occupant dynamics, but ***k*** is important in determining early response differences between males and females. (***k*** = seat stiffness, ***j*** = frame rotation stiffness; stiff seats have *k = 40 kN/m* and *j = 1.8°/kN.*) Viano DC. Seat influences of female neck responses in rear crashes: A reason why women have higher whiplash rates. Traffic Injury Prevention 2003; 4:228–239.

§ 2:28 Variables affecting injury—Gender variability in whiplash injuries—Gender and facet joint

The lack of adequate cartilage in females may expose the underlying adjacent subchondral bone to direct stresses during normal physiologic and traumatic loads. Yoganandan N, Knowles SA, M.S, Maiman DJ, Pintar FA. Anatomic Study of the Morphology of Human Cervical Facet Joint. Spine 2003; 28:2317–2323.

§ 2:29 Variables affecting injury—Gender variability in whiplash injuries—Gender and vertebral end plate

A mean compressive force of 754 N (± 445 N) was required before endplate failure. Trends toward increasing compressive loads were noted with decreasing endplate area and increasing bone mineral density. Increasing age (P = 0.0203), caudal vertebral level (P =0.0001), endplate burring (P =0.0068), and **female gender** (P = 0.0452) were associated with significantly lower endplate fracture loads in compression. Truumees E, Demetropoulos CK, Yang KH, Herkowitz HN. Failure of Human Cervical Endplates: A Cadaveric Experimental Model. Spine 2003;28:2204–2208.

The facet joint width is significantly greater in the upper cervical spine (UCS) than in the lower cervical spine (LCS). **The facet joint cartilage thickness is significantly greater in males than in females in both LCS and UCS**. The facet joint cartilage gap depends on the region of the spine (LCS vs. UCS), gender (male vs. female), and location (dorsal vs. ventral). Yoganandan N, Knowles SA, Maiman DJ, Pintar FA. Anatomic Study of the Morphology of Human Cervical Facet Joint. Spine 2003;28:2317–2323.

§ 2:30 Variables affecting injury—Gender variability in whiplash injuries—Gender in Diffuse Noxious Inhibitory Control (DNIC)

Our results indicate that DNIC effects on experimental wind-up of second pain are gender specific, with **women generally lacking this pain-inhibitory mechanism**. Staud R, Robinson ME, Vierck Jr CJ, Price DD. Diffuse noxious inhibitory controls (DNIC) attenuate temporal summation of second pain in normal males but not in normal females or fibromyalgia patients. Pain 2003;101: 167–174.

§ 2:31 Variables affecting injury—Gender variability in whiplash injuries—Gender and pain

Several factors have been proposed to account for the differences observed between men and women in pain perception. Our results permit us to believe that testosterone plays a protective role in pain perception. Moreover, the female hormones act mainly on pain inhibition mechanisms (interphase), suggesting that the prevalence of **certain chronic pain conditions in women could be related to a deficit of these pain inhibitory mechanisms** rather than an increased nociceptive activity. Gaumond I, Arsenault P, Marchand S. Specificity of female and male sex hormones on excitatory and inhibitory phases of formalin-induced nociceptive responses. Brain Res. 2005 Aug 2;1052(1):105–11.

§ 2:32 Whiplash mechanism of injury testing

Below are a series of articles published by noted authors from the Biomechanics Research Laboratory at the Yale University School of Medicine and the Department of Neurosurgery at the Medical College of Wisconsin. Each of these research institutions are leaders in this area of testing.

§ 2:33 Whiplash mechanism of injury testing—Yale University School of Medicine

Previous clinical studies have identified the cervical facet joint, including the capsular ligaments, as sources of pain in whiplash patients. The goal of this study was to determine whether whiplash caused increased capsular ligament laxity by applying quasi-static loading to whiplash-exposed and control capsular ligaments.

Average elongation of the whiplash-exposed capsular ligaments was significantly greater than that of the control ligaments at tensile forces of 0 and 5 N. No significant differences between spinal levels were observed.

Capsular ligament injuries, in the form of increased laxity, may be one component perpetuating chronic pain and clinical instability in whiplash patients.

Ivancic PC, Ito S, Tominaga Y, Rubin W, Coe MP, Ndu AB, Carlson EJ, Panjabi MM. Whiplash causes increased laxity of cervical capsular ligament. Clin Biomech (Bristol, Avon). 2008 Feb;23(2):159–65.

Side impact may cause neck and upper extremity pain, paresthesias, and impaired neck motion.

Soft tissue injury was defined as a significant increase ($p < 0.05$) in the average intervertebral flexibility above the baseline 2 g impact. The injury threshold was the lowest T1 horizontal peak acceleration that caused the injury.

The injury threshold acceleration was 6.5 g, with injuries occurring at C4-C5 through C7-T1 in flexion, axial rotation, or left lateral bending. After 8 g, three-plane injury was observed at C4-C5 and C6-C7, whereas two-plane injury occurred at C3-C4 in flexion and left lateral bending and at C5-C6 and C7-T1 in axial rotation and left lateral bending.

Side impact caused multiplanar injuries at C3-C4 through C7-T1 and significantly greater injury at C6-C7, as compared with head-forward rear impact.

Maak TG, Ivancic PC, Tominaga Y, Panjabi MM. Side impact causes multiplanar cervical spine injuries. J Trauma. 2007 Dec;63(6):1296–307.

Most previous studies have investigated ligament mechanical properties at slow elongation rates of less than 25 mm/s.

To determine the tensile mechanical properties, at a fast elongation rate, of intact human cervical anterior and posterior longitudinal, capsular, and interspinous and supraspinous ligaments, middle-third disc, and ligamentum flavum.

Highest average peak force, up to 244.4 and 220.0 N in the ligamentum flavum and capsular ligament, respectively, were significantly greater than in the anterior longitudinal ligament and middle-third disc. Highest peak elongation reached 5.9 mm in the intraspinous and supraspinous ligaments, significantly greater than in the middle-third disc. Highest peak energy of 0.57 J was attained in the capsular ligament, significantly greater than in the anterior longitudinal ligament and middle-third disc. Average stiffness was generally greatest in the ligamentum flavum and least in the intraspinous and supraspinous ligaments. For all ligaments, peak elongation was greater than average physiological elongation computed using the mathematical model.

Comparison of the present results with previously reported data indicated that high-speed elongation may cause cervical ligaments to fail at a higher peak force and smaller peak elongation and they may be stiffer and absorb less energy, as compared with a slow elongation rate. These comparisons may be useful to clinicians for diagnosing cervical ligament injuries based upon the specific trauma.

Ivancic PC, Coe MP, Ndu AB, Tominaga Y, Carlson EJ, Rubin W, Dipl-Ing FH, Panjabi MM. Dynamic mechanical properties of intact human cervical spine ligaments. Spine J. 2007 Nov-Dec;7(6):659–65.

The goal of the present study was to determine the dynamic sagittal flexibility coefficients, including coupling coefficients, throughout the human cervical spine using rear impacts.

A biofidelic whole cervical spine model (n=6) with muscle force replication and surrogate head was rear impacted at 5 g peak horizontal accelerations of the T1 vertebra within a bench-top mini-sled. The dynamic main and coupling sagittal flexibility coefficients were calculated at each spinal level, head/C1 to C7/T1.

Head/C1 was significantly more flexible than all other spinal levels. The cervical spine was generally more flexible in posterior shear, as compared to axial compression. The coupling coefficients indicated that extension moment caused coupled posterior shear translation while posterior shear force caused coupled extension rotation. The present results may be used towards the designs of anthropometric test dummies and mathematical models that better simulate the cervical spine response during dynamic loading.

Ivancic PC, Ito S, Panjabi MM. Dynamic sagittal flexibility coefficients of the human cervical spine. Accid Anal Prev. 2007 Jul;39(4):688–95

Elongation-induced vertebral artery (VA) injury has been hypothesized to occur during nonphysiological coupled head motions during automobile impacts. Although previous work has investigated VA elongation during head-turned and head-forward rear impacts, no studies have performed similar investigations for frontal or side impacts.

The present study quantified dynamic VA elongations during simulated frontal and side automotive collisions, and compared these data with corresponding physiological limits.

A biofidelic whole cervical spine model with muscle force replication and surrogate head underwent simulated frontal impacts (n=6) of 4, 6, 8, and 10 g or left side impacts (n=6) of 3.5, 5, 6.5, and 8 g.

Average (SD) maximum physiological VA elongation was 7.1 (3.2) mm, measured during intact flexibility testing. Average peak dynamic elongation of right VA during left side impact, up to 17.4 (2.6) mm, was significantly greater (p<.05) than physiological beginning at 6.5 g, whereas the highest average peak VA elongation during frontal impact was 2.5 (2.4) mm, which did not exceed the physiological limit. Side impact, as compared with frontal impact, caused earlier occurrence of average peak VA elongation, 113.8 (13.5) ms versus 155.0 (46.2) ms, and higher average peak VA elongation rate, 608.8 (99.0) mm/s versus 130.0 (62.9) mm/s. Elongation-induced VA injury is more likely to occur during side impact as compared with frontal impact.

Carlson EJ, Tominaga Y, Ivancic PC, Panjabi MM. Dynamic vertebral artery elongation during frontal and side impacts. Spine J. 2007 Mar-Apr;7(2):222–8

The potential increased severity of C3–4 through C6–7 injury resulting from head-turned, as compared with head-forward, rear impact may result in more severe acute symptoms of radicular irritation, including increased dermatomal pain, paresthesias, numbness, and weakness. This increase in nerve injury and symptom severity may also lead to a worse clinical prognosis, including increased chronic radicular symptoms. Head-turned rear impact causes ganglion compression in nonstenotic C5–6 and C6–7 foramina, and the injury risk greatly increases and extends to the C3–7 foramina and nerve roots, in cases involving a stenotic foramen. **Greater potential for ganglion compression injury** existed at C3–4 and C4–5 during head-turned rear impact than **during head-forward rear impact**. **Potential ganglion compression can occur in patients with a non-stenotic foramen at C5–6 and**

C6–7; in patients with a stenotic foramen the injury risk greatly increases and spreads to include C3–4 through C6–7, as well as C4–5 through C6–7 nerve roots. **"Chronic radicular symptoms reported by whiplash-injured patients may be caused by dynamic cervical ganglion or nerve root compressive injury or repeated and less severe compression due to cervical instability."** Tominaga Y, Maak TG, Ivancic PC, Panjabi MM, Cunningham BW. Head-turned rear impact causing dynamic cervical intervertebral foramen narrowing: implications for ganglion and nerve root injury. J Neurosurg Spine. 2006 May;4(5):380–7.

Head-turned whole cervical spine model was stabilized with muscle force replication and subjected to simulated rear impacts of increasing severity to identify and quantify cervical spine soft tissue injury and injury threshold acceleration for head-turned rear impact, and to compare these data with previously published head-forward rear and frontal impact results. Multiplanar flexibility testing evaluated any resulting injury. **Epidemiologically and clinically, head-turned rear impact is associated with increased injury severity and symptom duration, as compared to forward facing.** No biomechanical data appear to exist to explain this finding. Six human cervical spine specimens (C0–T1) with head-turned and muscle force replication were rear impacted at 3.5, 5, 6.5, and 8 g, and flexibility tests were performed before and after each impact. Soft tissue injury was defined as a significant increase ($P < 0.05$) in intervertebral flexibility above baseline. Injury threshold was the lowest T1 horizontal peak acceleration that caused the injury. The **injury threshold acceleration was 5 g** with injury occurring in extension or axial rotation at C3–C4 through C7–T1, excluding C6–C7. Following 8 g, 3-plane injury occurred in extension and axial rotation at C5–C6, while 2-plane injury occurred at C7–T1. **Head-turned rear impact caused significantly greater injury at C0–C1 and C5–C6, as compared to head-forward rear and frontal impacts, and resulted in multiplanar injuries at C5–C6 and C7–T1.** Panjabi MM, Ivancic PC, Maak TG, Tominaga Y, Rubin W. Multiplanar cervical spine injury due to head-turned rear impact. Spine. 2006 Feb 15;31(4):420–9.

Alar, transverse, and apical ligament strains were studied during simulated head-turned rear impact to quantify the alar, transverse, and apical ligament strains during head-turned rear impacts of increasing severity, to compare peak strains with baseline values, and to investigate injury mechanisms. Clinical and epidemiologic studies have documented upper cervical spine ligament injury due to severe whiplash trauma. There are no previous biomechanical studies investigating injury mechanisms during head-turned rear impacts. Whole cervical spine specimens (C0–T1) with surrogate head and muscle force replication were used to simulate head-turned rear impacts of 3.5, 5, 6.5, and 8 g horizontal accelerations of the T1 vertebra. The peak ligament strains during impact were compared ($P < 0.05$) to baseline values, obtained during a noninjurious 2 g acceleration. The highest right and left alar ligament average peak strains were 41.1% and 40.8%, respectively. The highest transverse and apical ligament average strain peaks were 17% and 21.3%, respectively. There were no significant increases in the average peak ligament strains at any impact acceleration compared with baseline. The alar, transverse, and apical ligaments are not at risk for injury due to head-turned rear impacts up to 8 g. **The upper cervical spine symptomatology reported by whiplash patients may, therefore, be explained by other factors, including severe whiplash trauma in excess of 8 g peak acceleration and/or other impact types, e.g., offset, rollover, and multiple collisions.** Maak TG, Tominaga Y, Panjabi MM, Ivancic PC. Alar, transverse, and apical ligament strain due to head-turned rear impact. Spine. 2006 Mar 15;31(6):632–8.

Dynamic intervertebral foramen narrowing during simulated rear impact. Significant increases ($P < 0.05$) in average peak foraminal width narrowing above baseline were observed at C5–C6 beginning with 3.5 g impact. No significant increases in average peak foraminal height narrowing were observed, while average peak foraminal areas were significantly narrower than baseline at C4–C5 at 3.5, 5, and 6..5 g. The present results indicated that the **highest potential for ganglia compression injury was at the lower cervical spine, C5–C6 and C6–C7. Acute ganglia compression may produce a sensitized neural response to repeat compression, leading to chronic radiculopathy following rear impact.** Panjabi MM, Maak TG, Ivancic PC, Ito S. Dynamic intervertebral foramen narrowing during simulated rear impact. Spine. 2006 Mar 1;31(5):E128–34.

A rotated head posture at the time of vehicular rear impact has been correlated with a higher incidence and greater severity of chronic radicular symptoms than accidents occurring with the occupant facing forward. No studies have been conducted to quantify the dynamic changes in foramen dimensions during head-turned rear-impact collisions. The objectives of this study were to quantify the changes in foraminal width, height, and area during head-turned rear-impact collisions and to determine if dynamic narrowing causes potential cervical nerve root or ganglion impingement. The authors subjected a whole cervical spine model with muscle force replication and a surrogate head to simulated head-turned rear impacts of 3.5, 5, 6.5, and 8 g following a noninjurious 2 g baseline acceleration. Continuous dynamic foraminal width, height, and area narrowing were recorded, and peaks were determined during each impact; these data were then statistically compared with those obtained at baseline. The authors observed significant increases ($p < 0.05$) in mean peak foraminal width narrowing values greater than baseline values, of up to 1.8 mm in the left C5–6 foramen at 8 g. At the right C2–3 foramen, the mean peak dynamic foraminal height was significantly narrower than baseline when subjected to rear-impacts of 5 and 6.5 g, but no significant increases in foraminal area were observed. Analysis of the results indicated that the greatest potential for cervical ganglion compression injury existed at C5–6 and C6 7. Greater potential for ganglion compression injury existed at C3–4 and C4–5 during head-turned rear impact than during head-forward rear impact. Extrapolation of present results indicated **potential ganglion compression in patients with a non-stenotic foramen at C5–6 and C6–7**; in patients with a stenotic foramen the injury risk greatly increases and spreads to include the C3–4 through C6–7, as well as C4–5 through C6–7 nerve roots. Ivancic PC, Ito S, Tominaga Y, Carlson EJ, Rubin W, Panjabi MM. Effect of rotated head posture on dynamic vertebral artery elongation during simulated rear impact. Clin Biomech (Bristol, Avon). 2006 Mar;21(3):213–20.

Spinal canal narrowing during simulated frontal impact. Between 23 and 70% of occupants involved in frontal impacts sustain cervical spine injuries, many with neurological involvement. It has been hypothesized that cervical spinal cord compression and injury may explain the variable neurological profile described by frontal impact victims. The goals of the present study, using a biofidelic whole cervical spine model with muscle force replication, were to quantify canal pinch diameter (CPD) narrowing during frontal impact and to evaluate the potential for cord compression. The biofidelic model and a sled apparatus were used to simulate frontal impacts at 4, 6, 8, and 10 g horizontal accelerations of the T1 vertebra. The CPD was measured in the intact specimen in the neutral posture (neutral posture CPD), under static sagittal pure moments of 1.5 Nm (pre-impact CPD), during dynamic frontal impact (dynamic impact CPD), and again under static pure moments following each impact (post-impact CPD). Frontal impact caused significant (P<0.05) dynamic CPD narrowing at C0-dens, C2–C3, and C6–C7. The narrowest dynamic CPD was observed at C0-dens during the 10 g impact and was 25.9% narrower than the corresponding neutral posture CPD. Interpretation of the present results indicate that the **neurological symptomatology reported by frontal impact victims is most likely not due to cervical spinal cord compression. Cord compression due to residual spinal instability is also not likely**. Ivancic PC, Panjabi MM, Tominaga Y, Pearson AM, Elena Gimenez S, Maak TG. Spinal canal narrowing during simulated frontal impact. Eur Spine J. 2006 Jun;15(6):891–901.

Spinal canal narrowing during simulated whiplash. Spinal cord injuries are uncommon in whiplash patients, although such injuries have been reported in those with narrow canals. It has been hypothesized that increased cerebral spinal fluid pressure during whiplash could injure neural tissues. The biofidelic model and a bench-top whiplash apparatus were used to simulate whiplash at 3.5, 5, 6.5, and 8 g accelerations of the T1 vertebra. The CPD was measured in the intact specimen in the neutral posture (neutral posture CPD) and under a 1.5 Nm static extension load (pre-whiplash CPD), during simulated whiplash (dynamic whiplash CPD), and again under a 1.5 Nm extension load following each whiplash simulation (post-whiplash CPD). The average dynamic whiplash CPDs were significantly narrower (P < 0.05) than the corresponding pre-whiplash CPDs at accelerations of 3.5 g and above. The narrowest CPD was observed at C5–C6 during the 6.5 g simulation and was 3.5 mm narrower than the neutral posture CPD. In general, the average post-whiplash CPDs were not significantly narrower than the corresponding pre-whiplash CPDs. **Spinal cord injury during whiplash is unlikely in patients with average normal canal diameters.** Cord compression following whiplash due to physiologic extension loading is not likely. **Previous clinical studies have found that whiplash patients with narrow canals may be at risk of injury, and our results do not disprove it.** Ito S, Panjabi MM, Ivancic PC, Pearson AM. Spinal canal narrowing during simulated whiplash. Spine. 2004 Jun 15;29(12):1330–9.

The potential "increased severity of C3–4 through C6–7 injury resulting from head-turned rear impact, as compared with head-forward rear impact, may result in more severe acute symptoms of radicular irritation, including increased dermatomal pain, paresthesias, numbness, and weakness." This "increase in nerve injury and symptom severity may also lead to a worse clinical prognosis, including increased chronic radicular symptoms." Head-turned rear impact causes ganglion compression in nonstenotic C5–6 and C6–7 foramina, and the injury risk greatly increases and extends to the C3–7 foramina and nerve roots, in cases involving a stenotic foramen. "The greater potential severity of ganglion injury observed as a result of head-turned compared with head-forward rear impact is supported by clinical and epidemiological observations." **"Chronic radicular symptoms reported by whiplash-injured patients may be caused by dynamic cervical ganglion or nerve root compressive injury or repeated and less severe compression due to cervical instability."** Tominaga Y, Maak TG, Ivancic PC, Panjabi MM, Cunningham BW. Head-turned rear impact causing dynamic cervical intervertebral foramen narrowing: implications for ganglion and nerve root injury. J Neurosurg Spine. 2006 May;4(5):380–7.

The **Intervertebral Neck Injury Criterion** (IV-NIC) is based on the hypothesis that intervertebral motion beyond the physiological limit may injure spinal soft tissues during whiplash, while the Neck Injury Criterion (NIC) hypothesizes that sudden changes in spinal fluid pressure may cause neural injury. Goals of the present study, using a biofidelic whole cervical spine model with muscle force replication, were to correlate IV-NIC with soft-tissue injury, determine the IV-NIC injury threshold, and compare IV-NIC and NIC. Using a bench-top apparatus, rear-impacts were simulated at 3.5, 5, 6.5, and 8 g horizontal accelerations of the T1 vertebra. Pre- and post-whiplash flexibility tests measured the soft tissue injury threshold, i.e. significant increases in the intervertebral neutral zone (NZ) or range of motion (ROM) above corresponding baseline values. Extension IV-NIC peaks correlated well with NZ and ROM increases at C0–C1 and at C3–C4 through C7–T1 ($r=0.64$ and 0.62 respectively, $p<0.001$). Average IV-NIC injury thresholds (95% confidence limits) varied among the intervertebral levels and ranged between 1.5 (1.1, 1.9) at C5–C6 and 3.4 (2.4, 4.4) at C7–T1. **The NIC injury threshold was 8.7** (7.7, 9.7) m2/s2, substantially less than the proposed threshold of 15 m2/s2. Results support the use of IV-NIC for determining the cervical spine injury threshold and injury severity. Advantages of IV-NIC include the ability to predict the intervertebral level, mode, severity, and time of the cervical spine soft-tissue injury. Panjabi MM, Ito S, Ivancic PC, Rubin W. Evaluation of the intervertebral neck injury criterion using simulated rear impacts. J Biomech. 2005 Aug;38(8):1694–701.

The Intervertebral Neck Injury Criterion (IV-NIC) is based on the hypothesis that dynamic intervertebral motion beyond physiological limits may injure soft tissues. In contrast, the Neck Injury Criterion (NIC) hypothesizes that sudden change in spinal fluid pressure may cause neural injuries. The goals of this study, using the biofidelic whole human cervical spine model with muscle force replication, were to determine the IV-NIC injury threshold due to frontal impact at each intervertebral level, and to compare the IV-NIC and NIC in determining injury. Using a bench-top apparatus, frontal impacts were simulated at 4, 6, 8, and 10 g horizontal accelerations of the T1 vertebra. Pre- and post-trauma flexibility testing measured the soft tissue injury; that is, a significant increase ($p < 0.05$) in neutral zone or range of motion at any intervertebral level, above the corresponding physiological limit. **Results indicated that the soft tissue injury occurred due to flexion mode of injury and its threshold was 8 g.** The average IV-NIC injury threshold (95% confidence interval) was 2.0 (1.2–2.8) at C4–C5 and 2.3 (1.6–3.0) at C6–C7, while the average NIC injury threshold was 18.4 (17.9–19.0) m(2)/s(2). The NIC injury threshold was reached significantly earlier than all the IV-NIC injury thresholds, demonstrating that the NIC may be unable to predict facet and soft tissue injury caused by non-physiologic inververtebral rotation. Ivancic PC, Ito S, Panjabi MM, Pearson AM, Tominaga Y, Wang JL, Gimenez SE. Intervertebral neck injury criterion for simulated frontal impacts. Traffic Inj Prev. 2005 Jun;6(2):175–84.

The average dynamic **whiplash spinal canal pinch diameters** (CPDs) were significantly narrower ($P < 0.05$) than the corresponding pre-whiplash CPDs at accelerations of 3.5 g and above. The narrowest CPD was observed at C5–C6 during the 6.5 g simulation and was 3.5 mm narrower than the neutral posture CPD. In general, the average post-whiplash CPDs were not significantly narrower than the corresponding pre-whiplash CPDs. Spinal cord injury during whiplash is unlikely in patients with average normal canal diameters. Cord compression following whiplash due to physiologic extension loading is not likely. **Previous clinical studies have found that whiplash patients with narrow canals may be at risk of injury, and our results do not disprove it.** Ito S, Panjabi MM, Ivancic PC, Pearson AM. Spinal canal narrowing during simulated whiplash. Spine. 2004 Jun 15;29(12):1330–9.

Clinical studies have documented **acute intervertebral disc injury** and accelerated disc degeneration in whiplash patients, although there has been no biomechanical investigation of the disc injury mechanisms. A bench-top sled was used to simulate whiplash at 3.5, 5, 6.5, and 8 g using six specimens. The 30 degrees and 150 degrees fiber strains, disc shear strains, and axial disc deformations during whiplash were compared with the sagittal physiologic levels. Increases over sagittal physiologic levels ($P < 0.05$) were first observed during the **3.5 g** simulation. Peak fiber strain was greatest in the posterior 150 degrees fibers (running posterosuperiorly), reaching a maximum of 51.4% at C5–C6 during the 8 g simulation. Peak disc shear strain was also greatest at the posterior region of C5–C6, reaching a maximum of 1.0 radian due to posterior translation during the 8 g simulation. **Axial deformation at the anterior disc region exceeded physiologic levels at 3.5 g and above**, while axial deformation at the **posterior region exceeded physiologic limits only at C5–C6 at 6.5 g and 8 g.** The **cervical intervertebral discs may be at risk for injury** during whiplash because of excessive 150 degrees fiber strain, disc shear strain, and anterior axial deformation. Panjabi MM, Ito S, Pearson AM, Ivancic PC. Injury mechanisms of the cervical intervertebral disc during simulated whiplash. Spine. 2004 Jun 1;29(11):1217–25.

Cervical spine instability may result from automotive collisions. No previous studies have quantified soft tissue injuries due to **frontal impact**. Six human cervical specimens (occiput-T1) with muscle force replication were subjected to frontal impacts of 4, 6, 8, and 10 g. Before frontal impact, baseline flexibility data were collected following a 2 g simulation. Flexibility parameters of total (flexion plus extension) neutral zone (NZ), flexion NZ, total range of motion (ROM), and flexion ROM were obtained following each impact and compared with baseline flexibility. Injury was a significant increase ($P < 0.05$) in intervertebral flexibility due to frontal impact over baseline. Injury threshold was the lowest T1 peak acceleration that caused injury. **The injury threshold acceleration was 8 g**, as determined by significant increases of 12.6 to 51.4% over the baseline flexibility, in the C4–C5 total NZ, and the C6–C7 total NZ, flexion NZ, total ROM, and flexion ROM. Following 10 g, significant increases in flexibility parameters were observed at C2–C3, C3–C4, C4–C5, C6–C7, and C7–T1. Middle (C2–C3 to C4–C5) and lower (C6–C7 and C7–T1) cervical spine were at risk for injury during frontal impacts, for the experimental conditions studied. Pearson AM, Panjabi MM, Ivancic PC, Ito S, Cunningham BW, Rubin W, Gimenez SE. Related Articles, Frontal impact causes ligamentous cervical spine injury. Spine. 2005 Aug 15;30(16):1852–8.

Whiplash has been simulated using mathematical models, whole cadavers, volunteers, and WCSs. The measurement of injury (difference between pre-whiplash and postwhiplash flexibilities) is possible only using the WCS model. METHODS: Six WCS + MFR specimens (C0–T1) were incrementally rear-impacted at nominal T1 horizontal maximum accelerations of 3.5, 5, 6.5, and 8 g, and the changes in the intervertebral flexibility parameters of neutral zone and range of motion were determined. The injury threshold acceleration was the lowest T1 horizontal peak acceleration that caused a significant increase in the intervertebral flexibility. The first significant increase ($P < 0.01$) of 39.8% occurred in the C5–C6 extension neutral zone following the **5 g acceleration**. At higher accelerations, the injuries spread among the surrounding levels (C4–C5 to C7–T1). **A rear-end collision is most likely to injure the lower cervical spine by intervertebral hyperextension at a peak T1 horizontal acceleration of 5 g and above**. Ito S, Ivancic PC, Panjabi MM, Cunningham BW. Soft tissue injury threshold during simulated whiplash: a biomechanical investigation. Spine. 2004 Apr 23;29(9):979–87.

The whole cervical spine specimens with muscle force replication model and a bench-top trauma sled were used in an incremental trauma protocol to simulate whiplash of increasing severity. Peak facet joint compression (displacement of the upper facet surface towards the lower facet surface), facet joint sliding (displacement of the upper facet surface along the lower facet surface), and capsular ligament strains were calculated and compared to the physiologic limits determined during intact flexibility testing. Peak facet joint compression was greatest at C4–C5, reaching a maximum of 2.6 mm during the 5 g simulation. Increases over physiologic limits ($P < 0.05$) were initially observed during the 3.5 g simulation. In general, peak facet joint sliding and capsular ligament strains were largest in the lower cervical spine and increased with impact acceleration. Capsular ligament strain reached a maximum of 39.9% at C6–C7 during the 8 g simulation. **Facet joint components may be at risk for injury due to facet joint compression during rear-impact accelerations of 3.5 g and above**. Capsular ligaments are at risk for injury at higher accelerations. Pearson AM, Ivancic PC, Ito S, Panjabi MM. Facet joint kinematics and injury mechanisms during simulated whiplash. Spine. 2004 Feb 15;29(4):390–7.

A biofidelic model and a bench-top whiplash apparatus were used in an incremental rear-impact protocol (maximum 8 g) to simulate whiplash of increasing severity. To describe the spine curvature, the upper and lower cervical spine rotations were normalized to corresponding physiological limits. Average peak lower cervical spine extension first exceeded the physiological limits ($P<0.05$) at a horizontal T1 acceleration of 5 g. Average peak upper cervical spine extension exceeded the physiological limit at 8 g, while peak upper cervical spine flexion never exceeded the physiological limit. In the S-shape phase, lower cervical spine extension reached 84% of peak extension during whiplash. **Both the upper and lower cervical spine are at risk for extension injury during rear-impact**. Panjabi MM, Pearson AM, Ito S, Ivancic PC, Wang JL. Cervical spine curvature during simulated whiplash. Clin Biomech (Bristol, Avon). 2004 Jan;19(1):1–9.

Anterior longitudinal ligament (ALL) injuries following whiplash have been documented both in vivo and in vitro; however, ALL strains during the whiplash trauma remain unknown. A new in vitro whiplash model and a bench-top trauma sled were used in an incremental trauma protocol to simulate whiplash at 3.5, 5, 6.5 and 8 g accelerations, and peak ALL strains were determined for each trauma. Following the final trauma, the ALLs were inspected and classified as uninjured, partially injured or completely injured. Peak strain, peak intervertebral extension and increases in flexibility parameters were compared among the three injury classification groups. Peak ALL strains were largest in the lower cervical spine, and increased with impact acceleration, reaching a maximum of 29.3% at C6–C7 at 8 g. **Significant increases** ($P<0.05$) over the physiological strain limits first occurred at C4–C5 during the **3.5 g trauma** and spread to lower intervertebral levels as impact severity increased. The complete ligament injuries were associated with greater increases in ALL strain, intervertebral extension, and flexibility parameters than were observed at uninjured intervertebral levels ($P<0.05$). Ivancic PC, Pearson AM, Panjabi MM, Ito S. Injury of the anterior longitudinal ligament during whiplash simulation. Eur Spine J. 2004 Feb;13(1):61–8.

The hyper-extension hypothesis of injury mechanism was not supported by these studies. We found a distinct bi-phasic kinematic response of the cervical spine to whiplash trauma. In the first phase, the spine formed an S-shaped curve with flexion at the upper levels and hyper-extension at the lower levels. In the second phase, all levels of the cervical spine were extended, and the head reached its maximum extension. The occurrence of anterior injuries in the lower levels in the first phase was confirmed by functional radiography, flexibility tests and imaging modalities. The largest dynamic elongation of the capsular ligaments was observed at C6–C7 level during the initial **S-shaped phase of whiplash**. Similarly, the maximum elongation of the **vertebral artery** occurred during the S-shape phase of whiplash. We propose, based upon our experimental findings, that the lower cervical spine is injured in hyperextension when the spine forms an S-shaped curve. Further, this occurs in the first whiplash phase before the neck is fully extended. At higher trauma accelerations, there is a tendency for the injuries to occur at the upper levels of the cervical spine. Our findings provide truer understanding of whiplash trauma and may help in improving the diagnosis, treatment, and prevention of these injuries. Panjabi MM, Cholewicki J, Nibu K, Grauer JN, Babat LB, Dvorak J. Mechanism of whiplash injury. Clin Biomech (Bristol, Avon). 1998 Jun;13(4–5):239–249.

Instability of the cervical spine following whiplash trauma has been demonstrated in a number of studies. We hypothesized that, in patients with whiplash-associated disorder, rotation of the head would be accompanied by an earlier onset of neck muscle activity to compensate for intrinsic instability. The aim of the study was to examine the range of motion (RoM) of the cervical spine and the onset and activity of the sternocleidomastoid (SCM) muscles during axial rotation, in healthy control subjects and in patients with chronic whiplash-associated disorder. Forty-eight control subjects (42% male) and 46 patients (33% male) with chronic whiplash-associated disorder (symptoms lasting longer than 3 months) were examined. Cervical axial RoM differed significantly (P = 0.0001) between the groups, with the whiplash patients showing lower values (83 degrees +/- 30 degrees) than the healthy controls (137 degrees +/- 19 degrees). The whiplash patient group showed no evidence of the predicted earlier activation of SCM muscles. Many patients never reached the point in the RoM where SCM muscle activity rises steeply, as it does in the healthy controls (the 'elastic zone'), and their movements remained mostly within the region of low muscle activity (the 'neutral zone'). The whiplash patients appeared either unable or unwilling to drive the cervical spine into this region of high muscle activity, possibly because they were restricted by existing pain or fear of pain. Klein GN, Mannion AF, Panjabi MM, Dvorak J. Trapped in the neutral zone: another symptom of whiplash-associated disorder? Eur Spine J. 2001 Apr;10(2):141–8.

Symptoms often do not correlate to the clinical findings. It has been hypothesized that the long-term clinical symptoms associated with whiplash have their basis in mechanical derangement of the cervical spine caused at the time of trauma. Before such a hypothesis can be proven, one needs to document and quantify the soft tissue injuries of the cervical spine in whiplash. The purpose of the study was to quantify the mechanical changes that occur in the cervical spine specimen as a result of experimental whiplash trauma. Utilizing a whiplash trauma model, injuries to human cadaveric cervical spine specimens (C0–T1 or C0–C7) were produced by increasingly severe traumas. The flexibility tests determined the motion changes at each intervertebral level in response to 1.0 Nm pure flexion-extension moment. Parameters of range of motion (ROM) and neutral zone (NZ) were determined before and after each trauma. Significant flexibility increases first occurred in the lower cervical spine after 4.5-g rear-end (anteriorly directed) acceleration of the T1 vertebra. At this acceleration magnitude, extension ROM and NZ at C5–C6 increased ($P < 0.05$) by 98% and 160% respectively. There was also a tendency ($P < 0.1$) for the extension NZ at C0–C1 and C6–C7 levels to increase after the 6.5-g acceleration by 52% and 241% respectively. There were no such tendencies for the ROM parameter. **We have identified the threshold and sites of whiplash injury to the cervical spine**. This information should help the clinician make more precise diagnoses in the case of whiplash trauma patients. Panjabi MM, Nibu K, Cholewicki J. Whiplash injuries and the potential for mechanical instability. Eur Spine J. 1998;7(6):484–92.

This study reports a comprehensive data set describing head kinematic response to horizontal accelerations simulating whiplash. Seven isolated fresh human cervical spine specimens (C0 to T1 or C7), each carrying a surrogate head designed to represent a 50th percentile human head, were mounted on the sled and subjected to incremental trauma by horizontal sled accelerations of 2.5, 4.5, 6.5, 8.5, and 10.5 g. Sled and head kinematics were measured with potentiometers and accelerometers. The incremental sled accelerations resulted in average (standard deviations) sled velocity changes (delta V) ranging from 5.8 (0.2) to 15.8 (0.2) km/h. Generally, all the peak head kinematic parameters increased with increasing sled acceleration, except for the peak head angular displacement, which decreased. In the initial phase of a whiplash trauma, the head translated posteriorly with respect to T1, without rotation. In the later phase, the head rotated backwards, but much less than its physiological limit. Maximum head rotation of 31.5 (23.9) degrees occurred in a 2.5 g trauma class, and this was less than the maximum physiological head extension of 55.1 (13.3) degrees. Head kinematics expressed in the T1 or shoulder coordinate system is better suited to study potential neck injury in whiplash. Cholewicki J, Panjabi MM, Nibu K, Babat LB, Grauer JN, Dvorak J. Head kinematics during in vitro whiplash simulation. Accid Anal Prev. 1998 Jul;30(4):469–79.

Six occiput to T1 (or C7) fresh cadaveric human spines were studied. Physiologic flexion and extension motions were recorded with an Optotrak motion analysis system by loading up to 1.0 Nm. Specimens then were secured in a trauma sled, and a surrogate head was attached. Flags fixed to the head and individual vertebrae were monitored with high-speed cinematography (500 frames/sec). Data were collected for 12 traumas in four classes defined by the maximum sled acceleration. The trauma classes were 2.5 g, 4.5 g, 6.5 g, and 8.5 g. Significance was defined at $P < 0.01$. In the whiplash traumas, the peak intervertebral rotations of C6–C7 and C7–T1 significantly exceeded the maximum physiologic extension for all trauma classes studied. The maximum extension of these lower levels occurred significantly before full neck extension. In fact, the upper cervical levels were consistently in flexion at the time of maximum lower level extension. **In whiplash, the neck forms an S-shaped curvature, with lower level hyperextension and upper level flexion**. This was identified as the injury stage for the lower cervical levels. A subsequent C-shaped curvature with extension of the entire cervical spine produced less lower level extension. Grauer JN, Panjabi MM, Cholewicki J, Nibu K, Dvorak J. Whiplash produces an S-shaped curvature of the neck with hyperextension at lower levels. Spine. 1997 Nov 1;22(21):2489–94.

Vertebral artery (VA) stretch during trauma is a possible pathomechanism that could explain some aspects of the whiplash symptom complex. This study quantified the VA elongation during whiplash simulation using an in vitro model. Seven fresh human cadaveric specimens (occiput to C7 or T1) were carefully dissected, preserving the osteoligamentous structures. The right VA was replaced with a thin nylon-coated flexible cable. This cable was fixed at one end to the occipital bone and at the other end to a specially designed VA transducer. Physiological motion of the occiput and physiological elongation of the VA were measured with a standard flexibility test. Next the specimen was mounted on a specially designed sled and subjected to 2.5, 4.5, 6.5, and 8.5 g (1 g = 9.81 m/s2) horizontal accelerations. Elongation of the VA was continuously recorded from the start of the trauma. The average (standard deviation) physiological VA elongation was 5.8 (1.6) mm in left lateral bending and 4.7 (1.8) mm in left axial rotation. Flexion and extension did not result in any appreciable elongation of the VA. The maximum VA elongation during the whiplash trauma significantly correlated with the horizontal acceleration of the sled ($R2 = 0.7$, $P < 0.05$). The **VA exceeded its physiological** range by 1.0 (2.1), 3.1 (2.6), 8.9 (1.6), and 9.0 (5.9) mm in the 2.5-, 4.5-, 6.5-, and 8.5-g trauma classes respectively. Nibu K, Cholewicki J, Panjabi MM, Babat LB, Grauer JN, Kothe R, Dvorak J. Dynamic elongation of the vertebral artery during an in vitro whiplash simulation. Eur Spine J. 1997;6(4):286–9.

A functional rotatory computed tomography (CT) study of 423 whiplash patients with cervical spine soft-tissue injury was undertaken to determine its diagnostic value. The results are correlated with previous CT studies on normal subjects, and an evaluation of paradox motion, in which the lower vertebra rotates more than the vertebra immediately superior to it, is given. Asymmetrical left/right rotation reached the pathological value in 36% of the patient population at the level of C0–1. Twice as many patients had hypermobile rotation to the left as compared with the right, perhaps indicating that the right alar ligament is more often damaged in injuries involving the whiplash mechanism. A higher percentage of pathological values for hypermobile rotation was found at the level of C0–1 than at C1–2. Patients exhibiting paradox rotation had a significantly higher amount of rotation to the contralateral side than did those who exhibited no paradox rotation. **These findings validate the use of functional rotatory CT in the evaluation of soft-tissue damage of the upper cervical spine resulting from whiplash injury**. Antinnes JA, Dvorak J, Hayek J, Panjabi MM, Grob D. The value of functional computed tomography in the evaluation of soft-tissue injury in the upper cervical spine. Eur Spine J. 1994;3(2):98–101.

The aim of this study was to determine the clinical validity of functional flexion/extension radiographs of the cervical spine in a defined patient population. Sixty-four adults with functional disorders of the cervical spine underwent passive flexion/extension radiographic examinations. The radiographs were analyzed using a computer assisted method to calculate segmental motion parameters, such as rotations, translations, and centers of rotation. The patients were separated into three groups based on their specific functional disorders, and their motion parameters were compared with those of a healthy population. The three groups consisted of patients with degenerative changes, those with radicular syndrome, and those with whiplash trauma. Most of the patients displayed trends toward hypomobile segmental motion. This trend is displayed more substantially in the groups with degeneration and radicular syndrome. Hypomobility in segmental rotation was significant at C6–C7 for the degenerative and radicular groups. **The trauma group showed trends toward hypermobility in the upper and middle cervical levels**, and the locations of the centers of rotation were shifted in the anterior direction when compared with those of the healthy population. Dvorak J, Panjabi MM, Grob D, Novotny JE, Antinnes JA. Clinical validation of functional flexion/extension radiographs of the cervical spine. Spine. 1993 Jan;18(1):120–7.

The fiber orientation is dependent on the height of dens axis, mostly in the cranial caudal direction. In 12 specimens there was a ligamentous connection between dens and lateral mass of the atlas as a part of the alar ligament. In 2 specimens anterior atlanto-dental ligament was identified. The computerized tomographic (CT) images can clearly show alar ligaments in axial, coronal, and sagittal planes. The ligaments limit the axial rotation in the occipito-atlanto-axial complex (to the right by left alar and vice versa) as well as in side bending. The ligament is most stretched, and consequently most vulnerable, when the head is rotated and in addition flexed. This mechanism, common in whiplash injuries, could lead to irreversible overstretching or rupture of the ligaments especially as the ligaments consist of mainly collagen fibers. Dvorak J, Panjabi MM. Functional anatomy of the alar ligaments. Spine. 1987 Mar;12(2):183–9.

§ 2:34 Whiplash mechanism of injury testing—Medical College of Wisconsin

Recognizing the association of angular loading with brain injuries and inconsistency in previous studies in the application of the biphasic loads to animal, physical, and experimental models, the present study examined the role of the acceleration-deceleration pulse shapes on region-specific strains. An experimentally validated two-dimensional finite element model representing the adult male human head was used. The model simulated the skull and falx as a linear elastic material, cerebrospinal fluid as a hydrodynamic material, and cerebrum as a linear viscoelastic material.

The **falx cerebri**, so named from its sickle-like form, is a strong, arched fold of dura mater which descends vertically in the longitudinal fissure between the cerebral hemispheres.

The cerebrum was divided into 17 regions and peak values of average maximum principal strains were determined. In all simulations, the corpus callosum responded with the highest strains. Strains were the least under all simulations in the lower parietal lobes. In all regions peak strains were the same for both monophase pulses suggesting that the angular velocity may be a better metric than peak acceleration or deceleration. In contrast, for the biphasic pulse, peak strains were region- and pulse-shape specific. Peak values were lower in both biphasic pulses when there was no time separation between the pulses than the corresponding monophase pulse. Increasing separation time intervals increased strains, albeit non-uniformly. Acceleration followed by deceleration pulse produced greater strains in all regions than the other form of biphasic pulse. Thus, **pulse shape appears to have an effect on regional strains in the brain**.

Yoganandan N, Li J, Zhang J, Pintar FA, Gennarelli TA. Influence of angular acceleration-deceleration pulse shapes on regional brain strains. J Biomech. 2008;41(10):2253–62.

Clinical literature consistently identifies women as more susceptible to trauma-related neck pain, commonly resulting from soft tissue cervical spine injury. Structural gender differences may explain altered response to dynamic loading in women leading to increased soft tissue distortion and greater injury susceptibility.

Previous studies investigating male and female vertebral and vertebral body geometry demonstrated female vertebral dimensions were smaller. However, populations were not size matched and parameters related to biomechanical stability were not reported.

Two volunteer subsets were size matched based on sitting height and head circumference. All geometrical measures were greater in men for both subsets. Vertebral width and disc-facet depth were significantly greater in men. Additionally, segmental support area, combining interfacet width and disc-facet depth, was greater in men, indicating more stable intervertebral coupling. Present results of decreased linear and areal cervical dimensions leading to decreased column stability may partially explain **increased traumatic injury rates in women**.

Stemper BD, Yoganandan N, Pintar FA, Maiman DJ, Meyer MA, DeRosia J, Shender BS, Paskoff G. Anatomical gender differences in cervical vertebrae of size-matched volunteers. Spine. 2008 Jan 15;33(2):E44–9.

Biomechanical studies using postmortem human subjects (PMHS) in lateral impact have focused primarily on chest and pelvis injuries, mechanisms, tolerances, and comparison with side impact dummies. A paucity of data exists on the head-neck junction, i.e., forces and moments, and cranial angular accelerations. The objective of this study was to determine lateral impact-induced three-dimensional temporal forces and moments at the head-neck junction and cranial linear and angular accelerations from sled tests using PMHS and compare with responses obtained from an anthropomorphic test device (dummy) designed for lateral impact. Following initial evaluations, PMHS were seated on a sled, restrained using belts, and lateral acceleration was applied. Specimens were instrumented with a pyramid-shaped nine-accelerometer package to record cranial accelerations. A sled accelerometer was used to record the input acceleration. Radiographs and computed tomography scans were obtained to identify pathology. A similar testing protocol was adopted for dummy tests. Results indicated that profiles of forces and moments at the head-neck junction and cranial accelerations were similar between the two models. However, peak forces and moments at the head-neck junction were lower in the dummy than PMHS. Peak cranial linear and angular accelerations were also lower in the dummy than in the PMHS. Fractures to the head-neck complex were not identified in PMHS tests. **Peak cranial angular accelerations were suggestive of mild traumatic brain injury with potential for loss of consciousness**. Findings from this study with a limited dataset are valuable in establishing response corridors for side impacts and evaluating side impact dummies used in crashworthiness and safety-engineering studies

Yoganandan N, Pintar FA, Zhang J, Stemper BD, Philippens M. Upper neck forces and moments and cranial angular accelerations in lateral impact. Ann Biomed Eng. 2008 Mar;36(3):406–14.

While lateral impact sled studies have been conducted to determine injuries, injury mechanisms, and derive human tolerance using post mortem human subject (PMHS) for the chest and pelvis regions of the human body, there is a paucity of three-dimensional (3-D) motions at high-speeds. Since out-of-position occupants respond with 3-D motions even under pure frontal and lateral impacts, it is important to determine such kinematics at high-speeds in the temporal domain. Consequently, the objective of the study was to determine lateral impact-induced 3-D temporal motions at 1,000 frames per sec. PMHS were screened, seated on a sled, restrained using belt systems, and 13.5 g lateral impact acceleration was applied. Retroreflective photographic markers were placed at various locations including the head, first thoracic vertebra, sacrum, dorsal spine, and sled. 3-D coordinates of the anatomical locations of PMHS, fiducially placed markers, and sled were obtained pretest and post test. Kinematics of the head with respect to sled, head with respect to first thoracic vertebra, and first thoracic vertebra with respect to sled in the Cartesian system of reference were determined using a nine-camera system. Head and first thoracic vertebral kinematic data are reported in the paper. 3-D motions induced from lateral impacts supplement sensor-based data for improved crashworthiness evaluations.

Yoganandan N, Pintar FA, Gennarelli TA. High-speed 3-D kinematics from whole-body lateral impact sled tests. Biomed Sci Instrum. 2007;43:40-5.

The objective of the present investigation is to determine localized brains strains in lateral impact using finite element modeling and evaluate the role of the falx. A two-dimensional finite element model was developed and validated with experimental data from literature. Motions and strains from the stress analysis matched well with experimental results. A parametric study was conducted by introducing flexible falx in the finite element model. For the model with the rigid falx, high strains were concentrated in the corpus callosum, whereas for the model with the flexible falx, high strains extended into the cerebral vertex. These preliminary findings indicate that the flexibility of falx has an effect on regional brain strains in lateral impact.

Li J, Zhang J, Yoganandan N, Pintar F, Gennarelli T. Regional brain strains and role of falx in lateral impact-induced head rotational acceleration. Biomed Sci Instrum. 2007;43:24–9.

This paper presents a survey of side impact trauma-related biomedical investigations with specific reference to certain aspects of epidemiology relating to the growing elderly population, improvements in technology such as side airbags geared toward occupant safety, and development of injury criteria. The first part is devoted to the involvement of the elderly by identifying variables contributing to injury including impact severity, human factors, and national and international field data. This is followed by a survey of various experimental models used in the development of injury criteria and tolerance limits. The effects of fragility of the elderly coupled with physiological changes (e.g., visual, musculoskeletal) that may lead to an abnormal seating position (termed out-of-position) especially for the driving population are discussed. Fundamental biomechanical parameters such as thoracic, abdominal and pelvic forces; upper and lower spinal and sacrum accelerations; and upper, middle and lower chest deflections under various initial impacting conditions are evaluated. Secondary variables such as the thoracic trauma index and pelvic acceleration (currently adopted in the United States Federal Motor Vehicle Safety Standards), peak chest deflection, and viscous criteria are also included in the survey. The importance of performing research studies with specific focus on out-of-position scenarios of the elderly and using the most commonly available torso side airbag as the initial contacting condition in lateral impacts for occupant injury assessment is emphasized.

Yoganandan N, Pintar FA, Stemper BD, Gennarelli TA, Weigelt JA. Biomechanics of side impact: injury criteria, aging occupants, and airbag technology. J Biomech. 2007;40(2):227–43

Reflex contraction did not substantially alter spinal kinematics; muscle contraction likely does not initiate in sufficient time to mitigate whiplash injuries that may occur during the retraction phase. Stemper BD, Yoganandan N, Rao RD, Pintar FA. Reflex muscle contraction in the unaware occupant in whiplash injury. Spine. 2005 Dec 15;30(24):2794–8; 2799 *(discussion).*

Due to the nominal effect of reflexive muscle contraction on segmental angulations and facet joint capsular ligament distractions during S-curvature, **it is unlikely that this contraction can alter the cervical kinematics responsible for whiplash injury**. Stemper BD, Yoganandan N, Pintar FA. Influence of muscle contraction on whiplash kinematics. Biomed Sci Instrum. 2004;40:24–9.

Shear and axial force, extension moment, and head angular acceleration increased with impact severity. Shear force was significantly larger than axial force ($p < 0.0001$). Shear force reached its maximum value at 46 msec. Maximum extension moment occurred between 7 and 22 msec after maximum shear force. Maximum angular acceleration of the head occurred 2 to 18 msec later. Maximum axial force occurred last (106 msec). All four kinetic components reached maximum values during cervical S-curvature, with maximum shear force and extension moment occurring before the attainment of maximum

S-curvature. Results of the present investigation indicate that **shear force and extension moment at the cervico-thoracic junction drive the non-physiologic cervical S-curvature responsible for whiplash injury and underscore the importance of understanding cervical kinematics and the underlying kinetics.** Stemper BD, Yoganandan N, Pintar FA. Kinetics of the head-neck complex in low-speed rear impact. Biomed Sci Instrum. 2003;39:245–50.

The presence of increased facet joint motions indicated that synovial joint soft-tissue components (i.e., synovial membrane and capsular ligament) sustain increased distortion that may subject these tissues to a greater likelihood of injury. **This finding is supported by clinical investigations in which lower cervical facet joint injury resulted in similar pain patterns due to the most commonly reported whiplash symptoms.** Stemper BD, Yoganandan N, Gennarelli TA, Pintar FA. Localized cervical facet joint kinematics under physiological and whiplash loading. J Neurosurg Spine. 2005 Dec;3(6):471–6.

A parametric study of increasing head restraint backset between 0 and 140mm was conducted using a comprehensively validated computational model. Head retraction values increased with increasing backset, reaching a maximum value of 53.5mm for backsets greater than 60mm. Segmental angulation magnitudes, greatest at levels C5–C6 and C6–C7, reached maximum values during the retraction phase and increased with increasing backset. Results were compared to a previously published head restraint rating system, wherein lower cervical extension magnitudes from this study exceeded mean physiologic limits for restraint positions rated good, acceptable, marginal, and poor. As head restraint contact was the limiting factor in head retraction and segmental angulations, the present study indicates that **minimizing whiplash injury may be accomplished by limiting head restraint backset to less than 60mm, either passively or actively after impact**. Stemper BD, Yoganandan N, Pintar FA. Effect of head restraint backset on head-neck kinematics in whiplash. Accid Anal Prev. 2006 Mar;38(2):317–23.

Anterior longitudinal ligament injuries in whiplash may lead to cervical instability. Injury to anterior spinal structures can result in clinical indications including cervical instability in extension, axial rotation, and lateral bending modes. In particular, the C5–C6 anterior longitudinal ligament sustained distraction magnitudes as high as 2.6mm during the retraction phase, corresponding to 56% of distraction necessary to result in ligament failure. Present results demonstrated that **anterior structures in the lower cervical spine may be susceptible to injury through excess distraction during the retraction phase of whiplash, which likely occurs prior to head restraint contact**. Susceptibility of these structures is likely due to non-physiologic loading placed on the cervical spinal column as the head translates posteriorly relative to the thorax. Stemper BD, Yoganandan N, Pintar FA, Rao RD. Anterior longitudinal ligament injuries in whiplash may lead to cervical instability. Med Eng Phys. 2006 Jul;28(6):515–24.

§ 2:35 Whiplash mechanism of injury testing—Medical College of Wisconsin—Abnormal posture and whiplash

The whiplash experiments in this study were collisions at less than 6 miles/hour. This study showed that pre-whiplash accident **straight or kyphotic curvatures of the cervical spine increase injury to the facet joint ligaments**. Specifically, **straight or kyphotic curvatures of the cervical spine increased cervical facet capsular ligament stretch by up to 70%.** Straight cervical spines and cervical kyphosis affect injury mechanisms and lead to increased acute and chronic disorders. Pre-whiplash impact alignment of the cervical spine significantly affects injury mechanisms and severity of injury. **This study advanced the hypothesis that abnormal curvatures (straight or kyphotic) of the cervical column affect spinal kinematics during whiplash loading.** Specifically, compared to the normal lordotic curvature, abnormal curvatures altered facet joint ligament elongations. Under the normal posture, greatest elongations occurred in the dorsal anatomic region at the C2–C3 level and in the lateral anatomic region from C3–C4 to C6–C7 levels. Stemper BD, Yoganandan N, Pintar FA. Effects of abnormal posture on capsular ligament elongations in a computational model subjected to whiplash loading. J Biomech. 2005 Jun;38(6):1313–23.

§ 2:36 Whiplash mechanism of injury testing—Medical College of Wisconsin—Gender and region-dependent kinematics

Localized facet joint kinematics resulting from whiplash acceleration were analyzed in the dynamic domain during the time of cervical S-curvature using intact head and neck specimens and a pendulum mini-sled loading apparatus. To determine the effects of gender, impact severity, cervical level, and anatomic joint region on shear and distraction motion of lower cervical facet joints. Clinical and experimental studies identify cervical facet joints to be a likely location of whiplash injury. **Epidemiologic studies report that female occupants sustain a greater percentage of whiplash injuries**. Previous experimental studies have not analyzed facet joint motion as a function of variables such as gender. Intact head and neck complexes were subjected to whiplash acceleration using a pendulum mini-sled apparatus at four impact severities. Facet joint kinematics were analyzed using digital high-resolution video at 1000 frames per second during the time of maximum cervical S-curvature. Shear and distraction motions were analyzed in the ventral and dorsal joint regions from C4–C5 to C6–C7 levels. Analysis of variance techniques were used to analyze biomechanical data. Intact head and neck complexes sustained cervical S-curvature during whiplash loading. Lower cervical facet joints demonstrated dorsally directed shear motion with distraction in the ventral and compression in the dorsal regions of the joint. Magnitudes of distraction and compression were significantly lower than shear motion ($P < 0.05$). Facet joint shear and distraction motion increased with impact severity. Lower cervical facet joint shear and distraction motions in female specimens were greater than in male specimens. This difference reached statistical significance at C4–C5 ($P < 0.05$). **Secondary to whiplash loading, lower cervical facet joints responded with a shear plus distraction mechanism in the anatomic ventral and shear plus compression mechanisms in the dorsal region. Injury to the ventral region stems from tensile failure of the joint capsule. Injury to the dorsal region stems from pinching of the joint capsule or synovial fold and contact between subchondral bone of superior and inferior facet processes. Because excess spinal motion is biomechanically related to abnormalities and because lower cervical facet joints sustain greater motion in female specimens**, this population is more likely to be injured under whiplash loading. Potential contributors for the susceptibility of females to injury, including genotypic (apolipoprotein APOE-epsilon4), hormonal, structural, and tolerance factors, are discussed. Stemper BD, Yoganandan N, Pintar FA. Gender- and region-dependent local facet joint kinematics in rear impact: implications in whiplash injury. Spine. 2004 Aug 15;29(16):1764–71.

Clinical and epidemiological studies have frequently reported that female occupants sustain whiplash injuries more often than males. The current study was based on the hypothesis that segmental level-by-level cervical intervertebral motions in females are greater than in males during rear impact. The hypothesis was tested by subjecting 10 intact human cadaver head-neck complexes (five males, five females) to rear impact loading. Intervertebral kinematics were analyzed as a function of spinal level at the time of maximum cervical S-curve, which occurred during the loading phase. **Segmental angles were significantly greater ($p<0.05$) in female specimens at C2–C3, C4–C5, C5–C6, and C6–C7 levels**. Because greater angulations are associated with stretch in the innervated components of the cervical spinal column, these findings may offer a biomechanical explanation for the higher incidence of whiplash-related complaints in female patients secondary to rear impact acceleration. Stemper BD, Yoganandan N, Pintar FA. Gender dependent cervical spine segmental kinematics during whiplash. J Biomech. 2003 Sep;36(9):1281–9.

§ 2:37 Whiplash mechanism of injury testing—Medical College of Wisconsin—Validation of a head-neck computer model for whiplash simulation

A head-neck computer model was comprehensively validated over a range of rear-impact velocities using experiments conducted by the same group of authors in the same laboratory. Validations were based on mean +/- 1 standard deviation response curves, i.e. corridors. Global head-neck angle, segmental angle and local facet joint regional kinematic responses from the model fell within experimental corridors. This was true for all impact velocities (1.3, 1.8 and 2.6 m s(-1)). **The non-physiological S-curvature lasted approximately 100 ms.** The present, comprehensively validated model can be used to conduct parametric studies and investigate the effects of factors such as active sequential and parallel muscle contractions, thoracic ramping and local tissue strain responses, as a function of cervical level, joint region and impact velocity in whiplash injury assessment. Stemper BD, Yoganandan N, Pintar FA. Validation of a head-neck computer model for whiplash simulation. Med Biol Eng Comput. 2004 May;42(3):333–8.

Influence of muscle contraction on whiplash kinematics. It is unclear whether **reflexive muscle contraction in unaware occupants** can alter spinal kinematics to mitigate injury in the unaware occupant subjected to whiplash loading. Whiplash injury likely occurs during the non-physiologic S-curvature phase of spinal kinematics, present during the first 100 msec after the initiation of T1 acceleration. Experimental investigations using human volunteers have reported 45 to 60 msec delays prior to electrical activity of the sternocleidomastoid. The effects of reflexive contraction of the neck muscles were investigated using a validated head-neck computational model consisting of head, cervical spine, and first thoracic vertebra. Intervertebral discs, spinal ligaments, and facet joints were modeled using discrete elements. Passive and active musculature were incorporated using the Hill-type muscle model. The computational model was subjected to 2.6 m/sec rear impact velocity, applied to T1. Reflexive muscle contraction in the unaware occupant model was incorporated using a 54-msec muscle delay, 13-msec electromechanical delay, and an 81-msec muscle rise time. Results of the unaware occupant model were compared to the model exercised without muscle contraction. Reflexive muscle contraction altered segmental angulations by less than 10% and facet joint capsular ligament distractions by less than 16% during the time of maximum S-curvature. At the C5–C6 and C6–C7 levels, muscle contraction increased capsular ligament distractions. Due to the nominal affect of reflexive muscle contraction on segmental angulations and facet joint capsular ligament distractions during S-curvature, **it is unlikely that this contraction can alter the cervical kinematics responsible for whiplash injury**. Stemper BD, Yoganandan N, Pintar FA. Influence of muscle contraction on whiplash kinematics. Biomed Sci Instrum. 2004;40:24–9.

Kinetics of the head-neck complex in low-speed rear impact. A comprehensive characterization of the biomechanics of the cervical spine in rear impact will lead to an understanding of the mechanisms of whiplash injury. Cervical kinematics have been experimentally described using human volunteers, full-body cadaver specimens, and isolated and intact head-neck specimens. However, forces and moments at the cervicothoracic junction have not been clearly delineated. An experimental investigation was performed using ten intact head-neck complexes to delineate the loading at the base of the cervical spine and angular acceleration of the head in whiplash. A pendulum-minisled apparatus was used to simulate whiplash acceleration of the thorax at four impact severities. Lower neck loads were measured using a six-axis load cell attached between the minisled and head-neck specimens, and head angular motion was measured with an angular rate sensor attached to the lateral side of the head. Shear and axial force, extension moment, and head angular acceleration increased with impact severity. Shear force was significantly larger than axial force ($p < 0.0001$). **Shear force reached its maximum value at 46 msec. Maximum extension moment occurred between 7 and 22 msec after maximum shear force**. Maximum angular acceleration of the head occurred 2 to 18 msec later. Maximum axial force occurred last (106 msec). All four kinetic components reached maximum values during cervical S-curvature, with maximum shear force and extension moment occurring before the attainment of maximum S-curvature. **Results of the present investigation indicate that shear force and extension moment at the cervico-thoracic junction drive the non-physiologic cervical S-curvature responsible for whiplash injury** and underscore the importance of understanding cervical kinematics and the underlying kinetics. Stemper BD, Yoganandan N, Pintar FA. Kinetics of the head-neck complex in low-speed rear impact. Biomed Sci Instrum. 2003;39:245–50.

Intervertebral rotations as a function of rear impact loading. Rear impact loading of the cervical spine results in a complicated biomechanical problem due to the complex geometry and viscoelastic material properties of this anatomy. Although a number of investigations have been performed to understand the biomechanics of rear impact, the dependence of segmental kinematics on cervical level and input velocity has not been clearly outlined. An experimental investigation was performed for this purpose using 10 isolated head-neck specimens. Segmental motions of the cervical spine were obtained for levels C2–C3 to C6–C7 at rear impact velocities of 2.1, 4.6, 6.6, and 9.3 km/h. Increases in segmental motion from baseline kinematics were compared for the three higher velocity tests. Results indicated greater increase in magnitude of segmental motion for levels **C5–C6 and C6–C7** at higher input velocities than all other investigated levels. This finding helps to define the kinematics of the cervical spine leading to whiplash injury. Stemper BD, Yoganandan N, Pintar FA. Intervertebral rotations as a function of rear impact loading. Biomed Sci Instrum. 2002;38:227–31.

§ 2:38 Whiplash mechanism of injury testing—Medical College of Wisconsin—Whiplash injury determination with conventional spine imaging and cryomicrotomy

Soft tissue-related injuries to the cervical spine structures were produced by use of intact entire human cadavers undergoing rear-end impacts. Radiography, computed tomography, and cryomicrotomy techniques were used to evaluate the injury. To replicate soft tissue injuries resulting from single input of whiplash acceleration to whole human cadavers simulating vehicular rear impacts, and to assess the ability of different modes of imaging to visualize soft tissue cervical lesions. Whiplash-associated disorders such as headache and neck pain are implicated with soft tissue abnormalities to structures of the cervical spine. To the authors' best knowledge, no previous studies have been conducted to determine whether single cycle whiplash acceleration input to intact entire human cadavers can result in these soft tissue alterations. There is also a scarcity of data on the efficacy of radiography and computed tomography in assessing these injuries. Four intact entire human cadavers underwent single whiplash acceleration (3.3 g or 4.5 g) loading by use of a whole-body sled. Pretest and posttest radiographs, computed tomography images, and sequential anatomic sections using a cryomicrotome were obtained to determine the extent of trauma to the cervical spine structures. Routine radiography identified the least number of lesions (one lesion in two specimens). Although computed tomography was more effective (three lesions in two specimens), trauma was not readily apparent to all soft tissues of the cervical spine. Cryomicrotome sections identified structural alterations in all four specimens to lower cervical spine components that included **stretch and tear of the ligamentum flavum, anulus disruption, anterior longitudinal ligament rupture, and zygopophysial joint compromise with tear of the capsular ligaments**. These results clearly indicate that a single application of whiplash acceleration pulse **can induce soft tissue-related and ligament-related alterations to cervical spine structures**. The pathologic changes identified in this study support previous observations from human volunteers observations with regard to the location of whiplash injury and may assist in the explanation of pain arising from this injury. Although computed tomography is a better imaging modality than radiography, subtle but clinically relevant injuries may be left undiagnosed with this technique. The cryomicrotome technique offers a unique procedure to understand and compare soft tissue-related injuries to the cervical anatomy caused by whiplash loading. Recognition of these injuries may advance the general knowledge of the whiplash disorder. Yoganandan N, Cusick JF, Pintar FA, Rao RD. Whiplash injury determination with conventional spine imaging and cryomicrotomy. Spine. 2001 Nov 15;26(22):2443–8.

§ 2:39 Whiplash mechanism of injury testing—Medical College of Wisconsin—Whiplash syndrome: kinematic factors influencing pain patterns

Neck pain and headaches are the two most common symptoms of whiplash. The working hypothesis is that pain originates from excessive motions in the upper and lower cervical segments. The research design used an intact human cadaver head-neck complex as an experimental model. The intact head-neck preparation was fixed at the thoracic end with the head unconstrained. Retroreflective targets were placed on the mastoid process, anterior regions of the vertebral bodies, and lateral masses at every spinal level. Whiplash loading was delivered using a mini-sled pendulum device. A six-axis load cell and an accelerometer were attached to the inferior fixation of the specimen. High-speed video cameras were used to obtain the kinematics. During the initial stages of loading, a transient decoupling of the head occurs with respect to the neck exhibiting a lag of the cranium. The upper cervical spine-head undergoes local flexion concomitant with a lag of the head while the lower column is in local extension. This establishes a reverse curvature to the head-neck complex. With continuing application of whiplash loading, the inertia of the head catches up with the neck. Later, the entire head-neck complex is under an extension mode with a single extension curvature. **The lower cervical facet joint kinematics demonstrates varying local compression and sliding**. While the anterior- and posterior-most regions of the facet joint slide, the posterior-most region of the joint compresses more than the anterior-most region. These varying kinematics at the two ends of the **facet joint result in a pinching mechanism**. Excessive flexion of the posterior upper cervical regions can be correlated to headaches. **The pinching mechanism of the facet joints can be correlated to neck pain**. The kinematics of the soft tissue-related structures explain the mechanism of these common whiplash associated disorders. Yoganandan N, Pintar FA, Cusick JF. Biomechanical analyses of whiplash injuries using an experimental model. Accid Anal Prev. 2002 Sep;34(5):663–71.

The overall, local, and segmental kinematic responses of intact human cadaver head-neck complexes undergoing an inertia-type rear-end impact were quantified. High-speed, high-resolution digital video data of individual facet joint motions during the event were statistically evaluated. To deduce the potential for various vertebral column components to be exposed to adverse strains that could result in their participation as pain generators, and to evaluate the abnormal motions that occur during this traumatic event. The vertebral column is known to incur a nonphysiologic curvature during the application of an inertial-type rear-end impact. No previous studies, however, have quantified the local component motions (facet joint compression and sliding) that occur as a result of rear-impact loading. Intact human cadaver head-neck complexes underwent inertia-type rear-end impact with predominant moments in the sagittal plane. High-resolution digital video was used to track the motions of individual facet joints during the event. Localized angular motion changes at each vertebral segment were analyzed to quantify the abnormal curvature changes. Facet joint motions were analyzed statistically to obtain differences between anterior and posterior strains. The spine initially assumed an S-curve, with the upper spinal levels in flexion and the lower spinal levels in extension. The upper C-spine flexion occurred early in the event (approximately 60 ms) during the time the head maintained its static inertia. The lower cervical spine facet joints demonstrated statistically greater compressive motions in the dorsal aspect than in the ventral aspect, whereas the sliding anteroposterior motions were the same. **The nonphysiologic kinematic responses during a whiplash impact may induce stresses in certain upper cervical neural structures or lower facet joints, resulting in possible compromise sufficient to elicit either neuropathic or nociceptive pain**. These dynamic alterations of the upper level (occiput to C2) could impart potentially adverse forces to related neural structures, with subsequent development of a neuropathic pain process. The pinching of the lower facet joints may lead to potential for local tissue injury and nociceptive pain. Cusick JF, Pintar FA, Yoganandan N. Whiplash syndrome: kinematic factors influencing pain patterns. Spine. 2001 Jun 1;26(11):1252–8.

Whiplash injuries sustained during a rear-end automobile collision have significant societal impact. The scientific literature on whiplash loading is both diverse and confusing. Definitive studies are lacking to describe the local mechanisms of injury that induce either acute or chronic pain symptoms. A methodology has been presented to quantify the kinematics of the cervical spine components by inducing controlled whiplash-type forces to intact human head-neck complexes. The localized facet joint kinematics and the overall segmental motions of the cervical spine are presented. It is anticipated that the use of this methodology will assist in a better delineation of the localized mechanisms of injury leading to whiplash pain. Yoganandan N, Pintar FA, Klienberger M. Cervical spine vertebral and facet joint kinematics under whiplash. J Biomech Eng. 1998 Apr;120(2):305–7.

§ 2:40 Head position and impact direction in whiplash injuries

Whiplash patients who had been sitting with their **head/neck turned** to one side at the moment of collision more often had high-grade lesions of the alar and transverse ligaments ($p < 0.001$, $p = 0.040$, respectively). **Severe injuries to the transverse ligament and the posterior atlanto-occipital membrane were more common in front than in rear-end collisions** ($p < 0.001$, $p = 0.001$, respectively). In conclusion, the difference in MRI-verified lesions between WAD patients and control persons, and in particular the association with head position and impact direction at time of accident, indicate that these lesions are caused by the whiplash trauma. Kaale BR, Krakenes J, Albrektsen G, Wester K. Head position and impact direction in whiplash injuries: associations with MRI-verified lesions of ligaments and membranes in the upper cervical spine. J Neurotrauma. 2005 Nov;22(11):1294–302.

Elongation-induced vertebral artery injury is more likely to occur in those with rotated head posture at the time of rear impact, as compared to head-forward. Ivancic PC, Ito S, Tominaga Y, Carlson EJ, Rubin W, Panjabi MM. Effect of rotated head posture on dynamic vertebral artery elongation during simulated rear impact. Clin Biomech (Bristol, Avon). 2006 Mar;21(3):213–20.

Greater potential for ganglion compression injury existed at C3–4 and C4–5 during **head-turned rear impact** than during head-forward rear impact; potential ganglion compression occurred in patients with a non-stenotic foramen at C5–6 and C6–7. In patients with a stenotic foramen, the injury risk greatly increases and spreads to include the C3–4 through C6–7, as well as C4–5 through C6–7 nerve roots. Tominaga Y, Maak TG, Ivancic PC, Panjabi MM, Cunningham BW. Head-turned rear impact causing dynamic cervical intervertebral foramen narrowing: implications for ganglion and nerve root injury. J Neurosurg Spine. 2006 May;4(5):380–7.

Head-turned rear impact caused significantly greater injury at C0–C1 and C5–C6, as compared to head-forward rear and frontal impacts, and resulted in multiplanar injuries at C5–C6 and C7–T1. The injury threshold acceleration was 5 g with injury occurring in extension or axial rotation at C3–C4 through C7–T1, excluding C6–C7. Following 8 g, 3-plane injury occurred in extension and axial rotation at C5–C6, while 2-plane injury occurred at C7–T1. Panjabi MM, Ivancic PC, Maak TG, Tominaga Y, Rubin W. Multiplanar cervical spine injury due to head-turned rear impact. Spine. 2006 Feb 15;31(4):420–9.

The alar, transverse, and apical ligaments are not at risk for injury due to head-turned rear impacts up to 8 g. The upper cervical spine symptomatology reported by whiplash patients may, therefore, be explained by other factors, including severe whiplash trauma in excess of 8 g peak acceleration and/or other impact types, e.g., offset, rollover, and multiple collisions. Maak TG, Tominaga Y, Panjabi MM, Ivancic PC. Alar, transverse, and apical ligament strain due to head-turned rear impact. Spine. 2006 Mar 15;31(6):632–8.

Influence of the crash pulse shape on the peak loading and the injury tolerance levels of the neck in vitro low-speed side-collisions. The aim of the present in vitro study was to investigate the effect of the crash pulse shape on the peak loading and the injury tolerance levels of the human neck. In a custom-made acceleration apparatus, 12 human cadaveric cervical spine specimens equipped with a dummy head were subjected to a series of incremental side accelerations. While the duration of the acceleration pulse of the sled was kept constant at 120 ms, its shape was varied: Six specimens were loaded with a slowly increasing pulse, i.e., a low loading rate; the other six specimens with a fast increasing pulse, i.e., a high loading rate. The loading of the neck was quantified in terms of the peak linear and angular acceleration of the head, the peak shear force and bending moment of the lower neck, and the peak translation between head and sled. The shape of the acceleration curve of the sled only seemed to influence the peak translation between head and sled but none of the other four parameters. The neck injury tolerance level for the angular acceleration of the head and for the bending moment of the lower neck was almost identical for both the high and the low loading rate. In contrast, the injury tolerance level for the linear acceleration of the head and for the shear force of the lower neck was slightly higher for the low loading rate, as compared to the high loading rate. For the translation between head and sled, this difference was even statistically significant. Thus, **if the shape of the crash pulse is not known, solely the peak bending moment of the lower neck and the peak angular acceleration of the head seem to be suitable predictors for the neck injury risk** but not the peak shear force of the lower neck, the peak linear acceleration of the head, and the translation between head and thorax. Kettler A, Fruth K, Claes L, Wilke HJ. Influence of the crash pulse shape on the peak loading and the injury tolerance levels of the neck in in vitro low-speed side-collisions. J Biomech. 2006;39(2):323–9.

Intervertebral neck injury criterion for prediction of multiplanar cervical spine injury due to side impacts. Intervertebral Neck Injury Criterion (IV-NIC) is based on the hypothesis that dynamic three-dimensional intervertebral motion beyond physiological limits may cause multiplanar injury of cervical spine soft tissues. Using a biofidelic whole human cervical spine model with muscle force replication and surrogate head in simulated side impacts, the goals of this study were to correlate IV-NIC with multiplanar injury and determine IV-NIC injury threshold for each intervertebral level. Using a bench-top apparatus, side impacts were simulated at 3.5, 5, 6.5, and 8 g horizontal accelerations of the T1 vertebra. Pre- and post-impact flexibility testing in three-motion planes measured the soft tissue injury, i.e., significant increase ($p < 0.05$) in neutral zone (NZ) or range of motion (RoM) at any intervertebral level, above corresponding physiological limit. Results showed that IV-NIC in left lateral bending correlated well with total lateral bending RoM ($R = 0.61$, $P < 0.001$) and NZ ($R = 0.55$, $P < 0.001$). Additionally, the same IV-NIC correlated well with left axial rotation RoM ($R = 0.50$, $P < 0.001$). IV-NIC injury thresholds (95% confidence limits) varied among intervertebral levels and ranged between 1.5 (0.6–2.4) at C3–C4 and 4.0 (2.4–5.7) at C7–T1. IV-NIC injury threshold times were attained beginning at 84.5ms following impact. Present results suggest that **IV-NIC is an effective tool for determining multiplanar soft tissue neck injuries by identifying the intervertebral level, mode, time, and severity of injury**. Panjabi MM, Ivancic PC, Tominaga Y, Wang JL. Intervertebral neck injury criterion for prediction of multiplanar cervical spine injury due to side impacts. Traffic Inj Prev. 2005 Dec;6(4):387–97.

Side Impact Causes Multiplanar Cervical Spine injuries

Side impact caused multiplanar injuries at C3-4 through C7-T1 and significantly greater at C6-7 as compared with hear-forward rear impact.

The injuries caused by side impact were limited to C3-C4 through C7-T1 intervertebra1 levels.

Left lateral bending injuries caused by side impact may cause capsular ligament and lateral annular fiber and ruptures.

Maak TG, Ivancic PC, Tominaga Y, Panjabi MM. Side impact causes multiplanar cervical spine injuries. J Trauma. 2007 Dec;63(6):1296–307.

Correlation between neck injury risk and impact severity parameters in low-speed side collisions. In vitro acceleration study on human cadaveric cervical spine specimens was conducted to investigate the correlation between the risk to sustain a structural cervical spine injury and vehicle-related impact severity parameters. Impact severity parameters, such as the peak acceleration of the vehicle, its mean acceleration, and its velocity change, are often used to predict the whiplash injury risk or to objectify the patient's symptoms even though their correlation to injury is still not well understood. In a series of three in vitro experiments, a total of 18 human cadaveric cervical spine specimens were subjected to incremental side accelerations until structural injury occurred. While the duration of the acceleration pulse was kept constant throughout all three experiments, its shape was varied. **The injury risk to the cervical spine was predictable by the mean acceleration** of the sled and since the duration of the crash pulses was constant also by its velocity change but not by its peak acceleration. Kettler A, Fruth K, Hartwig E, Claes L, Wilke HJ. Correlation between neck injury risk and impact severity parameters in low-speed side collisions. Spine. 2004 Nov 1;29(21):2404–9.

Patterns of injury to restrained children in side impact motor vehicle crashes: the side impact syndrome. Injury patterns among children in frontal collisions have been well documented, but little information exists regarding injuries to children in side-impact collisions. Restrained children, 14-years-old or younger, admitted to the hospital for crash injuries were analyzed. Data concerning injuries, medical treatment, and outcome were correlated with crash data. Case reviews achieved consensus regarding injury contact points. Side impacts were compared with frontal impacts. These results were then compared with data from the National Automotive Sampling System. There were no differences between the groups with respect to age, sex, restraint type, or seat position. Compared with frontal crashes, children in side impacts were more likely to have an Injury Severity Score > 15 (odds ratio [OR], 3.1; 95% confidence interval [CI], 1.7–5.8) and were more likely to have Abbreviated Injury Scale score 2+

injuries to the head (OR, 2.5; 95% CI, 1.4–4.4), chest (OR, 4.0; 95% CI, 2.0–8.0), and cervical spine (OR, 3.7; 95% CI, 1.2–11.3). When compared with National Automotive Sampling System data, similar trends were seen regarding Abbreviated Injury Scale score 2+ injuries to the head, chest, and extremities. **In this study population, side impacts resulted in more injuries to the head, cervical spine, and chest.** Orzechowski KM, Edgerton EA, Bulas DI, McLaughlin PM, Eichelberger MR. Patterns of injury to restrained children in side impact motor vehicle crashes: the side impact syndrome. J Trauma. 2003 Jun;54(6):1094–101.

Chapter 3

Crash Study Comparisons

§ 3:1 Overview of chapter

Human crash studies are just that: vehicle collision tests involving live humans. These tests are designed mainly to measure movement of the subject, not to cause injury. The subjects are medically screened and sign a waiver prior to enrollment in the study. Obviously, the subjects are aware of what is to take place. Although there are no reported cases of chronic complaints following these tests, almost all of the tests do show some short-term complaints. Almost all of the tests have the subjects seated in an optimal position to resist injury. In most of the tests, there have been some modifications to the vehicles. Typically, only a few subjects are tested.

Most of the testing involves members of a society that investigate collisions. Some are employees of the business that conducted the tests; others are sponsored by insurance companies. See e.g., McConnell SAE 1993, 1995.

The most subjects in a crash-testing series is 42, with 21 male and 21 female participants. Test speeds were at 2.5 and 5.0 mph. Symptoms were produced in 29% at 2.5 mph; 38% at 5 mph experienced whiplash symptoms. Brault JR, Wheeler JB, Siegmund GP, Brault EJ. Clinical response of human subjects to rear-end automobile collisions. Arch Phys Med Rehabil. 1998 Jan;79(1):72–80.

Note that commentators of these types of tests have pointed out that factors other than selected peak kinematic responses influenced symptom production. **No one parameter was sufficiently strong to successfully predict symptoms.** Extrapolation of the current model outside these test conditions, injury types and injury severities may be inappropriate. **The results of this analysis were based on controlled human subjects tests using one vehicle, one seat, and one seated posture.** Siegmund GP, Brault JR, Wheeler JB. The relationship between clinical and kinematic responses from human subject testing in rear-end automobile collisions. Accid Anal Prev. 2000 Mar;32(2):207–17.

Variability in vehicle and dummy responses in rear-end collisions. The objective of this study was to quantify the occupant response variability due to differences in vehicle and seat design in low-speed rear-end collisions. Occupant response variability was quantified using a BioRID dummy exposed to rear-end collisions in 20 different vehicles. Vehicles were rolled rearward into a rigid barrier at 8 km/h, and the dynamic responses of the vehicle and dummy were measured with the head restraint adjusted to the upper most position. In vehicles not damaged by this collision, additional tests were conducted with the head restraint down and at different impact speeds. Despite a coefficient of variation (COV) of less than 2% for the impact speed of the initial 8 km/h tests, the vehicle response parameters (i.e., speed change, acceleration, restitution, bumper force) had COVs of 7 to 23%, and the dummy response parameters (head and T1 kinematics, neck loads, neck injury criterion (NIC), N(ij) and N(km)) had COVs of 14 to 52%. In five vehicles tested multiple times, a **head restraint in the down position significantly increased the peak magnitude of many dummy kinematic and kinetic response parameters**. Peak head kinematics and neck kinetics generally varied linearly with head restraint back set and height, although the neck reaction moment reversed and increased considerably if the dummy's head wrapped onto the top of the head restraint. **The results of this study support the proposition that the vehicle, seat, and head restraint are a safety system and that the design of vehicle bumpers and seats/head restraint should be considered together to maximize the potential reduction in whiplash injuries**. Siegmund GP, Heinrichs BE, Chimich DD, Lawrence J. Variability in vehicle and dummy responses in rear-end collisions. Traffic Inj Prev. 2005 Sep;6(3):267–77.

Human crash test studies show that there is complex motion.

Injuries do occur in speeds as low as 2.5 mph Delta-V. Although the symptoms only lasted for a short period of time, the subjects are pre-screened before they are allowed to participate in the study. Essentially, injury can occur at very low levels, and it is more of a consequence of the occupant than any measured vehicle parameter.

The larger retractions observed in surprised females likely produce larger tissue strains and may increase injury potential. **Aware human subjects may not replicate the muscle response, kinematic response, or whiplash injury potential of unprepared occupants in real collisions**. Siegmund GP, Sanderson DJ, Myers BS, Inglis JT. Awareness affects the response of human subjects exposed to a single whiplash-like perturbation. Spine. 2003 Apr 1;28(7):671–9

§ 3:2 Commonly cited defense studies

Below is a list of human crash tests commonly cited by the defense in soft tissue cases. These studies are discussed in more detail in later chapters of this text. Following this list is a table with an overview of the key findings from these studies.

1. Severy DM, Mathewson JH, Bechtol CO. Controlled Automobile Rear-End Collisions, An Investigation of Related Engineering and Medical Phenomena. Canadian Medical Journal 1955;11:152–184.

2. McConnell WE, Howard RP, Guzman HU, Bomar JB, Raddin JH, Benedict JV, Smith HL, Hatsell CP. Analysis of Human Test Subject Kinematic Responses to Low Velocity Rear-End Impacts: Vehicle and Occupant Kinematics: Simulation and Modeling (SP-975). Society of Automotive Engineers, 930889, Detroit, MI. 1993.

3. Szabo TJ and Welcher JB. Human subjects and electromyographic activity during low-speed rear impacts. SAE 962432, Society of Automotive Engineers, Warrendale PA, 1996

4. McConnell WE, Howard RP, Van Poppel J, et al. Human head and neck kinematics after low-velocity rear-end impacts—understanding "Whiplash." Society of Automotive Engineers 1995;952724.

5. Brault JR, Wheeler JB, Siegmund GP, Brault EJ. Clinical response of human subjects to rear-end automobile collisions. Arch Phys Med Rehabil. 1998 Jan;79(1):72–80.

6. West, DH et al. Low-speed rear-end collision testing using human subjects. Accident Reconstruction Journal, May/June 1993;5:22–26.

7. Siegmund, GP et al. Speed change of amusement park

bumper cars, Canadian Multidisciplinary Road Safety Conference VIII, June 14–16, 1993.

8. Siegmund, GP et al. Characteristics of specific automobile bumpers in low-velocity impacts. SAE 940916, Society of Automotive Engineers, Warrendale PA 1994.

9. Szabo, TJ et al. Human occupant kinematic response to low-speed rear-end impacts. SAE 940532, Society of Automotive Engineers, Warrendale, PA, 1994.

10. Rosenbluth W, Hicks L. Evaluating low-speed rear-end impact severity and resultant occupant stress parameters. J Forensic Sci. 1994 Nov;39(6):1393–424.

11. Bailey, MN et al. Data and methods for estimating the severity of minor impacts. SAE 950352, Society of Automotive Engineers, Warendale, PA 1995.

12. Castro WH, Schilgen M, Meyer S, Weber M, Peuker C, Wortler K. Do "whiplash injuries" occur in low-speed rear impacts? Eur Spine J. 1997;6(6):366–75.

13. Anderson RD, Welcher JB, Szabo TJ, Eubanks JJ, Haight WR. Effect of braking on human occupant and vehicle kinematics in low-speed rear-end collisions. SAE 980298, Society of Automotive Engineers, Detroit, MI, 1998.

§ 3:3 Commonly cited defense studies—Quick review of defense studies [grid]

Authors	Year of Study	Speed Change	Symptoms	Test Subjects
Severy [1]	1955	5.4 to 5.8 mph	None	Male
McConnell [2]	1993	2.5 to 5.0 mph	3 of the 4 developed transient neck and mild back pain at 4 and 5 mph	4 males
West [6]	1993	1.1 to 10.3 mph	Minor neck pain lasting 1 to 2 days	5 males
Siegmund [7]	1993	3.6 to 4.8 bumper cars	None	males

Authors	Year of Study	Speed Change	Symptoms	Test Subjects
Siegmund [8]	1994	1.0 to 5.5 mph	Subject dizzy for 15 minutes following 3.9 mph	males and one female
Szabo [9]	1994	5.0 mph	Transient headache and minor neck stiffness the morning after the test	3 males, 2 females
Rosenbluth [10]	1994	2.0 to 4.8 mph	None	1 male, 1 female
Bailey [11]	1995	1.1 to 5.5 mph	Twinge in neck at 4.3, headache after 3.6 and 4	9 males and fc males
McConnell [4]	1995	3.6 to 6.8 mph	Mild headache and neck pain lasting a few days	7 males
Szabo [3]	1996	4.6 to 6.2 mph and bumper cars	None	male and female
Castro [12]	1997	5.4 to 8.8 mph and 5.1 to 6.6 for bumper cars	Transient symptoms in 4 male, 1 female	14 male, 5 female
Brault [5]	1998	2.5 to 5.0 mph29% at 2.5 mph and 38% at 5.0 mph	Experienced whiplash symptoms	42 subjects, male and female

Authors	Year of Study	Speed Change	Symptoms	Test Subjects
Anderson [13]	1998	1.74 to 5.58 mph	Bilateral neck tenderness resolved in 3 days	male age 23

§ 3:4 "Real world" motor vehicle collision injury studies

Studies that evaluate real accidents may provide more reliable data. Below is an extensive list of such studies, followed by a chart with key findings.

1. Gotten N. Survey of one hundred cases of whiplash injury after settlement of litigation. JAMA 162(9):865–867, 1956.

2. Macnab I. Acceleration injuries of the cervical spine. J Bone Joint Surg 46A(8):1797–1799, 1964.

3. Hohl M. Soft-tissue injuries of the neck in automobile accidents. Factors influencing prognosis. J Bone Joint Surg Am. 1974 Dec;56(8):1675–82

4. Ellertsson AB, Sigurjóusson K, Thorsteinsson T. Clinical and radiographic study of 100 cases of whiplash injury. Acth Neurol Scand (Suppl) 67:269, 1978.

5. Norris SH, Watt I. The prognosis of neck injuries resulting from rear-end vehicle collisions. J Bone Joint Surg Br. 1983 Nov;65(5):608–11.

6. McKinney LA. Early mobilisation and outcome in acute sprains of the neck. BMJ. 1989 Oct 21;299(6706):1006–8.

7. Deans GT, McGalliard JN, Rutherford WH. Incidence and duration of neck pain among patients injured in car accidents. Br Med J (Clin Res Ed). 1986 Jan 11;292(6513):94–5.

8. Deans GT, Magalliard JN, Kerr M, Rutherford WH. Neck sprain—a major cause of disability following car accidents. Injury. 1987 Jan;18(1):10–2.

9. Miles KA, Maimaris C, Finlay D, Barnes MR. The incidence and prognostic significance of radiological abnormalities in soft tissue injuries to the cervical spine. Skeletal Radiol. 1988;17(7):493–6.

10. Maimaris C, Barnes MR, Allen MJ. 'Whiplash injuries' of the neck: a retrospective study. Injury. 1988 Nov;19(6):393–6.

11. Pearce JM. Whiplash injury: a reappraisal. J Neurol Neurosurg Psychiatry. 1989 Dec;52(12):1329–31.

12. Hodgson SP, Grundy M. Whiplash injuries: their long-term prognosis and its relationship to compensation. Neuro Orthop 1989;7:88–99.

13. Hildingsson C, Toolanen G. Outcome after soft-tissue injury of the cervical spine. A prospective study of 93 car-accident victims. Acta Orthop Scand. 1990 Aug;61(4):357–9.

14. Olsson I, Bunketorp O, Carlsson G, et al. An in-depth study of neck injuries in rear-end collisions. 1990 International IRCOBI Conference, Bron, Lyon, France, September 12–14, 1–15, 1990.

15. Pennie BH, Agambar LJ. Whiplash injuries. A trial of early management. J Bone Joint Surg Br. 1990 Mar;72(2):277–9.

16. Watkinson A, Gargan MF, Bannister GC. Prognostic factors in soft tissue injuries of the cervical spine. Injury. 1991 Jul;22(4):307–9.

17. Kischka U, Ettlin T, Heim S, Schmid G. Cerebral symptoms following whiplash injury. Eur Neurol. 1991;31(3):136–40.

18. Radanov BP, di Stefano G, Schnidrig A, Ballinari P. Role of psychosocial stress in recovery from common whiplash. Lancet. 1991 Sep 21;338(8769):712–5.

19. Ettlin TM, Kischka U, Reichmann S, Radii EW, Heim S, Wengen D, Benson DF. Cerebral symptoms after whiplash injury of the neck: a prospective clinical and neuropsychological study of whiplash injury. J Neurol Neurosurg Psychiatry. 1992 Oct;55(10):943–8.

20. Parmar HV, Raymakers R. Neck injuries from rear-impact road traffic accidents: prognosis in persons seeking compensation. Injury. 1993 Feb;24(2):75–8.

21. Robinson DD, Cassar-Pullicino VN. Acute neck sprain after road traffic accident: a long-term clinical and radiological review. Injury. 1993 Feb;24(2):79–82.

22. Hildingsson C, Wenngren BI, Bring G, Toolanen G. Oculomotor problems after cervical spine injury. Acta Orthop Scand. 1989 Oct;60(5):513–6.

23. Gargan MF, Bannister GC. The rate of recovery following whiplash injury. Eur Spine J. 1994;3(3):162–4.

24. Radanov BP, Di Stefano G, Schnidrig A, Sturzenegger M. Psychosocial stress, cognitive performance and disability after common whiplash. J Psychosom Res. 1993 Jan;37(1):1–10.

25. Radanov BP, Di Stefano G, Schnidrig A, Sturzenegger

M, Augustiny KF. Cognitive functioning after common whiplash. A controlled follow-up study. Arch Neurol. 1993 Jan;50(1):87–91.

26. Ryan GA, Taylor GW, Moore VM, Dolinis J. Neck strain in car occupants: injury status after 6 months and crash-related factors. Injury. 1994 Oct;25(8):533–7.

27. Jonsson H Jr, Cesarini K, Sahlstedt B, Rauschning W. Findings and outcome in whiplash-type neck distortions. Spine. 1994 Dec 15;19(24):2733–43.

28. Radanov BP, Sturzenegger M, De Stefano G, Schnidrig A. Relationship between early somatic, radiological, cognitive and psychosocial findings and outcome during a one-year follow-up in 117 patients suffering from common whiplash. Br J Rheumatol. 1994 May;33(5):442–8.

29. Di Stefano G, Radanov BP. Course of attention and memory after common whiplash: a two-years prospective study with age, education and gender pair-matched patients. Acta Neurol Scand. 1995 May;91(5):346–52.

30. Carlsson G, Nilsson S, Nilsson-Ehle A, et al. Neck injuries in rear-end car collisions: Biomechanical considerations to improve head restraints. Proceedings of the International IRCOBI/AAAM Conference on the Biomechanics of Impacts, Göteborg, Sweden, 277–289, 1995.

31. Spitzer WO, Skovron ML, Salmi LR, Cassidy JD, Duranceau J, Suissa S, Zeiss E. Scientific monograph of the Quebec Task Force on Whiplash-Associated Disorders: redefining "whiplash" and its management. Spine. 1995 Apr 15;20(8 Suppl):1S–73S.

32. Di Stefano G, Radanov BP. Course of attention and memory after common whiplash: a two-years prospective study with age, education and gender pair-matched patients. Acta Neurol Scand. 1995 May;91(5):346–52.

33. Borchgrevink GE, Lereim I, Royneland L, Bjorndal A, Haraldseth O. National health insurance consumption and chronic symptoms following mild neck sprain injuries in car collisions. Scand J Soc Med. 1996 Dec;24(4):264–71.

34. Mayou R, Bryant B. Outcome of 'whiplash' neck injury. Injury. 1996 Nov;27(9):617–23.

35. Squires B, Gargan MF, Bannister GC. Soft-tissue injuries of the cervical spine. 15-year follow-up. J Bone Joint Surg Br. 1996 Nov;78(6):955–7.

36. Pettersson K, Hildingsson C, Toolanen G, Fagerlund M, Bjornebrink J. Disc pathology after whiplash injury. A prospec-

tive magnetic resonance imaging and clinical investigation. Spine. 1997 Feb 1;22(3):283–7.

37. Karlsborg M, Smed A, Jespersen H, Stephensen S, Cortsen M, Jennum P, Herning M, Korfitsen E, Werdelin L. A prospective study of 39 patients with whiplash injury. Acta Neurol Scand. 1997 Feb;95(2):65–72.

38. Gargan M, Bannister G, Main C, Hollis S. The behavioural response to whiplash injury. J Bone Joint Surg Br. 1997 Jul;79(4):523–6.

39. Voyvodic F, Dolinis J, Moore VM, Ryan GA, Slavotinek JP, Whyte AM, Hoile RD, Taylor GW. MRI of car occupants with whiplash injury. Neuroradiology. 1997 Jan;39(1):35–40.

40. Borchgrevink GE, Stiles TC, Borchgrevink PC, Lereim I. Personality profile among symptomatic and recovered patients with neck sprain injury, measured by MCMI-I acutely and 6 months after car accidents. J Psychosom Res. 1997 Apr;42(4):357–67.

41. Borchgrevink GE, Kaasa A, McDonagh D, Stiles TC, Haraldseth O, Lereim I. Acute treatment of whiplash neck sprain injuries. A randomized trial of treatment during the first 14 days after a car accident. Spine. 1998 Jan 1;23(1):25–31.

42. Brison RJ, Hartling L, Pickett W. A prospective study of acceleration-extension injuries following rear-end motor vehicle collisions. J Musculoskletal Pain 2000; 8: 97–113.

43. Berglund A, Alfredsson L, Cassidy JD, Jensen I, Nygren A. The association between exposure to a rear-end collision and future neck or shoulder pain: a cohort study. J Clin Epidemiol. 2000 Nov;53(11):1089–94.

44. Bunketorp L, Nordholm L, Carlsson J. A descriptive analysis of disorders in patients 17 years following motor vehicle accidents. Eur Spine J. 2002 Jun;11(3):227–34.

45) Sterner Y, Toolanen G, Gerdle B, Hildingsson C. The incidence of whiplash trauma and the effects of different factors on recovery. J Spinal Dis Tech 16(2):195–199, 2002

46) Hartling L, Pickett W, Brison RJ. Derivation of a clinical decision rule for whiplash associated disorders among individuals involved in rear-end collisions. Accid Anal Prev 34(4):531–539, 2002.

47) Kasch H, Bach FW, Stengaard-Pedersen K, Jensen TS. Development in pain and neurologic complaints after whiplash. Neurology 60:743–761, 2003.

48) Ovadia D, Steinberg EL, Nissan M, Dekel S. Whiplash

injury-a retrospective study on patients seeking compensation. Injury 33:569–573, 2002.

49) Sterling M, Jull G, Vicenzino B, Kenardy J. Sensory hypersensitivity occurs soon after whiplash injury and is associated with poor memory. Pain 104:509–517, 2003.

50) Nederhand MJ, Hermens HJ, I Jzerman MJ, Turk DC, Zilvold G. Chronic neck pain disability due to an acute whiplash injury. Pain 102:63–71, 2003.

51) Bunketorp O, Jakobsson L, Norin H. Comparison of frontal and rear-end impacts for car occupants with whiplash-associated disorders: symptoms and clinical findings. Proceedings of the International IRCOBI Conference, Graz, Austria, September 22–24, 2004, 245–256.

52) Richter M, Ferrari R, Otte D, Kuensebeck HW, Blauth M, Krettek C. Correlation of clinical findings, collision parameters, and psychological factors in the outcome of whiplash associated disorders. J Neurol Neurosurg Psychiatry 2004 May;75(5):758–64.

53) Pettersson K, Brandstrom S, Toolanen G, Hildingsson C, Nylander PO. Temperament and character: prognostic factors in whiplash patients? Eur Spine J 2004 Aug;13(5):408–14.

§ 3:5 "Real world" motor vehicle collision injury studies—Quick review of real world studies [grid]

Authors	Year of Study	No. Studied	Type of Collisions	# Years Follow-up	% Chronic
Gotten [1]	1956	100	Mixed	>1	46
Macnab [2]	1964	266	Mixed	>2	45
Hohl [3]	1974	146	Mixed	>5	43
Ellertsson et al. [4]	1978	100	Rear	2	12
Norris and Watt [5]	1983	61	Rear	2	44–90
McKinney [6]	1989	167	Mixed	2	23–46
Ebbs et al. [7]	1986	137	Mixed	1	26
Deans et al. [8]	1987	137	Mixed	1	26
Miles et al [9]	1988	73	Mixed	2	29

Authors	Year of Study	No. Studied	Type of Collisions	# Years Follow-up	% Chronic
Maimaris et al. [10]	1988	102	Mixed	2	34
Pearce [11]	1989	100	Mixed	1	15
Hodgson and Grundy [12]	1989	40	Mixed	10–15	14–62
Hildingsson and Toolanen [13]	1990	93	Mixed	2	58
Olsson et al. [14]	1990	33	Rear	1	41
Pennie and Agambar [15]	1990	135	Mixed	1	13
Watkinson et al. [16]	1991	43	Rear	11	86
Kischka et al. [17]	1991	52	Mixed	>2	44; 61
Radanov et al. [18]	1991	78	Mixed	1	27
Ettlin et al. [19]	1992	21	Mixed	2	35; 41; 29
Parmar and Raymakers [20]	1993	100	Rear	8	55
Robinson & Cassar-Pullicino [21]	1993	21	–	10–19	86
Hildingsson et al. [22]	1993	38	Mixed	>1	45; 34
Gargan and Bannister [23]	1994	50	Rear	2	62
Radanov et al. [24]	1993	97	Mixed	1	27

Authors	Year of Study	No. Studied	Type of Collisions	# Years Follow-up	% Chronic
Radanov et al. [25]	1993	98	Mixed	1	32
Ryan et al. [26]	1994	29	Mixed	1	66
Jonsson et al. [27]	1994	50	Mixed	5	32
Radanov et al. [28]	1994	117	Mixed	1	24
Di Stefano et al. [29]	1995	117	Mixed	2	18
Ono and Kano [30]	1993	?	Mixed	?	15–20
Spitzer et al. [31]	1995	3,014	Mixed	6	?
Di Stefano et al. [32]	1995	117	Mixed	2	18
Borchgrevinck et al. [33]	1996	345	Rear	>2.5	58
Mayou and Bryant [34]	1996	57	Mixed	1	49
Squires et al. [35]	1996	40	Rear	15.5	70
Pettersson et al. [36]	1997	39	Mixed	2	45/44
Karsborg et al. [37]	1997	39	Mixed	0.6	71
Gargan et al. [38]	1997	52	Rear	2	64
Voyvodic et al. [39]	1997	29	?	0.5	62
Borchgrevink et al. [40]	1997	88	Mixed	1	28
Borchgrevink et al. [41]	1998	201	Mixed	0.5	41–66
Brison [42]	2000	380	Rear	2	36

Authors	Year of Study	No. Studied	Type of Collisions	# Years Follow-up	% Chronic
Berglund et al [43]	2000	138	Mixed	7	39.6
Bunkertorp et al [44]	2002	108	Mixed	17	55
Sterner et al. (45)	2002	296	Mixed	1.3	32
Hartling et al. (46)	2002	315	Rear	0.5	35
Ovadia et al. (47)	2002	866	Rear	2.7	69
Kasch et al. (48)	2003	141	Rear	1	74
Sterling et al. (49)	2003	76	Mixed	0.5	40
Nederhand et al. (50)	2003	92	Mixed	0.5	53
Bunketorp et al. (51)	2004	125	F/R22	1	19/28
Richter et al. (52)	2004	32	Mixed	0.5	34
Pettersson et al. (53)	2004	39	?	2	33

Chapter 4

Vehicle Damage & Occupant Injury

Whiplash is a mechanism of injury commonly associated with rear-impact vehicle collisions. To date, research has focused primarily on changes in velocity and acceleration as key factors for determining injuries due to whiplash mechanisms, but other characteristics of the acceleration pulse may be important. This study assessed whether the head acceleration response to whiplash-like perturbation profiles were affected by a change in the rate of the applied acceleration, or **jerk**. Twenty-one subjects were exposed to different low-velocity rear-impact whiplash-like perturbations using a precisely controlled robotic platform.

Results demonstrated that the jerk magnitude significantly affected forehead acceleration in the vertical and horizontal directions. Increasing the magnitude of the platform acceleration also differentially affected the horizontal and vertical forehead accelerations.

This indicates that the **level of jerk** influences the resulting head kinematics and should be considered when designing or interpreting experiments that are attempting to predict injury from whiplash-like perturbations.

Hynes LM, Dickey JP. The rate of change of acceleration: implications to head kinematics during rear-end impacts. Accid Anal Prev. 2008 May;40(3):1063–8.

Change of velocity (v), as an estimate of the impact severity, **was not related to residual problems**, neither after frontal (p=0.4), nor rear-end impacts (p=0.5), not even in subjects without any previous neck problems. A "stiff" impact pulse caused residual problems of non-minor grade in 20% of the subjects, without any difference between frontal and rear-end impacts.

Bunketorp O, Jakobsson L, Norin H. Comparison of frontal and rear-end impacts for car occupants with whiplash associated disorders: symptoms and clinical findings. IRCOBI Conference — Graz (Austria) September 2004:245–256.

§ 4:1 Vehicle damage threshold

The May 1, 1998 issue of Spine. (Freeman M, et. al. Spine, Volume 23, Number 9, 1998, p.1046) stated damage thresholds for some vehicles:

1980 Toyota Tercel	8.1 mph.
1977 Honda Civic	8.2 mph.
1980 Chevrolet Citation	8.4 mph.
1979 Pontiac Grand Prix	9.9 mph.
1979 Ford E-150 van	9.9 mph.
1981–1983 Ford Escorts	Withstood multiple impacts at 10 mph without sustaining vehicle damage.
1978 Honda Accord	11.0 mph.
1979 Ford F-250 pick-up	11.7 mph.
1983 Ford Thunderbird	12.1 mph.
1989 Chevrolet Citation	12.7 mph.

Crash tests at the Spine Research Institute of San Diego with more modern vehicles revealed the following damage thresholds:

1991 Lincoln	9.9 mph
1991 Honda Civic	7.2 mph
1989 Ford Tempo	7.0 mph
1992 Chrysler Le Baron	9.9 mph
1994 Hyundai Excel	7.2 mph
1992 Ford Taurus	7.7 mph
1996 Chevy Cavalier	5.9 mph
1994 Ford Taurus	7.5 mph
2000 Chevy Impala	8.7 mph

* multiple impacts without damage

See Croft AC, Herring P, Freeman MD, Haneline MT. The neck injury criterion: future considerations. Accid Anal Prev. 2002 Mar;34(2):247–55.

In appropriate circumstances, the accuracy of the defense investigators may be challenged. Often the investigator will not have inspected the vehicle. In an attempt to calculate the speed of the collision, the investigation may simply take a picture of the vehicle damage (or lack of) and relate the damage to a Delta-V. The accident reconstructionist's testimony may lack a proper foundation as in *Dunshee v. Douglas*, 255 N.W.2d 42 (Minn. 1977), in which the expert's testimony was based solely on photographs and blue prints and *Brock v. Artis*, Lake Circuit Court: Crown Point Indiana. No. 45C01-9602-CT-00344 (July 1998) in which the expert viewed photographs and repair estimate of plaintiff's vehicle.

Damage thresholds for most passenger vehicles is a closing speed of about **8–12 mph**. Freeman MD, Croft AC, Rossignol AM. "Whiplash associated disorders: redefining whiplash and its management" by the Quebec Task Force. A critical evaluation. Spine. 1998 May 1;23(9):1043–9.

§ 4:2 Vehicle damage threshold—No correlation with occupant injury

(1) The mean delta-V was 13 (<5-20) kph in frontal impacts and **8** (<5-30) kph in **rear-end** impacts. WAD grade II symptoms predominated in both groups at primary assessment. Head rotation at impact was predictive of more severe initial symptoms. Impact severity, determined by delta-V or property damage, was not predictive of neck pain or cervical range of motion (CROM). Indeed there was a trend towards an inverse relationship between delta-V and symptoms.

(2)

Sixty-nine subjects (55%) remained symptomatic at one year. Eighteen patients deteriorated between the first and last assessments, the index crash was thought to be the only possible cause of this deterioration in 15 of these cases.

The prevalence of residual problems was twice as high with rear-end crashes than frontal impacts. Age, weight, stature and prior neck symptoms did not influence outcome at one year. Females were more likely than males to have chronic symptoms. Other factors included high initial pain intensity, brachial radiations, reduced CROM (for women) and psychoneurosis.

Head rotation at impact was positively associated with chronic symptoms. Of 45 subjects with rotation 16 (36%) had non-minor symptoms after one year compared to13 (18%) of 71 without rotation (p=0.037). This association was less significant for rear impact crashes (p==0.18).

(3) **Delta-V was not significantly associated with symptom duration, regardless of vector**. Of 39 patients injured in MVC at delta-V less than 5 kph, eight (21%) had problems at one year. There was no difference in the prevalence of chronic symptoms according to delta-V below 26kph. The authors concluded '*we cannot specify a delta-V below which it is impossible to sustain a neck sprain with long term consequences*'. Case histories are presented for five previously healthy patients with significant symptoms at one year following low speed crashes.

This paper shows a high rate of persistent symptoms in patients injured in motor vehicle collisions. **Chronicity did not correlate with measures of impact severity**. A number of subjects remained symptomatic at one year following crashes with an estimated delta-V of 5 kph (3mph) or less. The data on crash severity may not be reliable, the authors relied on the subjective accounts of the injured parties. **There was no corroboration of delta-V by on-board crash pulse recorder in any of the rear-impact crashes**. However, there would be little advantage in subjects underestimating the crash severity or impact speed. The authors conclude that human factors (gender, pain intensity, brachial radiations and psychological distress) and kinematics (crash vector, head position) are more reliable predictors of chronic symptoms that estimate of impact speed. Indeed, in crashes causing speed changes of less than 26kph the relationship may be an inverse one.

Bunketorp O, Jakobsson L and Norin H. Comparison of frontal and rear-end impacts for car occupants with whiplash-associated disorders: Symptoms and clinical findings. Procedures of the International IRCOBI Conference, Gratz (Austria), Sept 2004: 245–256.

The Delta-V (change in velocity) in 70% of the collisions was 15 km/h (9.5 mph) or less. 27.2% were 8 km/h (5 mph) or less. Eichberger A, Geigl BC, Moser A, Fachbach B, Steffan H, Hell W, Langwieder K. Comparison of different car seats regarding head-neck kinematics of volunteers during rear end impact. IRCOBI Conference 1996: 199613-0011, pp.153–64.

Most injuries occur between 6–12 mph Delta-V in rear impact collisions. Hell W, Langwieder K, Walz F. Reported soft tissue neck injuries after rear-end car collisions. International Research Council on the Biomechanics of Impact (IRCOBI) Conference Proceedings. September 16–18, 1998, Göteborg, Sweden, 261–274.

A 1997 study showed the frequency of injured persons with different Delta-Vs differentiated by whiplash distortions and fractures/luxations. There were 1,238 whiplash distortions and 56 fractures. 23.9% of the whiplash distortions occurred with a Delta-V of 10 km/h (6 mph) or less, 33% with a Delta-V of 6–12 mph. An interesting note is that 8.8% of the fractures were with a Delta-V of 6 mph or less. The greatest percentage of fractures (25.7%) was with Delta-V between 31–40 km/h (19–25 mph). Otte D, Pohlemann T, Blauth M. Significance of soft tissue neck injuries AIS 1 in the accident scene and deformation characteristics of cars with a Delta-V up to 10 km/h. IRCOBI Conference, Hannover, September 1997. 1997-13-0017, pp.265–83.

A study with over 8,000 collisions showed a higher injury rate at lower speeds. Collisions with a **delta V under 9.3 mph had an injury rate of 36%,** and the injury rate for collisions with a **delta V over 9.3 mph was 20%.** Foret-Bruno JY, Dauvilliers F, Tarriere C: Influence of the seat and head rest stiffness on the risk of cervical injuries. 13th International Technical Conference on Experimental Safety Vehicles. S-8-W-19, 968–974, 1991.

Low speed motor vehicle crashes and whiplash-associated disorders

Whiplash injuries have increased in numbers during recent decades. The highest incidence rates of whiplash injury are found in low speed motor vehicle crashes during which many vehicles do not sustain significant property damage despite the fact that occupants may suffer personal injury. This article investigates the relationship between car crash velocity changes and residual vehicular damage in low speed crashes and personal injury thresholds. **It can be concluded that a personal injury threshold in relation to velocity change and property damage in low speed motor vehicle crashes cannot be established based on scientific evidence**.

Uhrenholt L, Gregersen M. [Low speed motor vehicle crashes and whiplash-associated disorders.] Ugeskr Laeger. 2008 Feb 25;170(9):713–715. *Danish.*

Auto insurers use a variety of techniques to control their losses, and one that has been widely employed since the mid-1990's is the Minor Impact Soft Tissue (MIST) segmentation strategy. MIST protocol dictates that all injury claims resulting from collisions producing US dollars 1000 or less in damage be "segmented", or adjusted for minimal compensation.

A limited correlation between crash severity and injury claims was found. We could not determine, however, whether this relationship held across all crash severities. Other studies provided conflicting results with regard to acute injury risk, but both found no statistically significant correlation between crash severity and long-term outcome.

A substantial number of injuries are reported in crashes of little or no property damage. **Property damage is an unreliable predictor of injury risk or outcome in low velocity crashes**. The MIST protocol for prediction of injury does not appear to be valid.

Croft AC, Freeman MD. Correlating crash severity with injury risk, injury severity, and long-term symptoms in low velocity motor vehicle collisions. Med Sci Monit. 2005 Oct;11(10):RA316–21

Delta-V (change and velocity) and Injuries

Most injuries occur between 6–12 mph Delta-V in rear impact collisions.

Hell W, Langwieder K, Walz F. Reported soft tissue neck injuries after rear-end car collisions. International Research Council on the Biomechanics of Impact (IRCOBI) Conference Proceedings. September 16–18, 1998, Göteborg, Sweden, 261–274.

The Delta-V (change in velocity) in 70% of the collisions was 15 km/h (9.5 mph) or less. 27.2% were 8 km/h (5 mph) or less.

Eichberger A, Geigl BC, Moser A, Fachbach B, Steffan H, Hell W, Langwieder K. Comparison of different car seats regarding head-neck kinematics of volunteers during rear end impact. IRCOBI Conference 1996: 199613-0011, pp.153–64.

There were 1,238 whiplash distortions and 56 fractures. **23.9%** of the whiplash distortions occurred with a **Delta-V 6 mph** or less, **33%** with a **Delta-V of 6–12 mph**.

An interesting note is that 8.8% of the fractures were with a Delta-V of 6 mph or less. The greatest percentage of fractures (25.7%) was with Delta-V between 19–25 mph.

Otte D, Pohlemann T, Blauth M. Significance of soft tissue neck injuries AIS 1 in the accident scene and deformation characteristics of cars with a Delta-V up to 10 km/h. IRCOBI Conference, Hannover, September 1997. 1997-13-0017, pp.265–83.

See the following studies regarding the correlation between damage to a vehicle and occupant injury:

Property damage is an unreliable predictor of injury risk or outcome in low velocity crashes. The MIST (minor impact soft tissue) protocol used by insurance companies for prediction of injury **does not appear to be valid**. Croft AC, Freeman MD. Correlating crash severity with injury risk, injury severity, and long-term symptoms in low velocity motor vehicle collisions. Med Sci Monit. 2005 Oct;11(10):RA316–21. Jackson R. The positive findings in alleged neck injuries. Am J Orthop. 1964 Aug-Sep;6:178–87.

The results of this study suggest that there is no established minimum threshold of significant spine injury. The greatest explanation for injury from traumatic loading of the spine is individual susceptibility to injury, an unpredictable variable. Freeman MD, Croft AC, Nicodemus CN, Centeno CJ, Elkins WL. Significant spinal injury resulting from low-level accelerations: a case series of roller coaster injuries. Arch Phys Med Rehabil. 2005 Nov;86(11):2126–30.

Robbins, M.C. Lack of Relationship Between Vehicle Damage and Occupant Injury. Society of Automotive Engineers, 1997;970494, Detroit, MI.

Evans RW. Some observations on whiplash injuries. Neurol Clin. 1992 Nov;10(4):975–97.

Hirsch SA, Hirsch PJ, Hiramoto H, Weiss A. Whiplash syndrome. Fact or fiction? Orthop Clin North Am. 1988 Oct;19(4):791–5.

Hijioka A, Narusawa K, Nakamura T. Risk factors for long-term treatment of whiplash injury in Japan: analysis of 400 cases. Arch Orthop Trauma Surg. 2001 Oct;121(9):490–3. (Treatment length with damage to 1/2 the vehicle is about the same with a vehicle with no damage.)

Olsson I, Bunketorp O, Carlsson G, et al.: An in-depth study of neck injuries in rear end collisions. 1990 International IRCOBI Conference, Bron, Lyon, France, September 12–14, 1–15, 1990.

Pennie B, Agambar L. Patterns of injury and recovery in whiplash. Injury. 1991 Jan;22(1):57–9.

Ryan GA, Taylor GW, Moore VM, Dolinis J. Neck strain in car occupants: injury status after 6 months and crash-related factors. Injury. 1994 Oct;25(8):533–7.

Ryan GA, Taylor GW, Moore VM, Dolinis J. Neck strain in car occupants. The influence of crash-related factors on initial severity. Med J Aust. 1993 Nov 15;159(10):651–6.

Sturzenegger M, DiStefano G, Radanov BP, Schnidrig A. Presenting symptoms and signs after whiplash injury: the influence of accident mechanisms. Neurology. 1994 Apr;44(4):688–93.

Kraft M, Kullgren A, Ydenius A, Tingvall C. Influence of crash pulse characteristics on whiplash associated disorders in rear impacts-Crash recording in real life impacts. Traffic Injury Prevention 2002;3:141–9.

Jackson, R. The positive findings in alleged neck injuries. American Journal of Orthopedics 1964;pp.178–187.

§ 4:3 Low incident of whiplash injuries in high-speed collisions

The injuries are different. Incidental neck symptoms in high energy trauma victims

We conducted a prospective study into the incidence of neck symptoms in victims of high energy trauma. Thirty consecutive patients were questioned regarding neck and jaw pain and stiffness initially and at six weeks. Despite suffering extensive skeletal injuries as a result of road traffic accidents, only two patients had such symptoms. We conclude that the incidence of 'whiplash' is surprisingly low in victims of high energy trauma.

Khan H, McCormack D, Burke J, McManus F. Incidental neck symptoms in high energy trauma victims. Ir Med J. 1997 Jun-Jul;90(4):143. Soft tissue neck symptoms following high-energy road traffic accidents

A total of 36 consecutive patients were recruited who had been involved in high-energy road traffic accidents and had chest, musculoskeletal, or abdominal injuries (ISS > 16) requiring admission for treatment, but who had no diagnosed injury of the cervical spine. Patients were asked in a nonspecific or leading manner at the time of admission and again at least 6 to 8 weeks post injury if they had any neck symptoms, headaches, or paresthesiae. Only 2 of the patients interviewed described any whiplash symptoms. All symptoms were resolved at the time of second interview.

Our study demonstrates a surprisingly low incidence of neck symptoms following high-energy road traffic accidents in which patients sustained unrelated injuries requiring treatment.

Malik H, Lovell M. Soft tissue neck symptoms following high-energy road traffic accidents. Spine. 2004 Aug 1;29(15):E315–7. Incidence and Outcome of Whiplash Injury After Multiple Trauma

Only 13 out of 101 patients (1 female/12 male) (13%) complained of whiplash injury. There was a significantly higher rate of neck pain at triage ($P < 0.001$) and higher combined mean of Abbreviated Injury Score of upper torso ($P < 0.0001$) in the study group, elucidating the cause of whiplash injury. The Neck Disability Index was <24 points, indicating only mild-to-moderate disability in these patients. Whiplash injury incidence in this study (13%) was similar to the incidence of neck pain in the general population.

The incidence of whiplash injury following polytrauma was found to be low in our study. There is no dose-response relation between magnitude of trauma severity and incidence of whiplash injury.

Giannoudis PV, Mehta SS, Tsiridis E. Incidence and Outcome of Whiplash Injury After Multiple Trauma. Spine. 2007 Apr 1;32(7):776–781

§ 4:4 Bumper damage as indicator of impact speed

Often the defense experts will attempt to determine the vehicle speed at impact by evaluating the bumper damage or known bumper impact standards. Attorneys attempting to challenge these opinions should know that bumper standards are designed to ensure that vehicle safety systems operate in a low-speed collision, not for occupant protection.

Another area of challenge occurs when the accident reconstructionist does not give the numbers and the equations used to determine the vehicle's change in velocity (Delta-V). The attorney should have the accident reconstructionist provide him with the calculations and how he derived the numbers. If the accident reconstructionist used a computer program, you should know that programs are based on collisions speeds of 20–50 mph. Even the creator of the CRASH program states that the program should not be used for collisions outside the rage of 10–40 mph Delta-V. See T. Day. Application and misapplication of computer programs for accident reconstruction. SAE 890738. The author of Traffic Accident Reconstruction, Volume 2, Lynn B. Fricke, said, "You might start to believe your answers are more accurate than they actually are, forgetting that many of the inputs are only slightly better than guesses. Clearly, this is a time to exercise caution and understand the limitation of your analysis" (pg. 68–27).

When Delta-V is estimated from bumper damage, counsel should read leading cases such as *Clemente v. Blumenberg*, 183 Misc. 2d 923, 705 N.Y.S.2d 792 (Sup 1999) or *Tittsworth v. Robinson* (No. 951742, September 13, 1996).

In *Clemente v. Blumenberg*, 183 Misc. 2d 923, 705 N.Y.S.2d 792 (Sup 1999), the engineer attempted to compute the change in velocity of the vehicles at impact by reviewing color photographs of the damaged portion of the two vehicles along with the repair bills for the vehicles, and comparing the cost of repair of the plaintiff's 1996 GMC Jimmy SUV with a chart entitled "Bumper Performance Repair Costs, 5 mph Crash Tests."

Since the plaintiff's repair bill for her 1996 GMC Jimmy was close to the $882 average cost of repair for a 1995 to 1997 GMC Jimmy SUV driven into a flat barrier at 5 mph, the engineer concluded that the change in velocity from the plaintiff's SUV, after being struck in the rear by the defendant's van, was 5 mph.

The Clemente court stated:

"Using repair costs and photographs as a method for calculating the change in velocity at impact is not a generally accepted method for computing speed or change in velocity between two vehicles after a rear end collision in any relevant field of engineering or under the laws of physics. Hence, under the Frye test of general acceptance, the opinion upon which it relies is inadmissible. Applying the Daubert/Kumho factors also found this methodology to be invalid. **The engineer acknowledged that this was a method that he developed. Indeed, the engineer when questioned by this court whether there was any literature supporting this method of calculating velocity claimed there was none."**

The likelihood that an individual will or will not sustain injury in a collision is simply not capable of being tested with any degree of scientific reliability, given the number of variables involved. Analyzing those features of a whiplash accident that might be responsible for development of persistent symptoms is difficult, since most biomechanical factors cannot be assessed with adequate accuracy in vivo in humans. The amount of damage to the automobile and the speed involved in the collision bear little relationship to the injury sustained by the cervical spine. See Sturzenegger M, DiStefano G, Radanov BP, Schnidrig A. Presenting symptoms and signs after whiplash injury: the influence of accident mechanisms. Neurology. 1994 Apr;44(4):688–93.

Overall, the movements of human volunteer occupants, even at very low severities, are too complex for a simple correlation between vehicle impact severity and single descriptors of occupant motion. See Bailey M. Assessment of impact severity in minor motor vehicle collisions. J Musculoskeletal Pain 1996;4(4):21–38.

In a personal injury action arising from a rear-end collision, the defendant offered expert testimony that the change in velocity of the plaintiff's vehicle caused by the collision was insufficient to cause the plaintiff's injuries. **The trial court excluded the evidence** under *People v. Kelly* (1976) 17 Cal.3d 24 (Kelly). We affirm.

Here, the delta v method is relatively new to the law, as we discuss in more detail in section V below. As Lotz testified, the studies on which he relied employed the scientific method. Finally, Lotz's testimony raises the dangers the Kelly test is designed to prevent: it is cloaked in scientific terminology such as "delta v" and "g forces" and bolstered by references to scientific studies the jury has no way to evaluate. (See Leahy, at pp. 606–607.)

Smith did not meet her burden of proof in the trial court of establishing that the delta v method is generally accepted in the relevant scientific community. Indeed, Smith barely presented any argument on the issue.

The scientific literature in the record, therefore, does not demonstrate that there is general acceptance in the scientific community of a particular correlation between change in velocity and probability of human injury. Rather, it appears that the relationship between these factors is currently the subject of experimentation and debate within the scientific community. It may be that the current studies are valid and the correlation will one day gain general acceptance in the community. However, until that occurs, expert testimony based on the experimental data is not admissible at trial.

Harrison v. Smith, 2008 Dist Appellate Court, Division Five, July 9, 2008.

§ 4:5 Bumper damage as indicator of impact speed—Accuracy of Accident Collision Reconstructionists (ACRs)

On the accuracy of the ACR measurements, see SAE paper 2002-01-0546, where some measurements are 2 standard deviations away from the mean. Estimates of EBS (equivalent barrier speed) from crush depth using 2 photographs. There was a wide variation of estimations of speed based on the damage of a vehicle based on looking at photographs.

Range	Number of ACR estimations
11–15 mph	- 5
16–20 mph	- 12
21–25 mph	- 18
26–30 mph	- 12
31–35 mph	- 3
41–45 mph	- 1

See Bartlett et al. Evaluating the uncertainty in various measurement tasks common to accident reconstruction. SAE 2002-01-0546.

§ 4:6 Crash pulse

The collision causes an impulse. This impulse is called a crash pulse. With no crush damage, a stiff vehicle with no damage has a different shape of crash pulse than a vehicle with crush damage. More energy will be transferred and less absorbed.

A formula used to determine acceleration involving velocity and crush: a = Vsup2/sup/2S

a = acceleration, Vsup2/sup = velocity squared, S = crush distance.

A stiffer vehicle increases peak accelerations to the occupant's head/neck and vehicle.

No damage can cause a different crash pulse. In fact, no damage suggests greater exchange of energy in the form of Delta-V. Crush means some energy is absorbed and a longer crush distance. A low crush distance value poses as great a danger as a high velocity value. Crush means longer impulse time and disperses energy.

V at 10 mph (4.46 m/sec), crush of 5 inches (0.127 m) = 8 Gs of acceleration.

V at 10 mph (4.46 m/sec), crush of 2 inches (0.0254 m) = 20 Gs of acceleration.

See Robbins. M.C. Lack of Relationship Between Vehicle Damage and Occupant Injury. Society of Automotive Engineers, 1997;970494, Detroit, MI.

Symptoms for more than 6 months may occur at a change of velocity below 10 km/h (6 mph), due to a relatively high mean acceleration. At low mean acceleration, when the change of velocity is relatively high, the risk of long-term consequences was low.

Kraft M, Kullgren A, Ydenius A, Tingvall C. Influence of crash pulse characteristics on whiplash associated disorders in rear impacts-Crash recording in real life impacts. Traffic Injury Prevention 2002;3:141–9.

§ 4:7 Crash pulse—Crash pulse recorders

In recent years, auto manufacturers have begun to install crash pulse recorders, also called event data recorders, to measure parameters of a vehicle collision. **These data recorders are for frontal impacts only at this time. Event data recorders can underestimate the speed change in low-speed collisions as high as 4 km/h.** See Lawrence JM, Wilkinson CC, King DJ, Heinrichs BE, Siegmund GP. The accuracy and sensitivity of event data recorders in low-speed collisions. SAE Technical paper 2002-01-0679.

The sensing and diagnostic module that records speed change can underestimate the actual collision speed change by as much as 44%. Correia JT, Ilidis KA, McCarron ES, Smolej MA. Utilizing data from automotive data recorders. Proceeding of the Canadian Multidisciplinary Road Safety Conference XII, London ON, 2001.

§ 4:8 Crash pulse—Shape of crash pulse

Volvo found that the shape of the acceleration pulse is significant because a more narrow pulse (acceleration occurring over less time) increases the relative movement of the lower cervical spine before the head contacts the headrest. Olsson I, et al. An in-depth study of neck injuries in rear end collisions. IRCOBI conference, September 12–14, 1990, Bron, Lyon, France, p.10; Eichberger A, et al. Evaluation of the applicability of the neck injury criterion (NIC) in rear impacts on the basis of human subject tests. IRCOBI conference, September 1998, Goteborg, Sweeden, p. 331.

A similar Delta-V can be generated by a variety of mean accelerations, pulse shapes, and peak accelerations. There is a great variation of acceleration pulses produced in rear impacts to cars manufactured during the 1990's. **Vehicles that perform well in a low-speed damage ability crash test are often those with a very stiff structure, and the acceleration pulse tends to be shorted and of a higher magnitude**. Linder A, Avery M, Krafft M, Kullgren A, Svensson MY. Acceleration pulses and crash severity in low velocity rear impacts: real world data and barrier tests. 17th ESV Conference, June 4–7,2001, Amsterdam, Netherlands, paper 216-O; Kraft M. When do AIS 1 neck injuries result in long-term consequences? Vehicle and human factors. Traffic Injury Prevention 2002;3:89–97.

The shape of the crash pulse influences the risk of long-term disability. The rate of change during the mid and last third of the crash pulse seem to be important. **A change of velocity of 3 mph or greater in a time span from 34 ms to 67 ms of the crash has a significantly larger chance of having long-term consequences**. Kullgren A, Krafft M, Nygren A, Tingvall C. Neck injuries in frontal impacts: influence of crash pulse characteristics on injury risk. Accid Anal Prev. 2000 Mar;32(2):197–205.

Factors other than selected peak kinematic responses influenced symptom production. No one parameter was sufficiently strong enough to successfully predict symptoms. **Extrapolation of the current model outside these test conditions, injury types and injury severities may be inappropriate**. The results of this analysis were based on controlled human subjects tests using one vehicle, one seat, and one seated posture. Siegmund GP, Brault JR, Wheeler JB. The relationship between clinical and kinematic responses from human subject testing in rear-end automobile collisions. Accid Anal Prev. 2000 Mar;32(2):207–17.

§ 4:9 Different cars and different neck injury factors

Not only the weight of the car involved in the collision, but the different cars have different injury risks. The rebound velocity of the occupant in a rear-end impact may be higher than the velocity of the vehicle. **The type of vehicle involve may have an injury risk of 4 times higher than another type of vehicle**. Koch M, Kullgren A, Lie A, Nygren A, Tingvall C. Soft tissue injury of the cervical spine in rear-end and frontal car collisions. IRCOBI 1995; 273–83.

The NIF (neck injury factor) of the worst car is 5.5 times higher than the best in this study. **This means that in the case of a rear end impact, the risk of neck injuries is 5.5 times higher for the worst than for the best car**. Eichberger et al. Comparison of different car seats regarding head-neck kinematics of volunteers during rear end impact. IRCOBI — 1996-13-0011, pp. 153–64.

§ 4:10 Injuries in low speed motor vehicle collisions

The Delta-V (change in velocity) in 70% of the collisions was 15 km/h (9.5 mph) or less. 27.2% were 8 km/h (5 mph) or less. Eichberger A, Geigl BC, Moser A, Fachbach B, Steffan H, Hell W, Langwieder K. Comparison of different car seats regarding head-neck kinematics of volunteers during rear end impact. IRCOBI Conference 1996: 199613-0011, pp.153–64.

Most injuries occur between 6–12 mph Delta-V in rear impact collisions. Hell W, Langwieder K, Walz F. Reported soft tissue neck injuries after rear-end car collisions. International Research Council on the Biomechanics of Impact (IRCOBI) Conference Proceedings. September 16–18, 1998, Göteborg, Sweden, 261–274.

A 1997 study showed the frequency of injured persons with different Delta-Vs differentiated by whiplash distortions and fractures/luxations. There were 1,238 whiplash distortions and 56 fractures. 23.9% of the whiplash distortions occurred with a Delta-V of 10 km/h (6 mph) or less, 33% with a Delta-V of 6–12 mph. An interesting note is that 8.8% of the fractures were with a Delta-V of 6 mph or less. **The greatest percentage of fractures (25.7%) was with Delta-V between 31–40 km/h (19–25 mph)**. Otte D, Pohlemann T, Blauth M. Significance of soft tissue neck injuries AIS 1 in the accident scene and deformation characteristics of cars with a Delta-V up to 10 km/h. IRCOBI Conference, Hannover, September 1997. 1997-13-0017, pp.265–83.

A study with over 8,000 collisions showed a higher injury rate at lower speeds. Collisions with a delta V under 9.3 mph had an injury rate of 36%, and the injury rate for collisions with a delta V over 9.3 mph was 20%. Foret-Bruno JY, Dauvilliers F, Tarriere C: Influence of the seat and head rest stiffness on the risk of cervical injuries. 13th International Technical Conference on Experimental Safety Vehicles. S-8-W-19, 968–974, 1991.

§ 4:11 Activities of daily living and injury threshold

A common study cited by the defense in lower speed automobile cases is the "Allen" study. In Allen, the authors compared the "G" forces in daily activities and attempted to make comparisons to whiplash. This study is riddled with problems, so much so that the appellate court in Colorado upheld the trial court decision not allowing the defense expert to testify, when the study was the basis for his opinion. **The defense uses the study to show that everyday activities generate the same forces from low-speed collisions and nobody can get hurt. The neck injury criterion of the tests conducted in this study would be close to 0**. Allen ME, Weir-Jones I, Motiuk DR, Flewin KR, Goring RD, Kobetitch R, Broadhurst A. Acceleration perturbations of daily living. A comparison to 'whiplash'. Spine. 1994 Jun 1;19(11):1285–90.

An Appellate Court addressed the Allen study for injury threshold: In *Schultz v. Wells* (Colorado Court of Appeals August 17, 2000, No. 99CA0688), the court ruled that **the force threshold for probability of injury demonstrated in the test results could not be used to "prove that a particular person was not injured or was likely not injured in this accident**." Defendant argued that daily living activities evidence would have been useful to the jury to get a sense of the practical significance of the horizontal G-forces sustained during the collision. The trial court, however, disagreed, and found that the list of representational horizontal G-forces did not take into consideration the entire mechanical movement of a body during a car collision, in that it did not address forces from other directions and the position of the body at the time of the accident.

The court specifically addressed the applicability of comparisons to the G-forces sustained while being hit in a carnival bumper car. The court acknowledged that such an activity is "somewhat similar" to a rear-end car accident, but noted that bumper cars is a game in which "a great deal of bracing action occurs."

Because of the lack of similarity between horizontal G-forces sustained during daily living activities and the numerous forces sustained during an unexpected rear-end automobile collision, evidence of the former would have been misleading. *Shultz Cf. Kling v. City and County of Denver*, 138 Colo. 567, 335, 335 P.2d 876 (1959). (To admit the results of an experiment, it is not necessary that the conditions be identical; it is "sufficient if there is a substantial similarity").

§ 4:12 Injury thresholds—Acceleration injury levels—Rear-end collision

At extremely low speeds of **1–2.5 mph**, neck injuries are possible if the headrest does not perform its protective function. Emori RI, Horiguchi J. Whiplash in low speed vehicle collisions. Detroit (MI): Society of Automotive Engineers, 9000542; 1990.

Injury below previously established 'tolerance' limits is possible, with some individuals being at risk from unexpected acceleration exposure above **around 2 to 5g**. Green NDC. Acute soft tissue neck injury from unexpected acceleration. Aviat Space Environ Med 2003; 74:1085–90.

Below are various studies at low thresholds:

3.5g (facet joint):

Pearson AM, Ivancic PC, Ito S. Panjabi MM. Facet Joint Kinematics and Injury Mechanisms During Simulated Whiplash. Spine 2004;29:390–397.

3.5g (cervical disc):

Panjabi MM, Ito S, Pearson AM, Ivancic PC. Injury Mechanisms of the Cervical Intervertebral Disc During Simulated Whiplash. Spine 2004;29:1217–1225.

3.5g (C4–5); 5.0g (C5–6); 6.5g (C6–7):

Ivancic PC, Pearson AM, Panjabi MM, Ito S. Injury of the anterior longitudinal ligament during whiplash simulation. Eur Spine J. 2004 Feb;13(1):61–8

4.5g (mechanical instability):

Panjabi MM, Nibu K, Cholewicki J. Whiplash injuries and the potential for mechanical instability. Eur Spine J. 1998;7(6) :484–92.

5g (soft tissue injury instability):

Ito S, Ivancic PC, Panjabi MM, Cunningham BW. Soft Tissue Injury Threshold During Simulated Whiplash: A Biomechanical Investigation. Spine 2004;29:979–987.

Delta-V of 8 km/h (5 mph) (cervical facet joint):

Siegmund GP, Myers BS, Davis MB, Bohnet HF, Winkelstein BA. Mechanical evidence of cervical facet capsule injury during whiplash. Spine 2001;26(19):2095–2101.

Delta-V of 5 mph (lumbar disc):

Bergman PC, Visarius H, Nolte LP, Prasad P. Viscoelastic shear responses of the cadaver and hybrid III lumbar spine. Proceedings of the 38th Stapp Car Crash Conference, SAE, Warrensale, PA. 1994;942205:438, fig. 41; Prasad P. Relationship between passenger car seat back strength and occupant injury severity in rear end collisions. Field and laboratory studies. SAE 1997;973343:438.

§ 4:13 Injury thresholds—Acceleration injury levels—Frontal impact

8g (soft tissue injury instability):

Pearson AM, Panjabi MM, Ivancic PC, Ito S, Cunningham BW, Rubin W, Gimenez SE. Frontal impact causes ligamentous cervical spine injury. Spine. 2005 Aug 15;30(16):1852–8.

4g (cervical disc C2–3); 10g (cervical disc C3–4, 5–6, 6–7):

Ito S, Ivancic PC, Pearson AM, Tominaga Y, Gimenez SE, Rubin W, Panjabi MM. Cervical intervertebral disc injury during simulated frontal impact. Eur Spine J. 2005 May;14(4):356–65; (Delta-V: 8.4 kph, 11.4 kph, 13.4 kph, and 13.8 kph), corresponding to the nominal maximum accelerations of 4g, 6g, 8g, and 10 g, respectively.

4g Supraspinous (SSL), interspinous ligaments (ISL), ligamentum flavum (LF):

Panjabi MM, Pearson AM, Ito S, Ivancic PC, Gimenez SE, Tominaga Y. Cervical spine ligament injury during simulated frontal impact. Spine. 2004 Nov 1;29(21):2395–403.

§ 4:14 Injury thresholds—Acceleration injury levels—Vehicle damage threshold

Damage thresholds for most passenger vehicles is a closing speed of about **8–12 mph**. Freeman MD, Croft AC, Rossignol AM. "Whiplash associated disorders: redefining whiplash and its management" by the Quebec Task Force. A critical evaluation. Spine. 1998 May 1;23(9):1043–9.

§ 4:15 Injury thresholds—Acceleration injury levels—Injury threshold

There were 932,000 riders of the Rattler roller coaster, estimated to represent between 300,000 and 600,000 individual riders. Based on injury incident reports and medical record review, it is estimated that there were a total of 656 neck and back injuries during the study period, with 39 considered significant by the study inclusion criteria. Seventy-two percent (28/39) of the injured subjects sustained a cervical disk injury; 71% of these injuries were at C5–6 (15 disk herniations, 5 symptomatic disk bulges), and 54% were at C6–7 (11 disk herniations, 4 symptomatic disk bulges). In the lumbar spine, the most frequent injury was a symptomatic disk bulge (20% of the cohort), followed by vertebral body compression fracture (18%), and L4–5 or L5–S1 disk herniation (13%). Accelerometry testing of passengers and train cars indicated a peak of 4.5 to 5 g of vertical or axial acceleration and 1.5 g of lateral acceleration over approximately 100ms (0.1s) on both. **The results of this study suggest that there is no established minimum threshold of significant spine injury. The greatest explanation for injury from traumatic loading of the spine is individual susceptibility to injury, an unpredictable variable.** Freeman MD, Croft AC, Nicodemus CN, Centeno CJ, Elkins WL. Significant spinal injury resulting from low-level accelerations: a case series of roller coaster injuries. Arch Phys Med Rehabil. 2005 Nov;86(11):2126–30.

Multiple databases were searched for studies comparing any of three dependent variables (injury risk, injury severity, or duration of symptoms) with structural damage in motor vehicle crashes of under 40 km/h (25 mph). A limited correlation between crash severity and injury claims was found, but it could not be determined whether this relationship held across all crash severities. Other studies provided conflicting results with regard to acute injury risk, but both found no statistically significant correlation between crash severity and long-term outcome. A substantial number of injuries are reported in crashes of little or no property damage. **Property damage is an unreliable predictor of injury risk or outcome in low velocity crashes.** The MIST (minor impact soft tissue) protocol used by insurance companies for prediction of injury **does not appear to be valid**. Croft AC, Freeman MD. Correlating crash severity with injury risk, injury severity, and long-term symptoms in low velocity motor vehicle collisions. Med Sci Monit. 2005 Oct;11(10):RA316–21.

§ 4:16 Frontal collision injury

The results of this study suggest that seatbelts alone or in combination with an airbag **increased the incidence of AIS1 spinal injuries**, but provide protection against more severe injury to all regions of the spine. Airbag deployment without seatbelt use did not show increased protection relative to unrestrained occupants.

Thoracolumbar region	AIS-1 Injury	Relative Risk	
	Delta–V	(9–15 mph)	(15 mph+)
Unrestrained		1.00	1.00
Seatbelt only		1.03	2.33
Airbag only		0.29	2.30
Airgbag and seat belt		0.90	3.78

In light of this research, consistent seatbelt use should still be encouraged to provide maximum protection in an MVC.

Reed MA, Naftel RP, Carter S, MacLennan PA, McGwin G Jr, Rue LW 3rd. Motor vehicle restraint system use and risk of spine injury. Traffic Inj Prev. 2006 Sep;7(3):256–63.

Airbag deployment does not appear to significantly reduce the risk of injury either alone or in combination with seat belts. Airbag deployment without associated seat belt use may increase the risk of lower extremity injury.

McGwin G Jr, Metzger J, Alonso JE, Rue LW 3rd. The association between occupant restraint systems and risk of injury in frontal motor vehicle collisions. J Trauma. 2003 Jun;54(6):1182–7.

The incidence of eye injuries in MVCs has progressively increased since 1998. Frontal air bag deployment was associated with a statistically significant, 2-fold (risk ratio, 2.13 [95% confidence interval, 1.56–2.91]) increased risk of eye injury, whereas seat belt use was associated with a 2-fold (risk ratio, 2.17 [95% confidence interval, 1.89–2.44]) reduced eye injury risk. In late-model vehicles, frontal air bags are the most common cause of MVC-related eye injury. Older age, female sex, seat position, vehicle weight, and collision severity were also associated with eye injury risk.

Seat belt use is the most effective means of occupant protection against Motor Vehicle Collision-related eye injury. For front-seated occupants in frontal collisions, the adverse effect of frontal air bags on the risk of eye injury should be considered against their protective effect for fatal injury.

McGwin G Jr, Owsley C. Risk factors for motor vehicle collision-related eye injuries. Arch Ophthalmol. 2005 Jan;123(1):89–95.

Analyses were performed examining the relationship between the estimated **delta V and any AIS $\geq$ 2 or any AIS $\geq$**

3 injury. Detailed crash investigation and clinical data were available on 407 children involved in 235 frontal crashes. The average delta V for all crashes was 29 ± 16.9 kph [18 ± 10.5 mph (range, 5–123 kph)]. Delta V was strongly and positively associated with the odds of both an AIS ≥ 2 and AIS ≥ 3 injury (P < 0.0001). The adjusted odds of at least one AIS ≥ 2 injury increased on average by 56% (95% confidence interval [CI], 33%–85%) for each 10 kph increase in delta V. Similarly, the adjusted odds of at least one AIS ≥ 3 injury increased on average by 67% (95% CI, 40%ndash;102%) for each 10 kph increase in delta V. The **delta V at which 50% of child occupants would be expected to sustain any AIS ≥ 2 injury was 37 kph [23.0 mph (95% CI, 32–45 kph)], and any AIS ≥ 3 injury was 63 kph [39.1 mph (95% CI, 51–∞ kph)]**. Delta V is strongly predictive of injury risk for child occupants for AIS injury 2 or 3.

Nance ML, Elliott MR, Arbogast KB, Winston FK, Durbin DR. Delta V as a predictor of significant injury for children involved in frontal motor vehicle crashes. Ann Surg. 2006 Jan;243(1):121–5.

§ 4:17 Side impact

Out of the 7812 crashes in the 1997–2004 weighted NASS files, AIS > or = 2 level injuries occurred to 5071 occupants. There were 3828 cases of torso-only airbags, 955 cases of torso-head bag combination, and 288 inflatable tubular structure/curtain systems. Side airbags were not attributed to be the cause of head or chest injury to any occupant at this level of severity. The predominance of torso-only airbags followed by torso-head airbag combination reflected vehicle model years and changing technology. Head and chest injuries were coupled for the vast majority of occupants with injuries to more than one body region. Comparing literature data for side impacts without side airbag deployments, **the presence of a side airbag decreased AIS=2 head, chest, and extremity injuries when examining raw data incidence rates**.

Yoganandan N, Pintar FA, Zhang J, Gennarelli TA. Lateral impact injuries with side airbag deployments—a descriptive study. Accid Anal Prev. 2007 Jan;39(1):22–7.

Lateral impact is an important independent risk factor for the development of traumatic brain injury after a serious motor vehicle crash. **Traumatic brain injuries incurred after lateral impact are more severe than those resulting from nonlateral impact.** Vehicle modifications that increase head protection could reduce crash-related severe traumatic brain injuries by up to 61% and prevent up to 2,230 fatal or critical traumatic brain injuries each year in the United States.

Bazarian JJ, Fisher SG, Flesher W, Lillis R, Knox KL, Pearson TA. Lateral automobile impacts and the risk of traumatic brain injury. Ann Emerg Med. 2004 Aug;44(2):142–52.

Field investigation of child restraints in side impact crashes.

Real world crashes involving children restrained in forward facing CRS in side impacts were analyzed from Partners for Child Passenger Safety, an on-going child specific crash surveillance system in which insurance claims are used to identify cases. In-depth crash investigations using standardized protocols were used to calculate the crash severity and determine the mechanisms and sources of the injuries sustained.

Cases of 32 children restrained in CRS in 30 side impact crashes were examined. Twenty-five percent sustained AIS 2+ injuries.

The most common injuries sustained by children restrained in CRS in side impact crashes were to the face, head, and lower extremity.

Characteristics of the crashes that appeared related to injury were intrusion that entered the child's occupant space or caused an interior part of the vehicle to enter the child's occupant space, forward component of the crash, and the rotation of the CRS, restrained by a seat belt, towards the side of the impact.

Arbogast KB, Ghati Y, Menon RA, Tylko S, Tamborra N, Morgan RM. Field investigation of child restraints in side impact crashes. Traffic Inj Prev. 2005 Dec;6(4):351–60.

Efficacy of side air bags in reducing driver deaths in driver-side collisions.

Side air bags, a relatively new technology designed to protect the head and/or torso in side-impact collisions, are becoming increasingly common in automobiles. Their efficacy in preventing US driver deaths among cars struck on the near (driver's) side was examined using data from the Fatality Analysis Reporting System and the General Estimates System. Risk ratios for driver death per nearside collision during 1999–2001 were computed for head/torso and torso-only side air bags in cars from model years 1997–2002, relative to cars without side air bags. Confounding was addressed by adjusting nearside risk ratios for front- and rear-impact mortality, which is unaffected by side air bags. Risk ratios were 0.55 (95% confidence interval: 0.43, 0.71) for head/torso air bags and 0.89 (95% confidence interval: 0.79, 1.01) for torso-only air bags. Risk was reduced when cars with head/torso air bags were struck by cars/minivans (significant) or pickup trucks/sport utility vehicles (nonsignificant). Risk was reduced in two-vehicle collisions and among male drivers and drivers aged 16–64 years.

Protective effects associated with torso-only air bags were observed in single-vehicle crashes and among male and 16- to 64-year-old drivers.

Head/torso side air bags appear to be very effective in reducing nearside driver deaths, whereas torso-only air bags appear less protective.

Braver ER, Kyrychenko SY. Efficacy of side air bags in reducing driver deaths in driver-side collisions. Am J Epidemiol. 2004 Mar 15;159(6):556–64.

Intervertebral Neck Injury Criterion (IV-NIC) is based on the hypothesis that dynamic three-dimensional intervertebral motion beyond physiological limits may cause multiplanar injury of cervical spine soft tissues.

Using a bench-top apparatus, side impacts were simulated at 3.5, 5, 6.5, and 8 g horizontal accelerations of the T1 vertebra. Pre- and post-impact flexibility testing in three-motion planes measured the soft tissue injury, i.e., significant increase ($p < 0.05$) in neutral zone (NZ) or range of motion (RoM) at any intervertebral level, above corresponding physiological limit.

The IV-NIC. The soft tissue injury criterion based upon the intervertebral rotation (IV-NIC) was defined as the dynamic intervertebral rotation, θdynamic, i,j(t), divided by the quasistatic physiological range of motion (RoM), θphysiological, i,j, where i is the intervertebral level, and j represents the plane of motion and where t is time.

Thus, the criterion is:IV — NICi, j (t) = θdynamic, i,j(t) / θphysiological, i,j

The principal mode of soft tissue injury was left lateral bending which produced coupled injuries in axial rotation, flexion, and extension. **The soft tissue injury threshold acceleration was 6.5 g**, as determined by significant increases above the corresponding baseline values in the flexion Neutral Zone and Range of Motion (C4-5, C5-6, C6-7).

Panjabi MM, Ivancic PC, Tominaga Y, Wang JL.

Intervertebral neck injury criterion for prediction of multiplanar cervical spine injury due to side impacts. Traffic Inj Prev. 2005 Dec;6(4):387–97.

Chapter 5

Common Symptoms

§ 5:1 Painful conditions

About 1/3 of the nociception (pain producing stimuli) goes up through the spinothalamic tract to the brain to be felt as pain. About 2/3 of the nociception goes to the brainstem areas, which may not be felt as pain.

Neck pain is the primary complaint from most whiplash injuries. In a 1996 study, **93.5% of the injured occupants had neck complaints**. Eichberger A, Geigl BC, Moser A, Fachbach B, Steffan H, Hell W, Langwieder K. Comparison of different car seats regarding head-neck kinematics of volunteers during rear end impact. IRCOBI Conference 1996: 1996-13-0011, pp.153–64.

With a whiplash injury, many symptoms can manifest. Doctors often think in terms of "syndromes." A syndrome is a pattern of symptoms (what the patient complains about) and signs (what the physician finds) that suggest the location of a disease process and, occasionally, its nature.

Symptoms from whiplash are varied and are variably combined in orthopedic, neurological, audiological, othorhiniolaryngological, equilibriometric, odontoiatric and/or neuropsychological manners. Cesarani A, Alpini R, Boniver R. eds. Whiplash injuries: diagnosis and treatment. New York: Springer; 1996.

Lesions and disorders from whiplash include neck pain, headache, post-concussion syndrome, shoulder pain, upper back pain, lower back pain, arm pain and paresthesia, jaw pain, ringing in the ears (tinnitus), chest pain, dysphagia, visual disturbance, auditory disturbance, balance disorders, cranial nerve palsies, dizziness, thoracic outlet syndrome, spinal cord injury, retrophyngeal hematoma, mediastinus, brain injury, hypothalamic-pituitary-thyroid disorder, cervical sympathetic disorder, menstrual disorder, occipital neuralgia, cervical dystonia, fibromyalgia, and posttraumatic stress disorder. Foreman SM, Croft AC eds. Whiplash injuries: The Cervical Acceleration/Deceleration Syndrome. 3 ed. Philadelphia: Lippincott Williams & Wilkins; 2002.

The delay in the onset of symptoms is common. **Even the Quebec Task Force indicated that there are delays in symptoms in 22% of the cases.** Spitzer WO, Skovron ML, Salmi LR, Cassidy JD, Duranceau J, Suissa S, Zeiss E. Scientific monograph of the Quebec Task Force on Whiplash-Associated Disorders: redefining "whiplash" and its management. Spine. 1995 Apr 15;20(8 Suppl):1S–73S.

The consequence of nerve root damage (from any cause) is known as a radiculopathy (Latin. radicula = little root; pathos = disease), whereas the syndrome of "myelopathy" (Greek. myelos = marrow, pertaining to the spinal cord, pathos = disease) results from spinal cord damage.

§ 5:2 Cervical radiculopathies

There are 7 cervical vertebrae and 8 cervical roots. The root number exiting between two vertebrae is always the number of the lower vertebra. For example, the C5 root exits between the C4–C5 vertebrae and would be affected by a C4/5 disc herniation; the C8 root exits between C7–T1 vertebrae and would be compressed by a C7/T1 disc.

Pain due to a C6 and C7 radiculopathy radiates from the neck and from around the shoulder into outer aspect of the arm and forearm. C6 radiculopathy may cause pain and numbness along the dorsal aspect of the thumb and index finger, C7 pain and paresthesia may radiate into the middle finger.

§ 5:3 Thoracic outlet syndrome

Note:

There are various names for thoracic outlet syndrome (TOS) including: cervical rib, scalenus anticus, costoclavicular, hyperabduction, pectoralis minor, bachiocephalic, and fractured clavicle-rib syndromes, nocturnal paresthetic brachialgia, and effort vein thrombosis. Common whiplash TOS symptoms include: nausea, dizziness, numbness, aching pain, disorientation, neck stiffness, arm heaviness, incapacitating headache, easy fatigability of the arm, tingling and numbness in the ulnar aspect of the hand. See Sanders, below.

Neck pain	90%
Paresthesia	90%
Arm pain	84%
Headaches	80%
Shoulder pain	75%
Arm weakness	47%
Chest pain	10%
Raynaud's Phenomenon	1–3%
Swelling	1–4%

Sanders RJ, Pearce WH. The treatment of thoracic outlet syndrome: a comparison of different operations. J Vasc Surg. 1989 Dec;10(6):626–34.

It is documented that whiplash trauma can cause TOS. Whiplash-caused TOS can cause long-term disabling symptom.

Whiplash injury patients occasionally do not respond to conventional treatment and become worse.

Arm pain and paresthesia following neck injury in motor vehicle accidents arise from irritable cervical neural tissues. Quintner JL. A study of upper limb pain and paraesthesiae following neck injury in motor vehicle accidents: assessment of the brachial plexus tension test of Elvey. Br J Rheumatol. 1989 Dec; 28(6):528–33.

In chronic whiplash patients, thoracic outlet syndrome was diagnosed in 31.6% of the cases. Magnusson T. Extracervical symptoms after whiplash trauma. Cephalalgia. 1994 Jun; 14(3):223–7; discussion 181–2.

Thoracic outlet syndrome (TOS) is a nonspecific label. When employing it, one should define the type of TOS as arterial TOS, venous TOS, or neurogenic TOS. Each type has different symptoms and physical findings by which the three types can easily be identified.

Neurogenic TOS (NTOS) is by far the most common, comprising well over 90% of all TOS patients. Arterial TOS is the least common accounting for no more than 1%. Many patients are erroneously diagnosed as "vascular" TOS, a nonspecific misnomer, whereas they really have NTOS. The Adson Test of noting a radial pulse deficit in provocative positions has been shown to be of no clinical value and should not be relied upon to make the diagnosis of any of the three types. The test is normal in most patients with NTOS and at the same time can be positive in many control volunteers. Arterial TOS is caused by emboli arising from subclavian artery stenosis or aneurysms. Symptoms are those of arterial ischemia and x-rays almost always disclose a cervical rib or anomalous first rib. Venous TOS presents with arm swelling, cyanosis, and pain due to subclavian vein obstruction, with or without thrombosis.

Neurogenic TOS is due to brachial plexus compression usually from scarred scalene muscles secondary to neck trauma, whiplash injuries being the most common. Symptoms include extremity paresthesia, pain, and weakness as well as neck pain and occipital headache. Physical exam is most important and includes several provocative maneuvers including neck rotation and head tilting, which elicit symptoms in the contralateral extremity; the upper limb tension test, which is comparable to straight leg raising; and abducting the arms to 90 degrees in external rotation, which usually brings on symptoms within 60 seconds.

Sanders RJ, Hammond SL, Rao NM. Diagnosis of thoracic outlet syndrome. J Vasc Surg. 2007 Sep;46(3):601–4.

§ 5:4 Thoracic outlet syndrome—Brachial plexus lesions

Note:

The article citations below give evidence of support for the "Double Crush Syndrome."

Our study shows that symptoms and signs attributable to stretching of the brachial plexus do occur after whiplash injury in a significant proportion of patients, and that the presence and the persistence of these symptoms and signs indicate an unfavorable prognosis. In addition to irritation of the scalene muscles, stretching of the brachial plexus secondary to trauma is being more commonly diagnosed. Tinel's sign over the brachial plexus was considered as marking the advance of a wave of regeneration or as a diminution of the threshold of nerve fibres to mechanical stimulus. Ide M, Ide J, Yamaga M, Takagi K. Symptoms and signs of irritation of the brachial plexus in whiplash injuries. J Bone Joint Surg Br. 2001 Mar;83(2):226–9.

Physical signs included: decreased range of movement of the neck; paraesthesiae in the upper arm; forearm and/or hand weakness; coldness, discoloration and hyperhydrosis in the upper limb; upper limb swelling; positive Tinel sign over the scalene muscles or in the supraclavicular fossa, the cubital tunnel, the radial nerve at the elbow and/ or the carpal tunnel; and discomfort with the maneuvers causing traction to the brachial plexus. A significant proportion of patients with irritation of the brachial plexus can have abnormal autonomic status, including neck and arm pain or numbness, headache, nausea, sleeplessness, general fatigue, hyperhydrosis and swelling of the hand. Ide M, Ide J, Yamaga M, Takagi K. Symptoms and signs of irritation of the brachial plexus in whiplash injuries. J Bone Joint Surg Br. 2001 Mar;83(2):226–9.

Brachial plexus irritation diagnosis was determined by: Persistent diffuse pain or paraesthesiae in the upper limb aggravated by carrying, lifting, overhead elevation or repetitive use of the arm. A positive Tinel sign over the brachial plexus at the scalene muscles or supraclavicular fossa. Reproduction of pain or paraesthesiae by maneuvers stressing the brachial plexus with the shoulder at 90° of abduction in external rotation, or with a traction maneuver. **Brachial plexus injury**

occurs often from whiplash. In this study it was found to be 37.8% of patients. **Delay onset for brachial plexus symptoms** is very common, with a mean of 6.7 days and some being delayed as long as **37 days**. Brachial plexus injury is not related to patient age (range 16–69 years) or to mechanism of injury. Brachial plexus injury is significantly more likely to occur in women compared to men (nearly twice as common). The brachial plexus injury and its associated symptoms involve the sympathetic portion of the autonomic nervous system. Postganglionic sympathetic efferents are termed gray rami because they are non-myelinated, and problems in these non-myelinated sympathetic fibers are not assessed with nerve conduction studies. Ide M, Ide J, Yamaga M, Takagi K. Symptoms and signs of irritation of the brachial plexus in whiplash injuries. J Bone Joint Surg Br. 2001 Mar;83(2):226–9.

When the nerve strain reached 8.1 ± 0.5% the muscle action potential was not evoked. Taki S, et al. In situ strain and stress of nerve conduction blocking in the brachial plexus. JOR 2002;20:1311–4.

The force leading to rupture of the brachial plexus ranged between 217.7N — 546.3N, stress values between 1.3 N/mm2 — 3.5 N/mm2. Mean elongation until rupture was 38.6%, ranging 19.6% — 58.8% of initial length. Zapalowicz K, Radek A. Mechanical properties of the human brachial plexus. Neur Neurochir 2000; Suppl 6:89–93.

§ 5:5 Reflex sympathetic dystrophy (complex regional pain syndrome)

Pain	93%
Hyperesthesia	75%
Hypesthesia	69%
Muscular incoordination	54%
Tremor	49%

Veldman PH, Reynen HM, Arntz IE, Goris RJ. Signs and symptoms of reflex sympathetic dystrophy: prospective study of 829 patients. Lancet. 1993 Oct 23;342(8878):1012–6.

§ 5:6 Post-concussion syndrome

Symptoms for post-concussion syndrome include:

- Light headedness
- Vertigo/dizziness
- Neck pain
- Headache
- Photophobia (affected by light)
- Phonophobia (affected by sounds)
- Tinnitus (ringing in the ears)
- Impaired memory
- Easy distractibility
- Impaired comprehension
- Forgetfulness
- Impaired logical thought
- Difficulty with new or abstract concepts
- Insomnia (difficulty in sleeping)
- Easy fatigability
- Apathy
- Outbursts of anger
- Mood swings
- Depression
- Loss of libido
- Personality change

Foreman SM, Croft AC, eds. Whiplash injuries: The Cervical Acceleration/Deceleration syndrome, 3 ed. Lippincott, Philadelphia, 2002. pg. 373

§ 5:7 Whiplash injuries and proprioceptive disturbance

A whiplash injury may produce a "proprioceptive" disturbance. Proprioception is the knowledge of where your body parts are. Proprioceptive receptors in the cervical spine play a key role in the Posture Control System (PCS)—the mechanism by which the body maintains balance and equilibrium.

In one test, patients wore a cervical range-of-motion device (CROM), and their heads were positioned at 30° of right rotation by the researcher. With the test subjects' eyes closed, the researcher positioned the patients' heads at 0°, and then instructed the patients to return to the 30° position three times, without opening their eyes. Five other test positions were evaluated as well, and the same test was given to eleven healthy control subjects. "The whiplash group averaged an absolute difference of 5.01° from their recorded angle measure compared with the true angle measure, whereas the control group averaged a 1.75° absolute difference." The authors concluded, "Individuals who have sustained a whiplash injury may have proprioceptive deficits that do not allow them accurately or reliably to calculate head position. This may be detrimental to their everyday function. **Rehabilitation after whiplash injury should focus not only on range of motion and strength but on postural awareness.**" See Loudon JK, Ruhl M, Field E. Ability to reproduce head position after whiplash injury. Spine. 1997 Apr 15;22(8):865–8.

Nontraumatic neck pain patients show little evidence of impaired cervicocephalic kinesthetic sensibility. Rix GD, Bagust J. Cervicocephalic kinesthetic sensibility in patients with chronic, nontraumatic cervical spine pain. Arch Phys Med Rehabil. 2001 Jul;82(7):911–9.

The proprioceptive deficit caused by a ligament injury rarely is due only to sensory and mechanical dysfunction of the ligament. **A ligament injury is often accompanied by damages to other joint structures, e.g. the joint capsule and menisci, implying that the disturbed sensory feedback from these structures is likely to contribute to the reported proprioceptive deficits.** Even in the cases of an isolated ligament injury, contributing effects from the surrounding tissue cannot be excluded, since the sprained or ruptured ligaments induce alterations of the normal biomechanics of the joint. Thereby, the loads imposed on different joint structures and muscles will change, causing altered sensory feedback from mechanoreceptors within and around the joints. See Sjolander P, Johansson H, Djupsjobacka M.

Spinal and supraspinal effects of activity in ligament afferents. J Electromyogr Kinesiol. 2002 Jun;12(3):167–76.

In conclusion, the study has found that balance deficits exist in both subjects with whiplash-associated disorders and idiopathic neck pain compared to controls; however, differences in balance strategies may exist between the neck pain groups. Overall, subjects who have experienced **trauma appear to have greater balance disturbances.**

Field S, Treleaven J, Jull G. Standing balance: A comparison between idiopathic and whiplash-induced neck pain. Man Ther. 2007 Feb 14

§ 5:8 Whiplash injuries and proprioceptive disturbance—Dizziness

Standing balance in persistent whiplash: a comparison between subjects with and without dizziness. The study's results indicated that the energy of the sway signal for comfortable stance tests was significantly greater in the group with dizziness compared with the group without dizziness. In the group without dizziness, the energy was greater than controls for all tests, but significantly different on selected tests. In selected tandem stance tests, subjects with dizziness were significantly less able to complete the test than subjects without dizziness and controls. These deficits could not be attributed to medications, compensation, anxiety, or age and are likely to be due to **disturbances to the postural control system possibly originating from abnormal cervical afferent input**. Treleaven J, Jull G, Lowchoy N. Standing balance in persistent whiplash: a comparison between subjects with and without dizziness. J Rehabil Med. 2005 Jul;37(4):224–9.

Smooth pursuit neck torsion test in whiplash-associated disorders: relationship to self-reports of neck pain and disability, dizziness and anxiety. The results provide further evidence of the usefulness of the **smooth pursuit neck torsion test** to identify eye movement disturbances in patients with whiplash, which are likely to be due to disturbed cervical afferentation. Treleaven J, Jull G, LowChoy N. Smooth pursuit neck torsion test in whiplash-associated disorders: relationship to self-reports of neck pain and disability, dizziness and anxiety. J Rehabil Med. 2005 Jul;37(4):219–23.

Symptoms of vertigo, dizziness, and visual disturbance are common after whiplash injuries, which may be due

to the proprioceptive functions of the cervical spine. There were significant differences between the two groups on reading behavior. The whiplash patients showed reading behaviors similar to children in the first three years of elementary school, while the control subjects showed behaviors in the high school range. The reading problems were found to be closely linked to problems with smooth pursuit. See Gimse R, Tjell C, Bjorgen IA, Saunte C. Disturbed eye movements after whiplash due to injuries to the posture control system. J Clin Exp Neuropsychol. 1996 Apr;18(2):178–86.

In another study, the stated objective was to see how different conditions influenced the results of a relatively new test called the Smooth Pursuit Neck Torsion test (the SPNT)-a test specifically designed to detect and diagnose cervical-related dizziness. The SPNT works by comparing the movement of the subject's eyes on a target in a neutral position and one in which the neck is experiencing torsion. A difference in eye movement between the torsion and neutral positions indicate that the postural control system is experiencing interference in the cervical spine. The only subjects that showed indications of cervical proprioceptive interference were the whiplash patients, and these results were highly significant statistically. The authors conclude that this proprioceptive interference may be caused by damage to the facet joints of the cervical spine—just as other researchers have recently concluded. "**The SPNT test therefore seems to be useful for diagnosing cervical dizziness, at least in patients with WAD having symptoms of dizziness, because it has a high sensitivity and specificity**." See Tjell C, Rosenhall U. Smooth pursuit neck torsion test: a specific test for cervical dizziness. Am J Otol. 1998 Jan;19(1):76–81.

§ 5:9 Whiplash injuries and proprioceptive disturbance—Cervical trauma and tremor

"Examination showed mild restriction of neck movements by pain and spasm in the trapeziae, worse on the right. Tone in the limbs was normal. There was slight weakness of hand grip and opponens pollicis on the right. Pin prick sensation was reduced in a C6 distribution in the hand. There was a 6–8 Hz action type tremor, particularly present when the right wrist was extended or flexed and also when the thumb was flexed." "**Plain cervical spine radiography showed loss of the normal curvature and MRI of the spine was normal**." Ellis SJ. Tremor and other movement disorders after whiplash type injuries. J Neurol Neurosurg Psychiatry. 1997 Jul;63(1):110–2.

The C6 distribution of symptoms is interesting, as most of the recent studies on whiplash show that this area of the cervical spine is most susceptible to trauma. Note that the author reported evidence of nerve root damage or spinal cord involvement in four of the six cases. Also, five of the six cases in this report were women, who are more likely to suffer from whiplash injury than men: "Idiopathic torsion dystonia and peripheral induced dystonia are reported to have a female preponderance."

Suggested criteria for determining whether movement disorders are trauma-related or not are: Injury must have been severe enough to cause local symptoms for two weeks . . . The onset of the movement disorder should be within a year of the injury . . . The movement disorder must have an anatomical association with the site of the injury. Jankovic J. Post-traumatic movement disorders: central and peripheral mechanisms.Neurology. 1994 Nov;44(11):2006–14.

Idiopathic torsion dystonia and peripheral induced dystonia are reported to have a female preponderance. This may reflect the higher incidence of joint laxity in the female population with a greater degree of flexion extension resulting from this type of injury. Larsson LG, Baum J, Mudholkar GS. Hypermobility: features and differential incidence between the sexes. Arthritis Rheum. 1987 Dec;30(12):1426–30.

Peripherial trauma can produce movement disorders. The pathophysiological mechanisms underlying these phenomena are not entirely known, but functional changes in afferent neuronal input to the spinal cord and secondary affection of higher brain stem and subcortical centers are probably involved. Nobrega JC, Campos CR, Limongi JC, Teixeira MJ, Lin TY. Movement disorders induced by peripheral trauma. Arq Neuropsiquiatr. 2002 Mar;60(1):17–20.

In a cross-sectional study 142 male and 139 female workers participated in a self-report questionnaire and a clinical examination. The aim of this study was to use the **cervicothoracic** ratio (CTR), a clinical method for measuring segmental mobility between C7 and T5, to evaluate the influence of segmental mobility in neck-shoulder pain and different subjectively experienced symptoms. The study showed that reduced relative mobility at levels C7-T1 and T1-T2 significantly predicted neck-shoulder pain and the symptom weakness in the hands. The strongest relationship between segmental mobility and symptoms was found among subjects classified as having an inverse C7-T1 function, defined as equal or less mobility in motion segment C7-T1 compared to T1-T2. Reduced mobility explained 14% of neck-shoulder pain and 15% of weakness in the hands. It is suggested that deviation from synchronous distribution of mobility between motion segments C7-T1 and T1-T2 might be a factor provoking **joint mechano receptors.**

Norlander S, Nordgren B. Clinical symptoms related to musculoskeletal neck-shoulder pain and mobility in the cervico-thoracic spine. Scand J Rehabil Med. 1998 Dec;30(4):243–51.

According to the authors' interpretation, lack of synchronous mobility distribution between adjacent motion segments might be a provoking factor. Inverse C7-T1 function predicts **neck-shoulder pain** related to the cervico-thoracic articulations and yields a positive predictive value of 84%.

Norlander S, Gustavsson BA, Lindell J, Nordgren B. Reduced mobility in the cervico-thoracic motion segment—a risk factor for musculoskeletal neck-shoulder pain: a two-year prospective follow-up study. Scand J Rehabil Med. 1997 Sep;29(3):167–74.

Assessments were performed at baseline and 3 and 9 months following randomization using a cervical range of motion instrument, the cervico-thoracic ratio, a Grippit, a visual analogue scale, a Painmatcher, and the Tampa Scale for Kinesiophobia. Women with whiplash-associated disorders seem to exhibit flexion **hypomobility in C7-T1**. The flexion mobility in C7-T1 was weakly, but significantly, correlated with **grip strength**. Neck pain may give rise to restricted range of motion.

Bunketorp Käll L. Assessment of motion in the cervico-thoracic spine in patients with subacute whiplash-associated disorders. J Rehabil Med. 2008 Jun;40(6):418–25.

§ 5:10 Chronic pain symptoms

Patients with chronic whiplash syndrome may have a generalized central hyperexcitability from a loss of tonic inhibitory input (disinhibition) and/or ongoing excitatory input. Dysfunction of the motor system may also occur, with or without pain. Davis C. Chronic pain/dysfunction in whiplash-associated disorders. J Manipulative Physiol Ther. 2001 Jan;24(1):44–51.

Studies on experimentally produced central hypersensitivity support three mechanisms; (1) maintenance of central hypersensitivity by ongoing peripheral nocicep-

tive input, (2) persistence of central hypersensitivity after resolution of primary peripheral event, and (3) imbalance of the descending modulation system. Curatolo M, Petersen-Felix S, Arendt-Nielsen L, Giani C, Zbinden AM, Radanov BP. Central hypersensitivity in chronic pain after whiplash injury. Clin J Pain. 2001 Dec;17(4):306–15.

Our findings suggest that **neurological dysfunction of whiplash may occur at several possible spinal cord localities** in the cutaneous silent period functional pathway. Lo YL, Tan YE, Fook-Chong S, Boolsambatra P, Yue WM, Chan LL, Tan SB. Role of spinal inhibitory mechanisms in whiplash injuries. J Neurotrauma. 2007 Jun;24(6):1055–67.

Electrophysiological analysis of the injury-induced increase in excitability of the flexion reflex shows that it in part arises from changes in the activity of the spinal cord. **The long-term consequences of noxious stimuli result, therefore, from central as well as from peripheral changes**. Woolf CJ. Evidence for a central component of post-injury pain hypersensitivity. Nature. 1983 Dec 15–21;306(5944):686–8.

Morphologic change in spinal cord dorsal horn lamina II occurs after partial dorsal root ganglion injury. This change may have significance in the pathogenesis of **chronic mechanical allodynia** after partial dorsal root ganglion injury. Nakamura SI, Myers RR. Injury to dorsal root ganglia alters innervation of spinal cord dorsal horn lamina involved in nociception. Spine. 2000 Mar 1;25(5):537–42.

We provide evidence for **spinal cord hyperexcitability** in patients with chronic pain after whiplash injury and in fibromyalgia patients. This can cause exaggerated pain following low intensity nociceptive or innocuous peripheral stimulation. Spinal hypersensitivity may explain, at least in part, pain in the absence of detectable tissue damage. Banic B, Petersen-Felix S, Andersen OK, Radanov BP, Villiger PM, Arendt-Nielsen L, Curatolo M. Evidence for spinal cord hypersensitivity in chronic pain after whiplash injury and in fibromyalgia. Pain. 2004 Jan;107(1–2):7–15.

Central hypersensitivity may explain exaggerated pain in the presence of minimal nociceptive input arising from minimally damaged tissues. This could account for pain and disability in the absence of objective signs of tissue damage in patients with whiplash.

Central hypersensitivity may provide a common neurobiological framework for the integration of peripheral and supraspinal mechanisms in the pathophysiology of chronic pain after whiplash. Therapy studies are needed. Curatolo M, Arendt-Nielsen L, Petersen-Felix S. Evidence, mechanisms, and clinical implications of central hypersensitivity in chronic pain after whiplash injury. Clin J Pain. 2004 Nov-Dec;20(6):469–76.

The authors found a **hypersensitivity** to peripheral stimulation in whiplash patients. Hypersensitivity was observed after cutaneous and muscular stimulation, at both neck and lower limb. Because hypersensitivity was observed in healthy tissues, it resulted from alterations in the central processing of sensory stimuli (central hypersensitivity). Central hypersensitivity was not dependent on a nociceptive input arising from the painful and tender muscles. Curatolo M, Petersen-Felix S, Arendt-Nielsen L, Giani C, Zbinden AM, Radanov BP. Central hypersensitivity in chronic pain after whiplash injury. Clin J Pain. 2001 Dec;17(4):306–15.

These findings suggest that those with persistent moderate/severe symptoms at 6 months display, soon after injury, generalised hypersensitivity suggestive of **changes in central pain processing mechanisms**. This phenomenon did not occur in those who recover or those with persistent mild symptoms. Sterling M, Jull G, Vicenzino B, Kenardy J. Sensory hypersensitivity occurs soon after whiplash injury and is associated with poor recovery. Pain. 2003 Aug;104(3):509–17.

Chronic neck pain of **whiplash** and non-traumatic origin appears to be unique in some respects. There appears to be different mechanisms involved. Guez M. Chronic neck pain. An epidemiological, psychological and SPECT study with emphasis on whiplash-associated disorders. Acta Orthop Suppl. 2006 Feb;77(320):preceding 1, 3–33.

The present study suggests **different pain mechanisms** in patients with chronic neck pain of non-traumatic origin compared to those with chronic neck pain due to a whiplash trauma. Sundstrom T, Guez M, Hildingsson C, Toolanen G, Nyberg L, Riklund K. Altered cerebral blood flow in chronic neck pain patients but not in whiplash patients: a 99mTc-HMPAO rCBF study. Eur Spine J. 2006 Aug;15(8):1189–95.

Both chronic whiplash-associated disorders and idiopathic neck pain groups were characterized by mechanical hyperalgesia over the cervical spine. Whiplash subjects showed additional **widespread hypersensitivity** to mechanical pressure and thermal stimuli, which was independent of state anxiety and may represent changes in central pain processing mechanisms. This may have implications for future treatment approaches.

Scott D, Jull G, Sterling M. Widespread sensory hypersensitivity is a feature of chronic whiplash-associated disorder but not chronic idiopathic neck pain. Clin J Pain. 2005 Mar-Apr;21(2):175–81.

Widespread pain was associated with negative consequences with respect to pain intensity, prevalence of other symptoms including depressive symptoms, some aspects of coping, life satisfaction and general health.

Peolsson M, Borsbo B, Gerdle B. Generalized pain is associated with more negative consequences than local or regional pain: a study of chronic whiplash-associated disorders. J Rehabil Med. 2007 Apr;39(3):260–8.

Based on the results of the present study, it reasonable to infer that a significant proportion of individuals with chronic neck pain in the general population were **originally injured in a motor vehicle accident**. Freeman MD, Croft AC, Rossignol AM, Centeno CJ, Elkins WL. Chronic neck pain and whiplash: a case-control study of the relationship between acute whiplash injuries and chronic neck pain. Pain Res Manag. 2006 Summer;11(2):79–83.

Women reported pain in the neck or shoulder more often before the accident and this was the only statistically significant predictor of chronic symptoms when analysed by logistic regression (odds ratio 4.5). To conclude, we found no evidence that the **different coping patterns during the early phase after a whiplash injury influenced the prognosis**. Kivioja J, Jensen I, Lindgren U. Early coping strategies do not influence the prognosis after whiplash injuries. Injury. 2005 Aug;36(8):935–40.

Some chronic painful conditions including e.g. fibromyalgia, whiplash associated disorders, endometriosis, and irritable bowel syndrome are associated with **generalized musculoskeletal hyperalgesia**. The aim of the present study was to determine whether generalized deep-tissue hyperalgesia could be demonstrated in a group of patients with chronic low-back pain with intervertebral disc herniation. Twelve patients with MRI confirmed lumbar intervertebral disc herniation and 12 age and sex matched controls were included. Subjects were exposed to quantitative nociceptive stimuli to the infraspinatus and anterior tibialis muscles. Mechanical pressure (thresholds and supra-threshold) and injection of hypertonic saline (pain intensity, duration, distribution) were used. Pain intensity to experimental stimuli was assessed on a visual analogue scale (VAS). Patients demonstrated significantly higher pain intensity (VAS), duration, and larger areas of pain referral following saline injection in both infraspinatus and tibialis anterior. The patients rated significantly higher pain intensity to supra-threshold mechanical pressure stimulation in both muscles. In patients, the pressure pain-threshold was lower in the anterior tibialis muscle compared to controls. In conclusion, **generalized deep-tissue hyperalgesia was demonstrated in chronic low-back pain patients** with radiating pain and MRI confirmed intervertebral disc herniation, suggesting that this **central sensitization** should also be addressed in the pain management regimes.

O'neill S, Manniche C, Graven-Nielsen T, Arendt-Nielsen L. Generalized deep-tissue hyperalgesia in patients with chronic low-back pain. Eur J Pain. 2007 May;11(4):415–20.

§ 5:11 Whiplash injury and eye movements—Overview

Brainstem, cerebellum and forebrain all contribute to control of eye movements via effects on CN nuclei III, IV, and VI. There are three main eye movements: 1) Horizontal, 2) Vertical and, 3) Vergence (defined below).

Below are more detail definitions relating to eye movements:

Saccades — rapid eye movements directed at targets in visual field.

Smooth pursuit (SP) — slower movements following objects in visual field.

Vergence — movements to maintain visual fixation on objects moving toward or away from viewer.

Convergence — produced by medial recti muscles (CN III) and divergence by lateral recti muscles (CN VI).

Reflex — including optokinetic nystagmus & vestibulo-ocular reflex.

Nystagmus — rhythmic form of reflex eye movement in one direction interrupted by fast saccade-like movement in the opposite direction (a few beats are normal when patient turns eyes far to side, continued beats or beats when eyes turned small amount is abnormal.

The MLF (medial longitudinal fasciculus) interconnects nuclei of III, IV, VI and vestibular nuclei.

§ 5:12 Whiplash injury and eye movements—Oculomotor Nucleus (CN III)

The nucleus is in the midbrain; it innervates four extraocular muscles and functions in most eye movements; it contains parasympathetic axons from Edinger-Westphal nucleus to ciliary ganglion which innervates pupillary constrictor muscles and ciliary muscle of the lens.

§ 5:13 Whiplash injury and eye movements—General whiplash studies and eye movement

Interaction between ocular stabilization reflexes in patients with whiplash injury. The automobile has become an increasingly more popular means of transport, which has led to an increasing number of rear-end collisions and has consequently resulted in more patients with whiplash-associated disorders (WADs). Recently, it was found that the gain of one of the ocular stabilization reflexes — the cervico-ocular reflex (COR) — is elevated in patients with whiplash injury. The COR responds to proprioceptive signals from the neck and acts in conjunction with the vestibulo-ocular reflex (VOR) and the optokinetic reflex (OKR) to preserve stable vision on the retina during head motion. Therefore, an investigation was conducted to determine whether the reported elevation of the COR in WADs is accompanied by changes in VOR or OKR. Eye movements of 13 patients and 18 age-matched healthy controls were recorded with an infrared eye-tracking device. Analysis confirmed a **significant increase in COR gain in whiplash patients**. Meanwhile, the VOR and OKR gains remained the same. No correlation was found between the gains of the reflexes in individual patients. This is in contrast to earlier observations in elderly subjects and subjects with labyrinthine defects, who showed increases in COR gain and decreases in VOR gain. **Impaired neck motion, altered proprioception of the neck, or disorganization in the process of VOR plasticity could explain the lack of change in VOR gain.** This leads to eye movement dysfunction in whiplash injury patients. Montfoort I, Kelders WP, van der Geest JN, Schipper IB, Feenstra L, de Zeeuw CI, Frens MA. Interaction between ocular stabilization reflexes in patients with whiplash injury. Invest Ophthalmol Vis Sci. 2006 Jul;47(7):2881–4.

The gain values of the COR were significantly increased in the patient population at a wide range of stimulus peak velocities with maximum difference at the lower frequencies. The cervico-ocular reflex (COR) gain appears to be a parameter that may permit an objective diagnosis of WAD. Kelders WP, Kleinrensink GJ, van der Geest JN, Schipper IB, Feenstra L, De Zeeuw CI, Frens MA. The cervico-ocular reflex is increased in whiplash injury patients. J Neurotrauma. 2005 Jan;22(1):133–7.

The results suggest that restricted cervical movements and changes in the quality of proprioceptive information from the cervical spine region affect voluntary eye movements. **A flexion/extension injury to the neck may result in dysfunction of the proprioceptive system. Oculomotor dysfunction after neck trauma might be related to cervical afferent input disturbances**. Heikkila HV, Wenngren BI. Cervicocephalic kinesthetic sensibility, active range of cervical motion, and oculomotor function in patients with whiplash injury. Arch Phys Med Rehabil. 1998 Sep;79(9):1089–94.

The smooth pursuit neck torsion test (SPNT) is thought to be a measure of neck afferent influence on eye movement control and is useful in assessing subjects with whiplash, especially those complaining of dizziness. **This study has determined that smooth pursuit neck torsion eye movement disturbances are present in patients with persistent neck pain following a whiplash injury and that disturbances are greater in those patients also reporting the symptom of dizziness in association with their pain.** Treleaven J, Jull G, LowChoy N. Smooth pursuit neck torsion test in whiplash-associated disorders: relationship to self-reports of neck pain and disability, dizziness and anxiety. J Rehabil Med. 2005 Jul;37(4):219–23.

Reduced smooth pursuit performance at one-year follow-up was associated with persistent neck pain.

Kongsted A, Jorgensen LV, Leboeuf-Yde C, Qerama E, Korsholm L, Bendix T. Are altered smooth pursuit eye movements related to chronic pain and disability following whiplash injuries? A prospective trial with one-year follow-up. Clin Rehabil. 2008 May;22(5):469–79.

Self-reports after whiplash often indicates associations with vertigo and reading problems. Neuropsychological and otoneurological tests were applied to a group of whiplash patients (n = 26) and to a carefully matched control group. The whiplash group deviated from the control group on measures of eye movements during reading, on smooth pursuit eye movements with the head in normal position, and with the body turned to the left or to the right. Clinical, caloric, and neurophysiological tests showed no injury to the vestibular system or to the CNS. Test results suggest that injuries to the neck due to whiplash can cause distortion of the posture control system as a result of disorganized neck proprioceptive activity. Gimse R, Tjell C, Bjorgen IA, Saunte C. Disturbed eye movements after whiplash due to injuries to the posture control system. J Clin Exp Neuropsychol. 1996 Apr;18(2):178–86.

Past studies examining whether or not cognitive changes actually have occurred as a result of a whiplash (WL) accident have produced varying results. The aim of this study was to identify possible cognitive dysfunctions in a group with persistent problems after whiplash due to injuries to the posture control system and related structures. The whiplash subjects (n = 23) were selected on the basis of their reduced gain in the Smooth Pursuit Neck Torsion test (SPNT). The WL group differed significantly from a closely matched control group on tests of learning and memory, and prolonged divided attention and concentration. After attempting to rule out other ways of interpreting these differences (such as pain, depression, medication, and premorbid health problems), these data were interpreted as lending support to the notion of a causal connection between the disturbed posture control system and some cognitive malfunctions. Gimse R, Bjorgen IA, Tjell C, Tyssedal JS, Bo K. Reduced cognitive functions in a group of whiplash patients with demonstrated disturbances in the posture control system. J Clin Exp Neuropsychol. 1997 Dec;19(6):838–49.

Oculomotor function was investigated in 39 patients with a previous soft-tissue injury of the cervical spine. The velocity, the accuracy, and the pattern of the eye movements were disturbed in 20 patients with chronic and disabling symptoms. Oculomotor function in the 19 asymptomatic patients did not differ from a control group. The oculomotor function seems to be impaired, possibly by brain stem lesions, in patients with chronic symptoms of whiplash injury of the cervical spine. Hildingsson C, Wenngren BI, Bring G, Toolanen G. Oculomotor problems after cervical spine injury. Acta Orthop Scand. 1989 Oct;60(5):513–6.

§ 5:14 Whiplash injury and eye movements—Forebrain control of eye movements

Multiple paths descend from forebrain and affect eye movements. These paths project either directly to brainstem nuclei involved with eye movements or relay via the superior colliculus. Frontal eye fields appear to be in area 6. FEF generates saccades in the contralateral direction via connections to contralateral PPRF. Parieto-occipital-temporal cortex functions in smooth pursuit eye movements in ipsilateral direction via connections with the vestibular nuclei, cerebellum, and PPRF. Inputs from visual cortex and visual association cortex influence FEF activity. The basal ganglia also appear to play a role in eye movements.

In the symptomatic group the pattern of eye movement disturbances together with normal performance in reflexive saccade tasks and impaired performance in the intentional saccade tasks, especially impaired inhibitory function, suggests dysfunction of prefrontal and frontal cortical structures. Mosimann UP, Muri RM, Felblinger J, Radanov BP. Saccadic eye movement disturbances in whiplash patients with persistent complaints. Brain. 2000 Apr;123 (Pt 4):828–35.

Chapter 6

Structures Injured

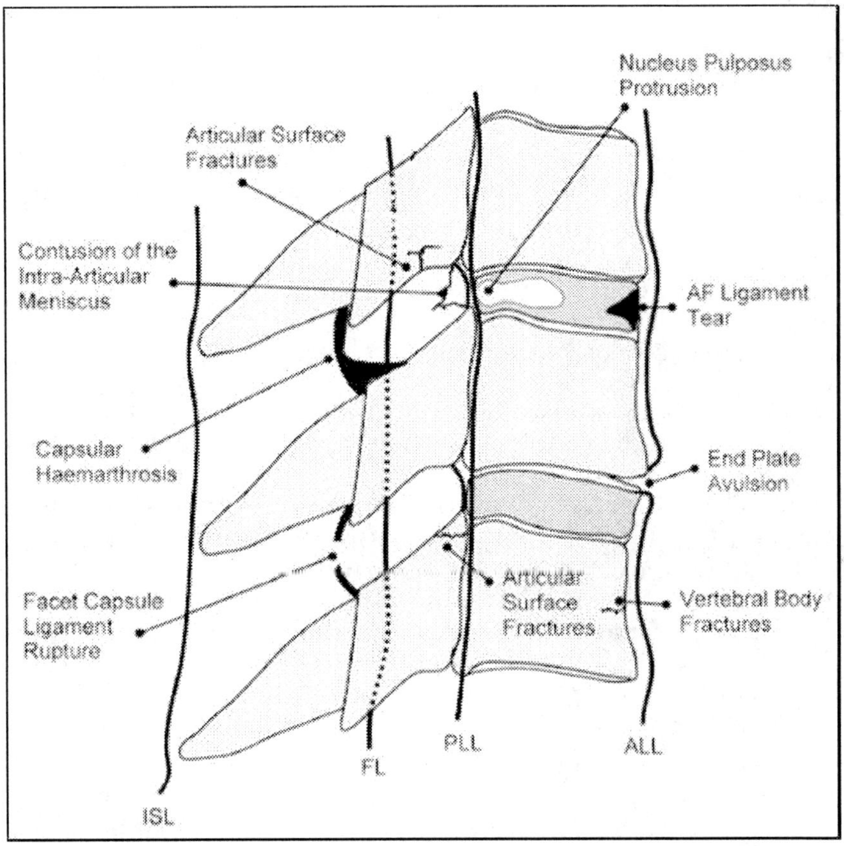

A lateral view of a section of the lower cervical spine showing possible whiplash associated injuries, adapted from Barnsley L, Lord S, Bogduk N. Whiplash injury. Pain. 1994 Sep;58(3):283–307.

§ 6:1 Ligaments—General structure and function

Ligaments, lying internal or external to the joint capsule, bind bone to bone and supply passive support and guidance to joints. They function to supplement active stabilizers (i.e. muscles) and bony geometry. Ligaments are generally named according to their position in the body (e.g. collateral) or according to their bony attachments. Collagen constitutes seventy percent of the dry weight of ligament, the majority being type I collagen, which is also found in tendon, skin and bone. Collagen has a relatively long turnover rate, its average half-life being 300 and 500 days, which is slightly longer than that of bone. **Therefore, several months may be required for a ligament to alter its structure to meet changes in physical loading conditions or to repair itself after injury**. Weiss JA, Gardiner JC. Computational Modeling of Ligament Mechanics. Critical Reviews in Biomedical Engineering 2001;29(4):1–70; Neuberger A, Slack HGB. Metabolism of collagen from liver, bone, skin, and tendon in normal rat. Biochem J 1953;53:47–52.

Ligaments are highly organized, dense, fibrous connective-tissue structures that provide stability to joints and participate in joint proprioception. Injuries to ligaments induce a healing response that is characterized by the formation of a scar. The scar tissue is weaker, larger and creeps more than normal ligament and is associated with an increased amount of minor collagens (types III, V and VI), decreased collagen cross-links and an increased amount of glycosaminoglycans. Studies have shown that certain surgical variables alter the healing of ligaments. Such factors include the size of gap between the healing ligament ends, the use of motion in a stable joint and the presence of multiple ligamentous injuries. Ligaments are composed primarily of water (approximately 70%), collagen (approximately 25%), other matrix components such as proteoglycans and fibronectin (approximately 4%) and cells (< 1%). Ligaments are less vascular than visceral organs. The pattern of ligament healing is qualitatively very similar to wound healing and culminates in the formation of a scar that bridges the torn tissue. After an injury to the ligament tissue, hemostasis is activated and a fibrin clot is formed within minutes. An inflammatory response ensues over the next 3 to 5 days, removing debris and attracting large numbers of angiogenic cells and fibroblasts. These cells begin to produce matrix, and formation of new tissue takes over as inflammation lessens over the next several weeks. In ligaments, collagen levels increase rapidly, reaching normal levels by 6 weeks. The collagen types are altered, with greater levels of types III, V and VI collagen ("minor collagens") and less type I collagen than normal. (Type I is still the most prevalent). Ligaments begin to resist appreciable forces, allowing biomechanical testing as early as 2 to 3 weeks after injury. The healing tissue is remodeled by cells over several months and years, leading to fewer cells and vessels, with better collagen alignment. Collagen types return closer to normal distribution, with type I increasing and most of the minor collagen types decreasing. **The structural strength and stiffness, stress and tissue quality continue to improve up to 12 months after injury, but after that time, only relatively small increases are made. However, the material properties of the ligament scar do not return to normal even after 2 years.** Hildebrand KA, Frank CB. Scar formation and ligament healing. Can J Surg. 1998 Dec;41(6):425–9.

The presence of peptidergic nerves suggests that ligaments may be susceptible to neurogenic inflammation and may be centers of articular nociception. McDougall JJ, Bray RC, Sharkey KA. Morphological and immunohistochemical examination of nerves in normal and injured collateral ligaments of rat, rabbit, and human knee joints. Anat Rec. 1997 May;248(1):29–39.

§ 6:2 Ligaments—General structure and function—Normal wound-healing phases

All forms of trauma, to any tissue, anywhere in the body, signal the reparative sequence to begin. The sequence of events is highly organized and predictable. One process is stimulated to begin, and its completion in turn signals another cellular response until the wound is bridged by scar. The ultimate goal in collagen research may be the discovery of healing without scar formation. Until then, to prevent scar formation is to prevent healing. **It is an inferior method compared with regeneration**, but it is the primary means of repair for all vertebrates. Special cells in our body respond to injury by forming a "collagenous glue." This body glue is called granulation scar tissue. The response to injury, either surgically or traumatically induced, is immediate. The wound then passes through three phases toward final repair: 1) the inflammatory phase, 2) the fibroplastic phase, and 3) the remodeling phase. The inflammatory phase prepares the area for healing, the fibroplastic phase rebuilds the structure, and the remodeling phase provides the final form. Hardy MA. The biology of Scar Formation. Physical Therapy 1989;69(12):1014.

§ 6:3 Ligaments—Ligaments of spine

The cervical spine without muscles acting to support it, buckles under very load compressive loads. **The loads to cause the buckling of the cervical spine are about one-fifth to one-quarter 10.5N (3.8) [2.4 lbs ± .85 lbs] the weight of the average head.** See Panjabi MM, Cholewicki J, Nibu K, Grauer J, Babat LB, Dvorak J. Critical load of the human cervical spine: an in vitro experimental study. Clin Biomech (Bristol, Avon). 1998 Jan;13(1):11–17.

Spine ligament strength varies in different specimens and in different ligaments. Most testing has been a quasi-static tension testing to failure. This is a slower rate than occurs in a whiplash event. See Myklebust JB, Pintar F, Yoganandan N, Cusick JF, Maiman D, Myers TJ, Sances A Jr. Tensile strength of spinal ligaments. Spine. 1988 May; 13(5):526–31; Przybylski GJ, Carlin GJ, Patel PR, Woo SL. Human anterior and posterior cervical longitudinal ligaments possess similar tensile properties. J Orthop Res. 1996 Nov;14(6):1005–8. Neumann P, Ekstrom LA, Keller TS, Perry L, Hansson TH. Aging, vertebral density, and disc degeneration alter the tensile stress-strain characteristics of the human anterior longitudinal ligament. J Orthop Res. 1994 Jan;12(1):103–12.

The ligamentum flavum has a specific and active role within the vertebral building, at the level of the spinal joints. Its characteristics described above confirm its neurological role especially for proprioceptive control. On the whole, this ligament is both mobilizing, stabilizing and adviser. The implications in spinal physiopathology are numerous. Viejo-Fuertes D, Liguoro JM, Vital JJ. Rombouts. Morphogenesis, anatomy and histology of the ligamentum flavum. Eur J Orthop Surg Traumatol 2000;10: 77–83; Viejo-Fuertes D, Liguoro D, Rivel J, Midy D, Guerin J. Morphologic and histologic study of the ligamentum flavum in the thoraco-lumbar region. Surg Radiol Anat. 1998;20(3):171–6.

§ 6:4 Ligaments—Alar and transverse ligaments (upper cervical spine)

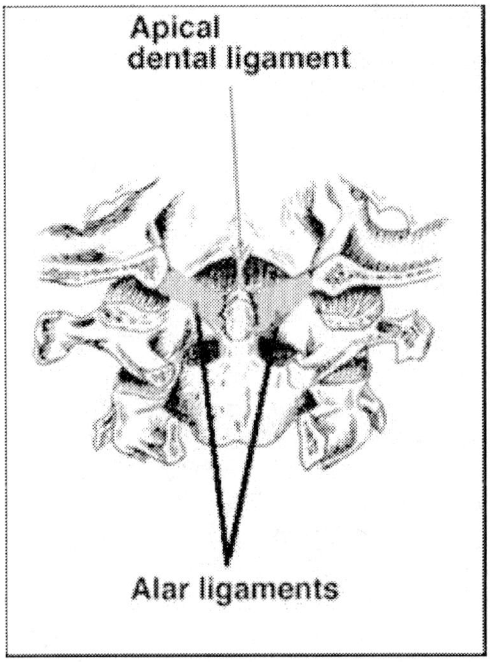

The alar ligaments connect the sides of the dens (on the axis, or the second cervical vertebra) to tubercles on the medial side of the occipital condyle. The alar ligament is also known as the "check ligament of the odontoid (dens)."

The greatest changes in motion occurred in axial rotation to the side opposite the transection. In the first group, left capsular transections resulted in a significant increase in axial rotation range of motion to the right of 1 degree. After the right capsular ligament was transected, there was a further significant increase of 1.8 degrees to the left and 1.0 degree to the right. Lateral bending to the left also increased significantly by 1.5 degrees after both ligaments were cut. In the second group, with the nonfunctional alar and transverse ligaments, transection of the left capsular ligament resulted in greater increases in range of motion: 3.3 degrees to the right and 1.3 degrees to the left. Lateral bending to the right also increased significantly by 4.2 degrees.

Crisco JJ 3rd, Oda T, Panjabi MM, Bueff HU, Dvorák J, Grob D. Transections of the C1-C2 joint capsular ligaments in the cadaveric spine. Spine. 1991 Oct;16(10 Suppl):S474–9.

MRI shows structural changes in ligaments and membranes after whiplash injury, and such lesions can be assessed with reasonable reliability. Lesions to specific structures can be linked with specific trauma mechanisms. There is a correlation between clinical impairment and morphologic findings.

Whiplash trauma can damage soft tissue structures of the upper cervical spine, particularly the **alar ligaments**. Structural lesions in this area contribute to the understanding of the chronic whiplash syndrome. Krakenes J, Kaale BR. Magnetic Resonance Imaging Assessment of Craniovertebral Ligaments and Membranes After Whiplash Trauma. Spine. 2006 Nov 15;31(24):2820–2826.

Whiplash trauma can result in injuries that are difficult to diagnose. Diagnosis is particularly difficult in injuries to the upper segments of the cervical spine (craniocervical joint [CCJ] complex). **Studies indicate that injuries in that region may be responsible for the cervicoencephalic syndrome, as evidenced by headache, balance problems, vertigo, dizziness, eye problems, tinnitus, poor concentration, sensitivity to light and pronounced fatigue.** Consequently, diagnosis of lesions in the CCJ region is important. Functional magnetic resonance imaging is a radiological technique that can visualize injuries of the ligaments and the joint capsules, and accompanying pathological movement patterns. Three severely injured patients that had been extensively examined without any findings of structural lesions were diagnosed by functional magnetic resonance imaging to have injuries in the CCJ region. These injuries were confirmed at surgery, and after surgical stabilization the medical condition was highly improved. It is important to draw attention to the urgent need to diagnose lesions and dysfunction in the CCJ complex and also improve diagnostic methods. Johansson BH. Whiplash injuries can be visible by functional magnetic resonance imaging. Pain Res Manag. 2006 Autumn;11(3):197–9.

If there is damage to the alar ligament, there can be long-term consequences. In the upper cervical spine there are the transverse and alar ligaments. The alar ligament is the weaker of the two ligaments. **The alar ligament, due to its lower strength and its axial direction of loading, might be prone to injury**. Panjabi MM, Crisco JJ 3rd, Lydon C, Dvorak J. The mechanical properties of human alar and transverse ligaments at slow and fast extension rates. Clin Biomech (Bristol, Avon). 1998 Mar;13(2):112–120; Dvorak J, Schneider E, Saldinger P, Rahn B. Biomechanics of the craniocervical region: the alar and transverse ligaments. J Orthop

Res. 1988;6(3):452–61.

Functional radiographs of anterior-posterior open mouth x-ray (APOM) with lateral bending or videoflouroscopy may show the movement of C1 on C2 and demonstrates the ligament stretching and or instability. Functional loss of the alar ligaments indicates a potential for rotatory instability, which, however, must be determined in conjunction with other clinical findings, such as neurological dysfunction, pain, and deformity. **The ligaments could be irreversibly overstretched or even ruptured when the head is rotated** and, in addition, flexed by impact trauma, especially in unexpected rear-end collisions. Panjabi M, Dvorak J, Crisco JJ 3rd, Oda T, Wang P, Grob D. Effects of alar ligament transection on upper cervical spine rotation. J Orthop Res. 1991 Jul;9(4):584–93; Saldinger P, Dvorak J, Rahn BA, Perren SM. Histology of the alar and transverse ligaments. Spine. 1990 Apr;15(4):257–61.

Specimens of the upper cervical spine were functionally examined by using radiography, cineradiography and computerized tomographic (CT) scan. The range of rotation was measured from CT images after maximal rotations to both sides. The left alar ligament was then cut and the examination repeated. The alar and transverse ligaments could be differentiated on CT images in axial, sagittal, and coronal views. Rotation at occiput-atlas was 4.35 degrees to the right and 5.9 degrees to the left, and at atlas-axis, it was 31.4 degrees to the right and 33 degrees to the left. After one-sided lesion of the alar ligament, there was an overall increase of 10.8 degrees or 30% of original rotation to the opposite side, divided about equally between the occiput-atlas and the atlas-axis. It is **concluded that a lesion (irreversible overstretching or rupture of alar ligaments) can result with instability of the upper cervical spine**. See Dvorak J, Panjabi M, Gerber M, Wichmann W. CT-functional diagnostics of the rotatory instability of upper cervical spine. 1. An experimental study on cadavers. Spine. 1987 Apr;12(3):197–205.

Among the WAD patients, **increasing severity of lesions to the alar ligaments was associated with a decrease in maximal flexion and rotation**. A similar pattern was seen for lesions to the transverse ligament, but the trend test was not significant. An abnormal posterior atlanto-occipital membrane was associated with shorter range of left rotation, with a significant trend test both in analyses with and without adjustment for lesions to other structures. No significant association was found in relation to lesions to the tectorial membrane, but very few persons had such lesions. **These find-**

ings indicate that soft tissue lesions may affect neck motion as reflected by Active Range Of Motion. However, since lesions to different structures seem to affect the same movement, AROM alone is not a sufficient indicator for soft-tissue lesions to specific structure in the upper cervical spine. Kaale BR, Krakenes J, Albrektsen G, Wester K. Active range of motion as an indicator for ligament and membrane lesions in the upper cervical spine after a whiplash trauma. J Neurotrauma. 2007 Apr;24(4):713–21.

§ 6:5 Joints

This study strongly indicates that whiplash trauma can damage the tectorial and **posterior atlanto-occipital membranes**; this can be shown on high-resolution MRI. Better knowledge of normal anatomical variations and improved image quality should increase the reliability of lesion classification. Krakenes J, Kaale BR, Moen G, Nordli H, Gilhus NE, Rorvik J. MRI of the tectorial and posterior atlanto-occipital membranes in the late stage of whiplash injury. Neuroradiology. 2003 Sep;45(9):585–91

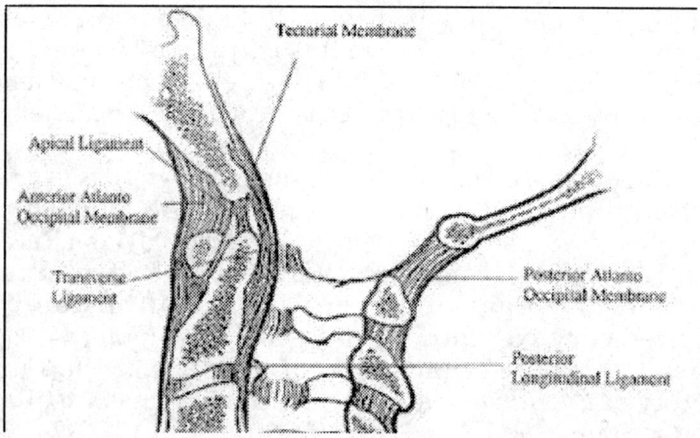

The tectorial membrane is a continuation of the posterior longitudinal ligament. It runs from the body of the axis, up over the posterior portion of the dens. It then makes a 45 degree angle in the anterior direction as it runs toward the attachment of the foramen magnum.

Ninety-two whiplash patients and 30 control persons, randomly drawn, were included. WAD patients reported significantly more pain and functional disability than the controls, both for total score and each of the ten single items. In the WAD patients, MRI lesions to the alar ligaments showed the most consistent association to the reported pain and disability. Lesions to other structures often occurred in combination with lesions to the alar ligaments. Lesions to the transverse ligament and to the posterior atlanto-occipital membrane also appeared to be related to the NDI score, although the association was weaker than for the alar ligament. The disability score increased with increasing number of abnormal (grade 2–3) structures. **These results indicate that symptoms and complaints among WAD patients can be linked with structural abnormalities in ligaments and membranes in the upper cervical spine, in particular the alar ligaments**. Kaale BR, Krakenes J, Albrektsen G, Wester K. Whiplash-associated disorders impairment rating: neck disability index score according to severity of MRI findings of ligaments and membranes in the upper cervical spine. J Neurotrauma. 2005 Apr;22(4):466–75.

Whiplash injuries can be visible by functional magnetic resonance imaging. Whiplash trauma can result in injuries that are difficult to diagnose, particularly in injuries to the upper segments of the cervical spine (craniocervical joint [CCJ] complex). Studies indicate that injuries in that region may be responsible for the cervicoencephalic syndrome, as evidenced by headache, balance problems, vertigo, dizziness, eye problems, tinnitus, poor concentration, sensitivity to light, and pronounced fatigue. Consequently, diagnosis of lesions in the CCJ region is important. Functional (kinematic) magnetic resonance imaging is a radiological technique that can visualize injuries of the ligaments and the joint capsules, and accompanying pathological movement patterns. Three severely injured patients that had been extensively examined without any findings of structural lesions were diagnosed by functional magnetic resonance imaging to have injuries in the CCJ region. These injuries were confirmed at surgery, and after surgical stabilization, the medical condition was highly improved. It is important to draw attention to the urgent need to diagnose lesions and dysfunction in the CCJ complex and also improve diagnostic methods. Johansson BH. Whiplash injuries can be visible by functional magnetic resonance imaging. Pain Res Manag. 2006 Autumn;11(3):197–9.

Comment:

The joint structures affect the muscles and the muscles affect the joints. In the joints there are large diameter and small diameter afferents. The nerve endings may be naked (free nerve endings) that can be nociceptive (transmit pain signals) or corpuscular endings transmitting mechanoreception. A cause of pain is an imbalance in mechanoreceptor input (larger diameter fiber input) into to small diameter fiber input (naked-free nerve endings). This is part of the basis of the "Gate Theory of Pain." If the muscles and/or the joints are injured and inflamed, this will have an imbalance in this system.

About 60% of the joint innervation may be classified as nociceptive. **Joint inflammation leads to the release of neuropeptides into the joint tissue and activates these "sleeping nociceptors."** See Heppelmann B. Anatomy and histology of joint innervation. J Peripher Nerv Syst. 1997;2(1):5–16.

A reflex connection exists between the receptors in the cervical facet joints and fusimotorneurons (muscle spindles). Thunberg J, Hellstrom F, Sjolander P, Bergenheim M, Wenngren B, Johansson H. Influences on the fusimotor-muscle spindle system from chemosensitive nerve endings in cervical facet joints in the cat: possible implications for whiplash induced disorders. Pain. 2001 Mar;91(1–2):15–22.

There is also a reflex connection between the TMJ nociceptors and the fusimotor-muscle spindle system of dorsal neck muscles. Hellstrom F, Thunberg J, Bergenheim M, Sjolander P, Djupsjobacka M, Johansson H. Increased intra-articular concentration of bradykinin in the temporomandibular joint changes the sensitivity of muscle spindles in dorsal neck muscles in the cat. Neurosci Res. 2002 Feb;42(2):91–9.

There are interactive responses between the structures of the joints: facets, disc, ligaments and multifitus muscle. Indahl A, Kaigle A, Reikeras O, Holm S. Electromyographic response of the porcine multifidus musculature after nerve stimulation. Spine. 1995 Dec 15;20(24):2652–58; Indahl A, Kaigle AM, Reikeras O, Holm SH. Interaction between the porcine lumbar intervertebral disc, zygapophysial joints, and paraspinal muscles. Spine. 1997 Dec 15;22(24):2834–40; Kang YM, Choi WS, Pickar JG. Electrophysiologic evidence for an intersegmental reflex pathway between lumbar paraspinal tissues. Spine. 2002 Feb 1;27(3):E56–63.

The nerve endings in the **outer annulus fibrosus of the disc**, in the **capsule of the zygapophysial joints**, and in the **ligaments** are most likely part of the proprioceptive system responsible for optimal recruitment of the paraspinal muscles. **Mechanical stimulation of the spinal viscoelastic tissues excites the muscles with higher excitation intensity when more than one tissue (e.g. ligaments and disc) is**

stimulated. See Holm S, Indahl A, Solomonow M. Sensorimotor control of the spine. J Electromyogr Kinesiol. 2002 Jun;12(3):219–34;

Proprioceptive information of even small movements of the intervertebral disks and vertebral bodies seems highly relevant for the control of muscle tone. Strasmann TJ, Feilscher TH, Baumann KI, Halata Z. Distribution of sensory receptors in joints of the upper cervical column in the laboratory marsupial monodelphis domestica. Anat Anz. 1999 Mar;181(2):199–206.

§ 6:6 Muscles

Muscles and ligaments work together to support the spine, hold it upright, and control movement during rest and activity. Muscle contractions are generally classified into three different types: **Concentric** (when muscle shortens to exert force); **Isometric** (when muscle exerts a force, but there is no movement in the limb); and **Eccentric** (contractions that occur in a muscle while it is lengthening). We rely on the latter type the most. For example, the biceps perform eccentric contractions when we lower a curl bar, in order to slow the descent of the bar. The muscle is getting longer, but it is still exerting force.

It is widely accepted that muscle strain injuries occur more frequently with eccentric muscle contractions. This may be due to the significantly greater force produced by these contractions as compared to concentric or isometric contractions. See Fox EL, Robinson S, Wiegman DL. Metabolic energy sources during continuous and interval running. J Appl Physiol. 1969 Aug;27(2):174–8.

Research supports denervation and/or traumatic processes (e.g. inflammatory response) as contributing to the development of muscular degeneration and higher pain and disability levels. The presence of fatty infiltrate was not featured in individuals with chronic insidious onset neck pain,[1] indicating that trauma related processes such as inflammation may play a role. Subjects with insidious neck pain demonstrated fat index scores that mirrored those previously reported

---

[Section 6:6]

[1]Elliott J, Jull G, Sterling M, Noteboom J, Darnell R, Galloway G. Fatty infiltrate in the cervical extensor muscles is not a feature of chronic insidious onset neck pain. Clin Radiol. 2008; 63(6):681–687.

for asymptomatic subjects[2] and they differed significantly on the sensory and psychological measures when compared to the group with chronic WAD. In the lower spine, Hodges et al[3] demonstrated rapid changes, including atrophy and fatty infiltration, in the segmental lumbar multifidus' cross-sectional area within 3 days following experimental lumbar disc and nerve lesion. Specifically, changes were observed in the ipsilesional, segmental multifidus following disc lesion. A different distribution was observed following nerve lesion to the medial branch of the dorsal ramus in which rapid atrophy and fatty infiltration occurred bilaterally at 3 segments caudal to the injury site. These findings provide evidence that rapid changes in multifidus occur following disc and nerve lesion but the resultant effects suggest differential mechanisms.

In WAD, we found signs of **generalized hypersensitivity** according to **Pain Pressure Thresholds**. The WAD group had significantly higher interstitial [IL-6] and [5-HT] in the trapezius than the CON. [Pyruvate] was overall significantly lower in WAD, and with lactate it showed another time-pattern throughout the test. In the multivariate regression analysis of pain intensity [5-HT] was the strongest regressor and positively correlated with pain intensity in WAD. In addition, blood flow, [pyruvate], and [potassium] influenced the pain intensity in a complex time dependent way. These findings may indicate that peripheral nociceptive processes are activated in WAD with generalized hypersensitivity for pressure and they are not identical with those reported in chronic work-related trapezius myalgia, which could indicate **different pain mechanisms**. Gerdle B, Lemming D, Kristiansen J, Larsson B, Peolsson M, Rosendal L. Biochemical alterations in the trapezius muscle of patients with chronic whiplash associated disorders (WAD) — A microdialysis study. Eur J Pain. 2007 Apr 23.

Skeletal muscle is striated (striped) in appearance. It is innervated under voluntary and non-voluntary control. Prior to a muscle contracting, a nerve impulse originates in the brain and cerebellum and travels through the spinal cord to the muscle. The tone of a muscle is set by the muscle spindle. **Monoaminergic descending pathways from brainstem**

---

[2]Elliott JM, Jull GA, Noteboom JT, Darnell R, Galloway GG, Gibbon WW. Fatty infiltration in the cervical extensor musculature in persistent whiplash: a MRI analysis. Spine. 2006;31(22):E847-855

[3]Hodges P, Holm AK, Hansson T, Holm S. Rapid atrophy of the lumbar multifidus follows experimental disc or nerve root injury. Spine. 2006 Dec 1;31(25):2926–33.

nuclei modulate the excitability of the circuits mediating group II muscle spindle input. Schieppati M, Nardone A, Cornoa S, Bove M. The complex role of spindle afferent input, as evidenced by the study of posture control in normal subjects and patients. Neurol Sci 2001; 22:S15–20.

The cervical muscles contract rapidly in response to impact and the potential exits for muscle injury due to lengthening contractions. Brault JR, Siegmund GP, Wheeler JB. Cervical muscle response during whiplash: evidence of a lengthening muscle contraction. Clin Biomech (Bristol, Avon). 2000 Jul;15(6):426–35.

The cervical facet capsule is at risk for injury due to eccentric muscle contractions. These forces can be as high as 66N (1 N = .225 lbs). This provides a possible mechanism for injury to the facet capsule ligament and the facet joint as a whole. Winkelstein BA, McLendon RE, Barbir A, Myers BS. An anatomical investigation of the human cervical facet capsule, quantifying muscle insertion area. J Anat. 2001 Apr;198(Pt 4):455–61.

There is a dual system for detection of changes in position of the cervical spine and head through muscles spindles and joint receptors. Joint movement is monitored and controlled by two sets of mechanoreceptors: muscle spindles and receptors in the joint capsules. See Gandevia SC, McCloskey DI. Joint sense, muscle sense, and their combination as position sense, measured at the distal interphalangeal joint of the middle finger. J Physiol. 1976 Sep;260(2):387–407. Hunt CC. Mammalian muscle spindle: peripheral mechanisms. Physiol Rev. 1990 Jul;70(3):643–63; Ferrell WR, Gandevia SC, McCloskey DI. The role of joint receptors in human kinaesthesia when intramuscular receptors cannot contribute. J Physiol. 1987 May;386:63–71. Johansson H, Sjolander P, Sojka P. Actions on gamma-motoneurones elicited by electrical stimulation of joint afferent fibres in the hind limb of the cat. J Physiol. 1986 Jun;375:137–52.

Muscle spindles have been demonstrated throughout the entire length of the intrinsic postvertebral muscles. **The location of muscle spindles in the suboccipital muscles differs from that of the cervical part of the extensor muscle mass.** Amonoo-Kuofi HS. The number and distribution of muscle spindles in human intrinsic postvertebral muscles. J Anat. 1982 Oct;135 (3):585–99.

Laminated corpusles are known to function as rapidly adapting mechanoreceptors, supplementing information supplied by muscle spindles to the central nervous system about position and movement of the cervical spine. **Most of the deep neck muscles are static muscles, and proprioceptive information of even small movements of the intervertebral disks and vertebral bodies seems highly relevant for the control of muscle tone**. Strasmann TJ, Feilscher TH, Baumann KI, Halata Z. Distribution of sensory receptors in joints of the upper cervical column in the laboratory marsupial monodelphis domestica. Anat Anz. 1999 Mar;181(2):199–206.

40% of the joint nerves show a low mechanical threshold during passive movements. 60% of the joint innervation may be classified as nociceptive. **Pathological conditions, like joint inflammation, activate the receptors.** Heppelmann B. Anatomy and histology of joint innervation. J Peripher Nerv Syst. 1997;2(1):5–16.

Chronic pain in fibromyalgia and whiplash groups was associated with significantly higher muscle tension than in pain-free controls. Biomechanical output was significantly lower in patients with pain. Elert J, Kendall SA, Larsson B, Mansson B, Gerdle B. Chronic pain and difficulty in relaxing postural muscles in patients with fibromyalgia and chronic whiplash associated disorders. J Rheumatol. 2001. Jun;28(6):1361–8.

Released by trauma or inflammatory injury, serotonin sensitizes muscle nociceptors to chemical and mechanical stimuli. Seratonin combined with bradykinin induces muscle hyperalgesia to pressure. These are peripheral mechanisms for muscle tenderness and hyperalgesia. Graven-Nielsen T, Mense S. The peripheral apparatus of muscle pain: evidence from animal and human studies. Clin J Pain. 2001 Mar;17(1):2–10.

Biopsies of ventral neck muscles (sternocleidomastoid, omohyoid, and longus colli) and dorsal neck muscles (rectus capitis posterior major, obliquus capitis inferior, splenius capitis, and trapezius) were taken from 64 patients who underwent spondylodesis for cervical dysfunction of different etiologies. **This strongly indicates that the transformations proceeded in the direction from "slow oxidative" to "fast glycolytic."** Uhlig Y, Weber BR, Grob D, Muntener M. Fiber composition and fiber transformations in neck muscles of patients with dysfunction of the cervical spine. J Orthop Res. 1995 Mar;13(2):240–9.

Central hypersensitivity is not dependent on a nociceptive input arising from the painful and tender

muscles. Curatolo M, Petersen-Felix S, Arendt-Nielsen L, Giani C, Zbinden AM, Radanov BP. Central hypersensitivity in chronic pain after whiplash injury. Clin J Pain. 2001 Dec;17(4):306–15.

A prospective study in 25 patients to identify whether those with prolonged symptoms following whiplash injury exhibit a rise in serum creatine kinase consistent with significant muscle damage at the time of injury. Transient rise in creatine kinase level was seen in only 2 of 25 patients, neither of whom complained of prolonged symptoms. Of the 8 patients who developed chronic symptoms following whiplash injury, none demonstrated a serum creatine kinase rise. **Prolonged symptoms following whiplash injury cannot be explained by biochemically measurable muscle damage.** Scott S, Sanderson PL. Whiplash: a biochemical study of muscle injury. Eur Spine J. 2002 Aug;11(4):389–92.

§ 6:7 Muscles—Effectiveness of treatment with anti-inflammatories or steroids

Stretch-induced muscle injuries or strains, muscle contusions, and delayed-onset muscle soreness (DOMS) are common muscle problems in athletes. Anti-inflammatory treatment is often used for the pain and disability associated with these injuries. The most recent studies on nonsteroidal anti-inflammatory drugs (NSAIDs) in strains and contusions suggest that the use of NSAIDs can result in a modest inhibition of the initial inflammatory response and its symptoms. However, this may be associated with some small, negative effects later in the healing phase. Corticosteroids have generally been shown to adversely affect the healing of these acute injuries. Animal studies have suggested that anabolic steroids may actually aid in the healing process, but clinical studies are not yet available, and the exact role of these drugs has yet to be determined. **Studies on anti-inflammatory treatment of DOMS have yielded conflicting results. However, the effect of NSAIDs on DOMS appears small at best. Future research may have to focus on different aspects of these injuries as the emphasis on anti-inflammatory treatment has yielded somewhat disappointing results.** See Almekinders LC. Anti-inflammatory treatment of muscular injuries in sport. An update of recent studies. Sports Med. 1999 Dec;28(6):383–8.

§ 6:8 Muscles—EMG studies measuring surface muscles

Note:

The Kumar-Ferrari-Narayan studies have been questioned in published commentary. See 14:23, infa.

Contrary to a popular notion, head rotation or trunk flexion at the time of impact are factors that probably reduce injury risk. This data adds to attempts to approach an understanding of the human response to more complex scenarios of low-velocity road collisions. Kumar S, Ferrari R, Narayan Y. Kinematic and electromyographic response to whiplash-type impacts. Effects of head rotation and trunk flexion: summary of research. Clin Biomech (Bristol, Avon). 2005 Jul;20(6):553–68.

Compared to what is known for EMG responses with an occupant in the neutral posture, the right sternocleidomastoid (usually the most active muscle in a left lateral collision) was significantly less-active with trunk flexion than with neutral posture conditions ($P<0.01$). **In the absence of bodily impact, the flexed trunk posture does not produce a biomechanical response that would increase the likelihood of cervical muscle injury in low velocity lateral impacts, and may lessen the risk of injury for some muscles.** Kumar S, Ferrari R, Narayan Y, Vieira ER. Cervical muscle response to trunk flexion in whiplash-type lateral impacts. Exp Brain Res. 2005 Jul 21;:1–7.

Because the muscular component of the head-neck complex plays a role in the abatement of impact at higher acceleration levels, they are likely a primary site of injury in the whiplash phenomenon in rear collisions. **More specifically, when a rear impact is offset to the subject's left, it results in not only increased electromyographic generation in both sternocleidomastoids, but the splenius capitis contralateral to the direction of impact offset also bears part of the force of the neck perturbation. Expecting or being aware of imminent impact also plays a role in reducing muscle responses in low-velocity offset rear impacts.** Kumar S, Ferrari R, Narayan Y. Electromyographic and kinematic exploration of whiplash-type rear impacts: effect of left offset impact. Spine J. 2004 Nov–Dec;4(6):656–65; discussion 666–8.

The EMG response to a right anterolateral impact is highly dependent on the head position. The sternocleidomastoid responsible for the direction of head rotation and the trapezius ipsilateral to the direction of head rotation generate the most EMG activity. Kumar S, Ferrari R, Narayan Y. Analysis of right anterolateral impacts: the effect of head rotation on the cervical muscle whiplash response. J Neuroengineering Rehabil. 2005 May 31;2(1):11.

In the absence of bodily impact, the flexed trunk posture appears to produce a biomechanical response that would probably decrease the likelihood of cervical muscle injury in low velocity posterolateral impacts. Kumar S, Ferrari R, Narayan Y. Effect of trunk flexion on cervical muscle EMG to rear impacts. J Orthop Res. 2005 May 19;

When the subject sits with trunk flexed out of neutral posture at the time of an anterolateral impact, the cervical muscle response is reduced compared with anterolateral impacts with the trunk in neutral posture. Kumar S, Ferrari R, Narayan Y, Vieira ER. Effect of trunk flexion on the occupant neck response to anterolateral whiplash impacts. Am J Phys Med Rehabil. 2005 May;84(5):346–54.

If the head is rotated out of neutral posture at the time of rear impact, the injury risk tends to be greater for the sternocleidomastoid muscle contralateral to the side of rotation. Measures to prevent whiplash injury may have to account for the asymmetric response because many victims of whiplash are expected to be looking to the left or right at the time of collision. Kumar S, Ferrari R, Narayan Y. Looking away from whiplash: effect of head rotation in rear impacts. Spine. 2005 Apr 1;30(7):760–8.

Direction of impact is a factor in determining the muscle response to whiplash, but head rotation at the time of impact is also important in this regard. More specifically, when a rear impact is left posterolateral, it results in increased EMG generation mainly in the contralateral sternocleidomastoid, as expected, but head rotation at the same time in this type of impact reduces the EMG response of the cervical muscles. Muscle injury seems less likely under these conditions in low-velocity impacts. Kumar S, Ferrari R, Narayan Y. Effect of head rotation in whiplash-type rear impacts. Spine J. 2005 Mar–Apr;5(2):130–9.

Compared to a lateral impact with the volunteer's head in the neutral position, a lateral impact with head rotation to either right or left may reduce the muscle response. **Further studies are needed to determine whether or not head rotation at the time of lateral impact reduces overall injury risk.** Kumar S, Ferrari R, Narayan Y. Cervical muscle response to head rotation in whiplash-type left lateral impacts. Spine. 2005 Mar 1;30(5):536–41.

Expecting or being aware of imminent impact may play a role in reducing muscle responses in low-velocity impacts. Kumar S, Ferrari R, Narayan Y. Electromyographic and kinematic exploration of whiplash-type neck perturbations in left lateral collisions. Spine. 2004 Mar 11;29(6):650–9.

This approach involves the use of four levels of very-low to low velocity impacts to describe the kinematics of the head and the EMG response of cervical muscles in response to acceleration, but avoids any discernible risk of injury. This allows researchers to determine the cervical muscle response under many different scenarios, including varying direction of impact, awareness of impending impact, and others, without subjecting volunteers to any discernible risk. An initial series of results of impacts from eight directions is presented here, and these reveal that **the cervical response to whiplash-type impacts is modified by impact awareness, muscles studied, and direction of impact.** This will hopefully improve the understanding of the human response to low-velocity whiplash impacts. Kumar S, Ferrari R, Narayan Y. Kinematic and electromyographic response to whiplash loading in low-velocity whiplash impacts—a review. Clin Biomech (Bristol, Avon). 2005 May;20(4):343–56.

Frontal impacts tend to generate the most muscle activity in the ipsilateral trapezius muscle, increasing the risk of their injury. Kumar S, Ferrari R, Narayan Y. Turning away from whiplash. An EMG study of head rotation in whiplash impact. J Orthop Res. 2005 Jan;23(1):224–30.

Because the muscular component of the head-neck complex likely plays a central role in the abatement of higher acceleration levels, it may be a primary site of injury in the whiplash phenomenon in lateral collisions, and specifically, the splenius capitis muscle contralateral to the side of impact is most likely to be injured. Being aware of an impact may reduce the degree of head perturbation. Kumar S, Ferrari R, Narayan Y. Cervical muscle response to whiplash-type right lateral impacts. Spine. 2004 Nov 1;29(21):E479–87.

Head rotation in a right posterolateral impact modifies the cervical response mainly by generating an asymmetry in the paired sternocleidomastoid electromyograms. This may asymmetrically affect the risk of injury to the sternocleidomastoids. An understanding of the muscular response to rear-impacts of different types and the effect of head rotation at the time of impact is relevant to understanding the mechanism of acute whiplash injury and may be helpful to develop targeted treatments and preventative measures. Kumar S, Ferrari R, Narayan Y. Cervical muscle response to posterolateral impacts—effect of head rotation. Clin Biomech (Bristol, Avon). 2004 Nov;19(9):899–905.

More specifically, **when a frontal impact is offset to the subject's left, it not only results in increased EMG generation in both trapezii, but the splenius capitis contralateral to the direction of impact also bears part of the force of the neck perturbation.** Expecting or being aware of imminent impact may play a role in reducing muscle responses in low-velocity anterolateral impacts. Kumar S, Ferrari R, Narayan Y. Electromyographic and kinematic exploration of whiplash-type left anterolateral impacts. J Spinal Disord Tech. 2004 Oct;17(5):412–22.

Head rotation in a right posterolateral impact modifies the cervical response mainly by generating an asymmetry in the paired sternocleidomastoid electromyograms. This may asymmetrically affect the risk of injury to the sternocleidomastoids. An understanding of the muscular response to rear-impacts of different types and the effect of head rotation at the time of impact is relevant to understanding the mechanism of acute whiplash injury and may be helpful to develop targeted treatments and preventative measures. Kumar S, Ferrari R, Narayan Y. Cervical muscle response to right posterolateral impacts. Clin Biomech (Bristol, Avon). 2004 Jul;19(6):543–50.

In response to right anterolateral impacts, muscle responses were greater with higher levels of acceleration, and more specifically, when a frontal impact is offset to the subject's right, it results in not only increased EMG generation in the contralateral trapezius, but the splenius capitis contralateral to the direction of impact also bears part of the force of the neck perturbation. Expecting or being aware of imminent impact plays a role in reducing muscle responses in low-velocity anterolateral impacts. Kumar S, Ferrari R, Narayan Y. Cervical muscle response to whiplash-type right anterolateral impacts. Eur Spine J. 2004 Aug;13(5):398–407.

If the head is rotated out of neutral posture at the time of rear impact, the injury risk tends to be greater for the sternocleidomastoid muscle contralateral to the side of rotation.

Measures to prevent whiplash injury may have to account for the asymmetric response because many victims of whiplash are expected to be looking to the left or right at the time of collision. Kumar S, Ferrari R, Narayan Y. Looking away from whiplash: effect of head rotation in rear impacts. Spine. 2005 Apr 1;30(7):760–8.

Direction of impact is a factor in determining the muscle response to whiplash, but head rotation at the time of impact is also important in this regard. More specifically, **when a rear impact is left posterolateral, it results in increased EMG generation mainly in the contralateral sternocleidomastoid, as expected, but head rotation at the same time in this type of impact reduces the EMG response of the cervical muscles.** Muscle injury seems less likely under these conditions in low-velocity impacts. Kumar S, Ferrari R, Narayan Y. Effect of head rotation in whiplash-type rear impacts. Spine J. 2005 Mar–Apr;5(2):130–9.

Compared to a lateral impact with the volunteer's head in the neutral position, a lateral impact with head rotation to either right or left may reduce the muscle response. Further studies are needed to determine whether or not head rotation at the time of lateral impact reduces overall injury risk. Kumar S, Ferrari R, Narayan Y. Cervical muscle response to head rotation in whiplash-type left lateral impacts. Spine. 2005 Mar 1;30(5):536–41.

Overall, a right lateral impact with head rotation to either right or left appears to reduce the activity and thus the risk of muscle injury, perhaps because of "bracing" by muscles actively producing rotation or because of greater spinal stability from other structures when the head is in the rotated position. Kumar S, Ferrari R, Narayan Y. Cervical muscle response to head rotation in whiplash-type right lateral impacts. J Manipulative Physiol Ther. 2005 Jul–Aug;28(6):393–401.

Note:

In this article the authors discuss making a linear relationship of a minor collision of 1.5 mph and doing a linear extrapolation to indicate injury. It should be noted that Mertz and Patrick in their SAE paper (1967) attempted to extrapolate their data to show that an injury would occur in a 44 mph collision. Linear extrapolations in biological organisms are dubious especially on the issue of pain.

The muscle responses were greater with higher levels of acceleration, particularly the trapezius in frontal impacts. **Since the muscular components play a significant and central role in head/neck complex motion abatement at higher levels of acceleration, it may be a primary site of injury at low velocity whiplash phenomenon.** Kumar S, Narayan Y, Amell T. Analysis of low velocity frontal impacts. Clin Biomech (Bristol, Avon). 2003 Oct;18(8):694–703. (Note: An understanding of the pattern of biomechanical loading may assist in a more specific treatment of the patient injured in a low velocity frontal impact.)

There was a modest correlation between EMG of the investigated muscles and force (r=0.15–0.76, P<0.01). EMG output was, for example, approximately 66% higher in flexion than in extension (while force output was roughly 30% less in flexion than extension) — thus relatively more muscle activity was required in flexion than extension to generate a given force. The intermediate positions (i.e. anterolateral flexion) revealed force/EMG ratio scores that were intermediate in relation to the force/EMG ratios for pure flexion and pure extension. **The cervical muscle strength and cervical muscle EMG are therefore dependent on the direction of effort.** Kumar S, Narayan Y, Amell T, Ferrari R. Electromyography of superficial cervical muscles with exertion in the sagittal, coronal and oblique planes. Eur Spine J. 2002 Feb;11(1):27–37.

§ 6:9 Muscles—Additional articles to consider relating to muscles and their activation

The significant changes observed in both muscle and kinematic variables by the **second perturbation** indicated that habituation was a potential confounder of whiplash injury studies using repeated perturbations of human subjects. Siegmund GP, Sanderson DJ, Myers BS, Inglis JT. Rapid neck muscle adaptation alters the head kinematics of aware and unaware subjects undergoing multiple whiplash-like perturbations. J Biomech. 2003 Apr;36(4):473–82.

The larger retractions observed in surprised females likely produce larger tissue strains and may increase injury potential. **Aware human subjects may not replicate the muscle response, kinematic response, or whiplash injury potential of unprepared occupants in real collisions.** Siegmund GP, Sanderson DJ, Myers BS, Inglis JT. Awareness affects the response of human subjects exposed to a single whiplash-like perturbation. Spine. 2003 Apr 1;28(7):671–9.

Results of the unaware occupant model were compared to

the model exercised without muscle contraction. Reflexive muscle contraction altered segmental angulations by less than 10% and facet joint capsular ligament distractions by less than 16% during the time of maximum S-curvature. At the C5–C6 and C6–C7 levels, muscle contraction increased capsular ligament distractions. Due to the nominal affect of reflexive muscle contraction on segmental angulations and facet joint capsular ligament distractions during S-curvature, it is **unlikely that this contraction can alter the cervical kinematics responsible for whiplash injury.** Stemper BD, Yoganandan N, Pintar FA. Influence of muscle contraction on whiplash kinematics. Biomed Sci Instrum. 2004;40:24–9.

§ 6:10 Interevertebral disc

Fibrous Proteins of the Matrix. Collagen is the major insoluble fibrous protein in the extracellular matrix and in connective tissue. In fact, it is the single most abundant protein in the animal kingdom. **There are at least 16 types of collagen, but 80 – 90 percent of the collagen in the body consists of types I, II, and III.** At one time it was thought that all collagens were secreted by fibroblasts in connective tissue, but it is now known that numerous epithelial cells make certain types of collagens. The various collagens and the structures they form all serve the same purpose: to help tissues withstand stretching. **Intervertebral disc** is a highly specialized cartilaginous tissue, containing two genetic types of collagen (I and II). Analysis of peptides from a Cyanogen bromide (CNBr) digest of collagen showed that the proportions of I and II varied gradually and inversely across pig annulus fibrosus, with exclusively type I at the extreme outer edge and exclusively type II in the nucleus pulposus. Eyre DR, Muir H. Types I and II collagens in intervertebral disc. Interchanging radial distributions in annulus fibrosus. Biochem J. 1976 Jul 1;157(1):267–70.

Collagen has been isolated and purified from the pronase digest of the outer annulus fibrosus of degenerated and unaffected intervertebral discs obtained at necropsy. The mixture of different collagen types has been purified and fractionated by 2 subsequent DEAE-cellulose chromatographic procedures according to established methods. Collagen chain polymers were then isolated by molecular sieving. Their reduction with 2-mercaptoethanol followed by agarose chromatography resulted in the separation of three major peaks corresponding to gamma, beta, and alpha chains. Cyanogen bromide (CNBr) peptides and aminoacid analyses revealed the identity of the isolated alpha-chain as alpha 1 (III). Further support for this finding was obtained by immunofluorescence. It is suggested that **the presence of collagen type III in the outer anulus fibrosus may be related to intervertebral disc prolapse**. Adam M, Deyl Z. Degenerated annulus fibrosus of the intervertebral disc contains collagen type II. Ann Rheum Dis. 1984 Apr;43(2):258–63.

Complete human intervertebral discs with their adjacent vertebral bodies were fixed, decalcified, and embedded in paraffin. The intervertebral disc and its adjacent structures were reviewed in their entirety on one histologic slide. Monoclonal antibodies against human Types I, II, and III collagen were used for immunohistochemistry. A comparative analysis based on both immunohistochemical and histologic evaluation was performed. Type I collagen was seen abundantly in the outer zone and outer lamellas of the inner zone of the anulus fibrosus. On longitudinal sections, the Type I collagen distribution took the shape of a wedge. On horizontal sections, the Type I collagen positive area took the shape of a ring that was wider anteriorly than posteriorly. **This suggests that the three-dimensional shape of the Type I collagen-positive tissue in the anulus fibrosus can be described by a donut that is wider anteriorly than posteriorly.** Type II collagen was present in the entire inner of the anulus fibrosus but not in the outer zone. It was also found in the cartilaginous endplates. Type III collagen showed some codistribution with Type II collagen, particularly in pericellular locations in areas of spondylosis, which was noted at the endplates, vertebral rim, and insertion sites of the anulus fibrosus. **These observations on the location of Types I and II collagen provide a more detailed structural definition of the anulus fibrosus, which may assist in further investigation of discal herniation.** Schollmeier G, Lahr-Eigen R, Lewandrowski KU. Observations on fiber-forming collagens in the anulus fibrosus. Spine. 2000 Nov 1;25(21):2736–41.

The intervertebral disc is a highly organized matrix laid down by relatively few cells in a specific manner. The central gelatinous nucleus pulposus is contained within the more collagenous anulus fibrosus laterally and the cartilage end plates inferiorly and superiorly. The anulus consists of concentric rings or lamellae, with fibers in the outer lamellae continuing into the longitudinal ligaments and vertebral bodies. This arrangement allows the discs to facilitate movement and flexibility within what would be an otherwise rigid spine. At birth, the human disc has some vascular supply within both the cartilage end plates and the anulus fibrosus, but these vessels soon recede, leaving the disc with little direct blood supply in the healthy adult. **With increasing age, water is lost from the matrix, and the proteoglycan content also changes and diminishes. The disc — particularly the nucleus — becomes less gelatinous and more fibrous, and cracks and fissures eventually form.** More blood vessels begin to grow into the disc from the outer areas of the anulus. There is an increase in cell proliferation and formation of cell clusters, as well as an increase in cell death. The cartilage end plate undergoes thinning, altered cell density, formation of fissures, and sclerosis of the subchondral bone. These changes are similar to those seen in degenerative disc disease, causing discussion as to whether aging and degeneration are separate processes or the same process occurring over a different timescale. Additional disorders involving the intervertebral disc can demonstrate other changes in morphology. Discs from patients with spinal deformities such as scoliosis have ectopic calcification in the cartilage end plate and sometimes in the disc itself. Cells in these discs and cells from patients with spondylolisthesis have been found to have very long cell processes. Cells in herniated discs appear to have a higher degree of cellular senescence than cells in nonherniated discs and produce a greater abundance of matrix metalloproteinases. The role that abnormalities play in the etiopathogenesis of different disorders is not always clear. Disorders may be caused by a genetic predisposition or a tissue response to an insult or altered mechanical environment. Whatever the initial cause, **a change in the morphology of the tissue is likely to alter the physiologic and mechanical functioning of the tissue**. Roberts S, Evans H, Trivedi J, Menage J. Histology and pathology of the human intervertebral disc. J Bone Joint Surg Am. 2006 Apr;88 Suppl 2:10–4.

The prevalence of cervical disc herniations in asymptomatic subjects of less than 40 years of age is 3% to 10% and increases to 20% in subjects up to 54 years of age. The prevalence increases with age from 5% to 35% in subjects between 40 and 60 years of age. D'Antoni AV, Croft AC. Prevalence of herniated intervertebral discs of the cervical spine in asymptomatic subjects using MRI scans: a qualitative systematic review. J Whiplash & Related Disorders 2006;5(1):5–13.

The results suggest a mechanism of force balancing in lordotic postures under static loads, whereas flexed postures produce large increases to the tensile forces in the region of the posterior anulus.

Hedman TP, Fernie GR. Mechanical response of the lumbar spine to seated postural loads. Spine. 1997 Apr 1;22(7):734–43.

Discogenic pain criteria — Lumbar Disc. For the diagnosis of discogenic pain, criteria A, B, C, and D must each be satisfied:

A. Stimulation of the target disc reproduces concordant pain.

B. The pain that is reproduced is registered as at least 7 on a 10-point visual analog scale or equlivant scale.

C. The pain is reproduced at a pressure:

i. less than 50psi, or

ii. Less than 15 psi, above the opening pressure.

D. Stimulation of adjacent discs provides controls such that:

D. when only one adjacent disc can be stimulated,

i. that disc is painless, or

ii. pain from that disc is not concordant and is reproduced at a pressure greater than 15 psi above the opening pressure.

when two adjacent discs can be stimulated,

i. both discs are painless, or

ii. one disc is painless, and

iii. if the other disc is painful, that pain not concordant and is produced at pressure greater than 15 psi above the opening pressure.

Unequivocal Discogenic Pain

A. stimulation of the target disc reproduces concordant pain
B. that pain is registered as at least 7 on a 10-point visual analog scale
C. that pain is reproduced at a pressure of less that 15 psi above the opening pressure
D. stimulation of two adjacent discs does not produce pain at all

Definite or Highly Probable Discogenic Pain

A. stimulation of the target disc reproduces concordant pain
B. that pain is registered as at least 7 on a 10-point visual analog scale
C. that pain is reproduced at a pressure of less that 15 psi above the opening pressure
D. stimulation of one adjacent discs does not produce pain at all

Definite Discogenic Pain

A. stimulation of the target disc reproduces concordant pain

B. hat pain is registered as at least 7 on a 10-point visual analog scale
C. that pain is reproduced at a pressure of less that 50 psi above the opening pressure
D. stimulation of two adjacent discs does not produce pain at all

Probable Discogenic Pain

A. stimulation of the target disc reproduces concordant pain
B. hat pain is registered as at least 7 on a 10-point visual analog scale
C. that pain is reproduced at a pressure of less that 50 psi above the opening pressure
D. stimulation of one adjacent disc does not reproduce pain at all, and stimulation of another adjacent disc produces pain at greater than 50 psi but that pain is not concordant

From Practice Guidelines for Spinal Diagnostic and Treatment Procedures. International Spine Intervention Society. Edited by Nikolai Bogduk 2004, p. 29.

Comment:

In soft tissue cases, defense experts may attempt to establish that a single event will not cause damage to a healthy disc, suggesting that, in live humans there are always pressures in the disc and that the disc is continually adapting to different pressures. See generally Adams MA, Hutton WC. The effect of fatigue on the lumbar intervertebral disc. J Bone Joint Surg Br. 1983 Mar;65(2):199–203.

Note that in Adams, forty-one cadaveric lumbar intervertebral joints from 18 spines were flexed and fatigue-loaded to simulate a vigorous day's activity. The joints were then bisected and the discs examined. Twenty-three out of 41 of the discs showed distortions in the lamellae of the annulus fibrosus, and, in a few of these, complete radial fissures were found in the posterior annulus. **Adams is used by the defense. They will state the disc can only get injured only after thousands of loads and flexion combined with compression pressures. Remember these are cadavers with no receptor activation, no inflammatory or immune response, etc.**

The following studies can be used to refute the findings addressed in the 1983 Adams paper: Disc failure in bending occurs through overstretching of the outer anulus in the vertical direction. **In life, the posterior elements may not adequately protect the posterior anulus from fatigue**

damage. Adams MA, Green TP, Dolan P. The strength in anterior bending of lumbar intervertebral discs. Spine. 1994 Oct 1;19(19):2197–203.

A *single application* of whiplash acceleration pulse can induce soft tissue-related and ligament-related alterations to cervical spine structures. Structural alterations in the lower cervical spine included stretch and tear of the ligamentum flavum, anulus disruption, anterior longitudinal ligament rupture, and zygopophysial joint compromise with tear of the capsular ligaments. Yoganandan N, Cusick JF, Pintar FA, Rao RD. Whiplash injury determination with conventional spine imaging and cryomicrotomy. Spine. 2001 Nov 15;26(22):2443–8.

In an analysis of real world impacts, an 8 km/h (5 mph) delta-v collision has been associated with a herniated cervical disc. Smith JJ. An analysis of 72 real world impacts-an initial investigation into injury and complaint factors. SAE technical paper 1999-01-0640.

Peak 150° fiber strains and **disc shear strains** exceeded sagittal physiologic levels at **3.5 g** and were greatest at the posterior region of C5–C6. **The cervical intervertebral disc may be at risk for injury during whiplash because of excessive 150° fiber strain, disc shear strain, and anterior axial deformation**. Panjabi MM, Ito S, Pearson AM, Ivancic PC. Injury Mechanisms of the Cervical Intervertebral Disc During Simulated Whiplash. Spine 2004;29:1217–1225.

§ 6:11 Interevertebral disc—Disc pressures in cervical spine

Cadaver specimens' flexion/extension pressures at the C5–6 disc produced pressures on the average of 0.23 MPa with a high of 0.53 MPa. Axial rotation pressures average 0.17 MPa with a high of 0.38 MPa. **With the addition of simulated muscle force, the pressures increase by 180% for flexion/extension and approximately 400% for axial rotation (1 MPa = 145 pounds/square inch; 0.1 MPa = 14.5 lbs).** Pospiech J, Stolke D, Wilke HJ, Claes LE. Intradiscal pressure recordings in the cervical spine. Neurosurgery. 1999 Feb;44(2):379–84;

Another study, on a limited number of cadavers, suggested that for every 1000N (225 pounds) of applied compression, the cervical disc pressure is approximately 3.75 MPa. (1 MPa = 145 pounds). **In this study, peak pressure was between 2.4 (348 lbs) and 3.5 MPa (507 lbs) under 800N (180 lbs) of**

compression. Cripton PA, Dumas GA, Nolte LP. A minimally disruptive technique for measuring intervertebral disc pressure in vitro: application to the cervical spine. J Biomech. 2001 Apr;34(4):545–9.

§ 6:12 Interevertebral disc—Disc pressures in lumbar spine

In the lumbar spine at the L4–5 disc in a live human volunteer, measurements were made of intradiscal pressure in different postures. **Relaxed sitting with a straight back produced intra-discal pressures of 0.45 to 0.50 MPa (0.1MPa = 14.5 pounds). Bending forward without arm support while seated increased the pressure to 0.83 MPa**. Wilke HJ, Neef P, Caimi M, Hoogland T, Claes LE. New in vivo measurements of pressures in the intervertebral disc in daily life. Spine. 1999 Apr 15;24(8):755–62.

Values for the rupture intradiscal pressure ranged from 750 kPa to 1300 kPa for neutral posture and the maximum in anterior flexion was 1177 kPa. 1 PSI = 6.89 kPa. Iencean SM. Lumbar intervertebral disc herniation following experimental intradiscal pressure increase. Acta Neurochir (Wien). 2000;142(6):669–76.

§ 6:13 Interevertebral disc—Cervical disc

Microdissection and histologic studies determine the innervation of the cervical intervertebral discs. The cervical sinuvertebral nerves were found to have an upward course in the vertebral canal, supplying the disc at their level of entry and the disc above. Branches of the vertebral nerve supplied the lateral aspects of the cervical discs. Histologic studies of discs obtained at operation showed the presence of nerve fibers as deeply as the outer third of the anulus fibrosus. **These anatomic findings provide the substrate for primary disc pain and the pain of provocation discography**. Bogduk N, Windsor M, Inglis A. The innervation of the cervical intervertebral discs. Spine. 1988 Jan;13(1):2–8.

Human cervical intervertebral discs are supplied with both nerve fibers and mechanoreceptors. **Nerves were seen throughout the anulus and most numerous in the middle third of the disc**. Mendel T, Wink CS, Zimny ML. Neural elements in human cervical intervertebral discs. Spine. 1992 Feb;17(2):132–5.

§ 6:14 Interevertebral disc—Internal disc disruption-anular tear

Comment:

Pain from the disc is from the disc itself and not on impingement upon the thecal sac (the covering of the nerve root/cord). The injury to the disc without herniation has been called an internal disc disruption or annular tear. Internal disc disruption is a painful entity that has been described and reported as annular fissures that distort the internal architecture of the disc. Externally the disc appears relatively intact and undeformed.

These results indicate that **disc disruption passing into the outer layers of the anulus, but not resulting in deformation of the outer anular wall, was as frequently associated with lower extremity pain as were discs with more severe disruption deforming the outer anular wall; however, they were associated with a greater degree of aching pain. These findings support that lower extremity pain may be referred from the disc.** See Ohnmeiss DD, Vanharanta H, Ekholm J. Degree of disc disruption and lower extremity pain. Spine. 1997 Jul 15;22(14):1600–5.

A clinical diagnosis of internal disc disruption, in absence of objective clinical findings, is extremely difficult. The only convincing means to establish the diagnosis is provocation discography. Unfortunately, this procedure is controversial, making the existence of internal disc disruption suspect. **Recent studies indicate the existence of a biochemical/ biomechanical model of discogenic pain, which explains the disabling low back pain in some subjects with no objective evidence of nerve-root compromise.** See Sehgal N, Fortin JD. Internal Disc Disruption and Low Back Pain. Pain Physician 2000; 3(2):143–157.

A disc does not have to impinge on the nerve root to cause back pain. Excitatory toxins/ neurotransmitters such as Glutamate may be causing the pain. Glutamate originating from degenerated disc may diffuse to the dorsal root ganglion and effect glutamate receptors and cause spinal pain. Harrington JF, Messier AA, Bereiter D, Barnes B, Epstein MH. Herniated lumbar disc material as a source of free glutamate available to affect pain signals through the dorsal root ganglion. Spine. 2000 Apr 15;25(8):929–36.

A diagnosis of internal disc disruption can be made in a significant proportion of patients with chronic low

back pain, but no conventional clinical test can discriminate patients with internal disc disruption from patients with other conditions. The diagnostic criteria for internal disc disruption were fully satisfied in 39% of patients. Schwarzer AC, Aprill CN, Derby R, Fortin J, Kine G, Bogduk N. The prevalence and clinical features of internal disc disruption in patients with chronic low back pain. Spine. 1995 Sep 1;20(17):1878–83.

§ 6:15 Interevertebral disc—Differences between cervical and lumbar discs

The cervical anulus fibrosus does not consist of concentric laminae of collagen fibers, as in lumbar discs. Instead, it forms a crescentic mass of collagen thick arteriorly and tapering laterally toward the uncinate processes. It is essentially deficient posterolaterally and is represented posteriorly only by a thin layer of paramedian, vertically orientated fibers. The anterior longitudinal ligament covers the front of the disc, and the posterior longitudinal ligament reinforces the deficient posterior anulus fibrosus with longitudinal and alar fibers. The three-dimensional architecture of the cervical anulus fibrosus is more like a crescentic anterior interosseous ligament than a ring of fibers surrounding the nucleus pulposus. **There is a difference between the cervical and lumbar discs.** *See* Mercer S, Bogduk N. The ligaments and annulus fibrosus of human adult cervical intervertebral discs. Spine. 1999 Apr 1;24(7):619–26.

§ 6:16 Interevertebral disc—Development of disc pain

Disc injury pain is not only an event but a process. After a trauma, the first stage is inflammation followed by cellular proliferation. The disc heals by scar tissue and not by regeneration of the original tissue. **Disc pain may not be immediate and can be delayed weeks before it becomes symptomatic. Jonsson reported that half of the disc herniation subjects developed pain within 6 weeks of injury**. Jonsson H Jr, Cesarini K, Sahlstedt B, Rauschning W. Findings and outcome in whiplash-type neck distortions. Spine. 1994 Dec 15; 19(24):2733–43.

Forces generated during simulated whiplash collision induce biphasic lumbar spinal motions (increased-decreased lordosis) of insufficient magnitude to cause bony injuries, but they may be sufficient to cause soft-tissue injuries. Fast A, Sosner J, Begeman P, Thomas MA,

Chiu T. Lumbar Spinal Strains Associated with Whiplash Injury: A Cadaveric Study. Am J Phys Med Rehabil. 2002 Sep;81(9):645–650.

It is true that many people have degeneration of their discs in the cervical spine and lumbar without symptoms. Matsumoto M, Fujimura Y, Suzuki N, Nishi Y, Nakamura M, Yabe Y, Shiga H. MRI of cervical intervertebral discs in asymptomatic subjects. J Bone Joint Surg Br. 1998 Jan;80(1):19–24; Jensen MC, Brant-Zawadzki MN, Obuchowski N, Modic MT, Malkasian D, Ross JS. Magnetic resonance imaging of the lumbar spine in people without back pain. N Engl J Med. 1994 Jul 14;331(2):69–73.

An injury to the disc will cause an inflammatory response. The inflammatory response is the first stage in the healing of tissues. The production of proinflammatory mediators within the nucleus pulposus may be a major factor in the genesis of a painful lumbar disc. Burke JG, Watson RW, McCormack D, Dowling FE, Walsh MG, Fitzpatrick JM. Intervertebral discs which cause low back pain secrete high levels of proinflammatory mediators. J Bone Joint Surg Br. 2002 Mar;84(2):196–201.

IL-1beta appeared to "sensitize" annulus cells to mechanical load. **This increased responsiveness to mechanical load in the face of inflammatory cytokines may imply that the sensitivity of annulus cells to shear increases during inflammation and may affect initiation and progression of disc degeneration.** Elfervig MK, Minchew JT, Francke E, Tsuzaki M, Banes AJ. IL-1beta sensitizes intervertebral disc annulus cells to fluid-induced shear stress. J Cell Biochem. 2001;82(2):290–8.

§ 6:17 Interevertebral disc—Discoligamentous injuries from whiplash

Cadavers subjected to "minor" collisions showed various injuries to the disc, facets and ligaments. Many of these injuries would not be detected on X-rays or CT scans. Deng B, Bergman PC, Yang KH, Tashman S, King AI. Kinematics of human cadaver cervical spine during low speed rear-end impacts. Stapp Car Crash Journal 2000;44:171–88; Yoganandan N, Pintar FA, Stemper BD, Schlick MB. Biomechanics of human occupants in simulated rear crashes: documentation of neck injuries and comparison of injury criteria. Stapp Car Crash Journal 2000; 44:189–204.

A rear-end crash causes a multi-axis loading event on

the spine. It is possible to herniate a cervical disc without contemporaneous fracture of any cervical vertebrae, no ligamentous damage, and with no degeneration as a contributing factor. Clemens HJ, Burow K. Experimental investigation injury mechanisms of cervical spine at frontal and rear-front vehicle impacts. Society of Automotive Engineers 1972; 72960.

Patients often develop neck pain and radiating arm pain secondary to a whiplash-type injury after a motor vehicle accident. The cervicalgia and brachialgia can often be progressive. The literature has supported that disc injuries are common secondary to motor vehicle collisions. Jonsson H Jr, Bring G, Rauschning W, Sahlstedt B. Hidden cervical spine injuries in traffic accident victims with skull fractures. J Spinal Disord. 1991 Sep;4(3):251–63; Davis SJ, Teresi LM, Bradley WG Jr, Ziemba MA, Bloze AE. Cervical spine hyperextension injuries: MR findings. Radiology. 1991 Jul;180(1):245–51; Hamer AJ, Gargan MF, Bannister GC, Nelson RJ. Whiplash injury and surgically treated cervical disc disease. Injury. 1993 Sep;24(8):549–50.

A high incidence of discoligamentous injuries was found in whiplash-type distortions. Most patients with severe persisting radiating pain had large disc protrusions on MRI that were confirmed on surgery. Jonsson H Jr, Cesarini K, Sahlstedt B, Rauschning W. Findings and outcome in whiplash-type neck distortions. Spine. 1994 Dec 15;19(24):2733–43.

Disc lesions are common in injured cervical spines where translation is much greater than in the lumbar spine, and these lesions are slow to heal. It is suggested that such injuries could cause the pain experienced by patients with neck sprain. Taylor JR, Twomey LT. Acute injuries to cervical joints. An autopsy study of neck sprain. Spine. 1993 Jul;18(9):1115–22.

Peak 150° fiber strains and disc shear strains exceeded sagittal physiologic levels at **3.5 g** and were greatest at the posterior region of C5–C6. Axial deformation at the anterior region of the disc exceeded sagittal physiologic limits at 3.5 g, while axial deformation at the posterior region exceeded physiologic limits only at 6.5 g and 8 g at C5–C6. Peak 150° fiber strain and disc shear strain occurred after peak intervertebral extension, demonstrating that posterior shearing continued after peak intervertebral extension and contributed considerably to the 150° fiber strain. **The cervical intervertebral disc may**

be at risk for injury during whiplash because of excessive 150° fiber strain, disc shear strain, and anterior axial deformation. Panjabi MM, Ito S, Pearson AM, Ivancic PC. Injury Mechanisms of the Cervical Intervertebral Disc During Simulated Whiplash. Spine 2004;29:1217–1225.

Peak disc shear strain and peak annular tissue strain during **frontal impact** exceeded ($p<0.05$) corresponding physiological limits at the C2–C3 intervertebral level, beginning at **4 g** and **6 g**, respectively. These subsequently spread throughout the entire cervical spine at 10 g, with the exception of C4–C5. The C5–C6 intervertebral level was at high risk for injury during both frontal and rear impacts, while during frontal impact, in addition to C5–C6, subfailure injuries were likely at superior intervertebral levels, including C2–C3. The disc injuries occurred at lower impact accelerations during rear impact as compared with frontal impact. The subfailure injuries of the cervical intervertebral disc that occur during frontal impact may lead to the chronic symptoms reported by patients, such as head and neck pain. Ito S, Ivancic PC, Pearson AM, Tominaga Y, Gimenez SE, Rubin W, Panjabi MM. Cervical intervertebral disc injury during simulated frontal impact. Eur Spine J. 2005 May;14(4):356–65.

§ 6:18 Interevertebral disc—Cartilaginous endplate in disc herniation

Cartilaginous endplate in cervical disc herniation is the predominant type of herniation in the cervical spine. Cervical intervertebral discs with herniation usually remain normal in height or change only slightly without abnormality in the Luschka joints. Luscha joints bear a part of axial load to the intervertebral disc. Disc degeneration may play a more important role in trauma in the production of herniation of the cervical spine. **Cervical disc herniation is rare under 30 years of age and the mean age is around 50 years.** Kokubun S, Sakurai M, Tanaka Y. Cartilaginous endplate in cervical disc herniation. Spine. 1996 Jan 15;21(2):190–5.

Minor damage to a vertebral body endplate leads to progressive structural changes in the adjacent intervertebral discs. Adams MA, Freeman BJ, Morrison HP, Nelson IW, Dolan P. Mechanical initiation of intervertebral disc degeneration. Spine. 2000 Jul 1; 25(13):1625–36.

Single photon emission computed tomography (SPECT)-based anomalies in the cervical spine of whiplash patients. In a series of 14 patients, approximately 70% had SPECT abnormalities. However, it's important to note that the VAS scores in these patients were quite high (7+), and the group should only be considered to be representative of late whiplash patients with moderate to severe pain. **The authors believe that the majority of the lesions represent fractures of end plates, which probably occur as a result of the high initial axial compression experienced during the initial phase of whiplash as the thoracic spine is flattened, and possibly made worse by subsequent shear effects and neck bending moments**. See Freeman MD, Sapir D, Boutselis A, Gorup J, Tuckman G, Croft AC, Centeno C, Phillips A. Whiplash injury and occult vertebral fracture: a case series of bone SPECT imaging of patients with persisting spine pain following a motor vehicle crash. Cervical Spine Research Society 29th Annual Meeting, Monterey, CA, Nov 29–Dec 1, 2001.

A chemotactic response to products of disc breakdown is responsible for the proliferation of vascularity and CGRP-containing sensory nerves found in the endplate region and vertebral body adjacent to degenerate discs. The neuropeptides substance P and CGRP have potent vasodilatory as well as pain-transmitting effects. The increase in sensory nerve endings suggests increase in blood flow, perhaps as an attempt to augment the nutrition of the degenerate disc. **The increase in the density of sensory nerves, and the presence of endplate cartilage defects, strongly suggest that the endplates and vertebral bodies are sources of pain; this may explain the severe pain on movement experienced by some patients with degenerative disc disease**. See Brown MF, Hukkanen MV, McCarthy ID, Redfern DR, Batten JJ, Crock HV, Hughes SP, Polak JM. Sensory and sympathetic innervation of the vertebral endplate in patients with degenerative disc disease. J Bone Joint Surg Br. 1997 Jan;79(1):147–53.

§ 6:19 Interevertebral disc—Traumatic disc injury and acceleration of disc disease and degeneration

Patients injured in such accidents develop spondylosis approximately six times more frequently than age and gender-matched controls, and in cases in which a loss of consciousness was reported, these patients were 10 times more likely to develop such degenerative changes. Hamer et al. provided further support for the connection between whiplash trauma and the progression of disc disease in their study in which they found that the incidence of whiplash in patients undergoing anterior cervical discectomy was twice that seen in the general population. They found that the mean age of the whiplashed surgical group was 45 +/- 12 years, whereas the mean age of the non-whiplashed surgical group was 55 +/- 14 years. See Hamer AJ, Gargan MF, Bannister GC, Nelson RJ. Whiplash injury and surgically treated cervical disc disease. Injury. 1993 Sep;24(8):549–50.

Other authors have found that patients with pre-existing spondylosis generally fared worse in whiplash (cervical acceleration/deceleration) injuries. Watkinson A, Gargan MF, Bannister GC. Prognostic factors in soft tissue injuries of the cervical spine. Injury. 1991 Jul;22(4):307–9; Parmar HV, Raymakers R. Neck injuries from rear impact road traffic accidents: prognosis in persons seeking compensation. Injury. 1993 Feb;24(2):75–8; *see also* Hohl M. Soft-tissue injuries of the neck in automobile accidents. Factors influencing prognosis. J Bone Joint Surg Am. 1974 Dec;56(8):1675–82.

Cervical instability was identified in 151 segments and correlated with Grade 1 and Grade 2 degeneration in the intervertebral discs ($P < 0.01$). Cervical segmental instability may indicate early degeneration of intervertebral disc in the cervical vertebrae. Translation of 3.5 mm or more, or more than 20% of sagittal plane displacement and/or more than 11°of relative sagittal plane angulation between vertebrae to be a sign of instability. These results provide the first comparison of the MRI assessment of disc degeneration with the conventional plain radiographic evaluation of segmental instability. In all intervertebral levels in the lower cervical spine, segmental instability was more often demonstrated in mildly degenerated discs than in normal and severely degenerated discs. The results support the hypothesis proposed by Kirkaldy-Willis and Farfan that segmental instability becomes more marked when the intervertebral disc is moderately degenerated. Dai L. Disc degeneration and cervical instability. Correlation of magnetic resonance imaging with radiography. Spine. 1998 Aug 15;23(16):1734–8.

§ 6:20 Facet joints

The presence of increased facet joint motions indicated that synovial joint soft-tissue components (i.e., synovial membrane and capsular ligament) sustain increased distortion that may subject these tissues to a greater likelihood of injury. This finding is supported by clinical investigations in which **lower cervical facet joint injury resulted in similar pain pat-**

terns due to the most commonly reported whiplash symptoms. Stemper BD, Yoganandan N, Gennarelli TA, Pintar FA. Localized cervical facet joint kinematics under physiological and whiplash loading. J Neurosurg Spine. 2005 Dec;3(6):471–6.

To define a relationship between mechanical properties at failure and a subfailure condition associated with pain for tension in the rat cervical facet capsular ligament. Tensile failure studies of the C6–C7 rat cervical facet capsular ligament were performed using a customized vertebral distraction device. Force and displacement at failure were measured, and stiffness and energy to failure were calculated. Vertebral motions and ligament deformations were tracked, and maximum principal strains and their directions were calculated. Mean tensile force at failure (2.96+/-0.69N) was significantly greater (p<0.005) than force at subfailure (1.17+/-0.48N). Mean ligament stiffness to failure was 0.75+/-0.27N/mm. Maximum principal strain at failure (41.3+/-20.0%) was significantly higher (p=0.003) than the corresponding subfailure value (23.1+/-9.3%). **This study determined that failure and a subfailure painful condition were significantly different in ligament mechanics and findings provide preliminary insight into the relationship between mechanics and pain physiology for this ligament.** Together with existing studies, these findings offer additional considerations for defining mechanical thresholds for painful injuries. Lee KE, Franklin AN, Davis MB, Winkelstein BA. Tensile cervical facet capsule ligament mechanics: failure and subfailure responses in the rat. J Biomech. 2006;39(7):1256–64.

To identify facet joint capsule receptors in the cervical spine and quantify their responses to capsular deformation. The response of mechanosensitive afferents in C5–C6 facet joint capsules to craniocaudal stretch (0.5 mm/s) was examined in anaesthetized adult goats. Capsular afferents were characterized into Group III and IV based on their conduction velocity. Two-dimensional strains across the capsules during stretch were obtained by a stereoimaging technique and finite element modeling. 17 (53%) Group III and 14 (56%) Group IV afferents were identified with low-strain thresholds of 0.107+/-0.033 and 0.100+/-0.046. A subpopulation of low-strain-threshold afferents had discharge rate saturation at the strains of 0.388+/-0.121 (n=9, Group III) and 0.341+/-0.159 (n=9, Group IV). Two (8%) Group IV units responded only to high strains (0.460+/-0.170); 15 (47%) Group III and 9

(36%) Group IV units could not be excited even by noxious capsular stretch. Simple linear regressions were conducted with capsular load and principal strain as independent variables and neural response of low-strain-threshold afferents as the dependent variable. Correlation coefficients (R2) were 0.73+/-0.11 with load, and 0.82+/-0.12 with principal strain. The stiffness of the C5–C6 capsules was 16.8+/-11.4 N/mm. **Results indicate that sensory receptors in cervical facet joint capsules are not only capable of signaling a graded physiological mechanical stimulus, but may also elicit pain sensation under excessive deformation.** Lu Y, Chen C, Kallakuri S, Patwardhan A, Cavanaugh JM. Neurophysiological and biomechanical characterization of goat cervical facet joint capsules. J Orthop Res. 2005 Jul;23(4):779–87.

Substance P (SP) contributes to the sensitization of a subpopulation of high-threshold articular afferents. Thus, this neuronal mediator released peripherally in response to an injury or acute inflammation causes considerable changes in the mechanosensitivity of this subpopulation of nociceptive joint afferents. Herbert MK, Schmidt RF. Sensitisation of group III articular afferents to mechanical stimuli by substance P. Inflamm Res. 2001 May;50(5):275–82.

Comment:

Each vertebra has two sets of facet joints. One pair faces upward (superior articular facet) and one downward (inferior articular facet). There is one joint on each side (right and left). Facet joints are hinge-like and link vertebrae together. They are located at the back of the spine (posterior). Facet joints are synovial joints. This means each joint is surrounded by a capsule of connective tissue and produces a fluid to nourish and lubricate the joint. The joint surfaces are coated with cartilage, allowing joints to move or glide smoothly (articulate) against each other. The facet capsule is ligament-like in composition and is partially covered and has insertions of the multifidus muscle. In the facet joint itself, there are three different types of synovial folds.

The components of the zygapophysial (facet) joint include the articular cartilage, synovial fluid, and synovial membrane. See Yoganandan N, Kumaresan S, Pintar FA. Biomechanics of the cervical spine Part 2. Cervical spine soft tissue responses and biomechanical modeling. Clin Biomech (Bristol, Avon). 2001 Jan;16(1):1–27.

In rear end impacts, axial compression together with shear force may be responsible for injuries to the cervi-

cal facet joints. The geometry of the cervical spine zygapophysial (facet) joints plays an important role. Cervical zygapophysial (facet) joint pain is common among patients with chronic neck pain after whiplash. Overall, the prevalence of cervical zygapophysial joint pain (C2–C3 or below) was 60% (95% confidence interval, 46%, 73%). The cervical zygapophysial joint pain is common among patients with chronic neck pain after whiplash. This nosologic entity has survived challenge with placebo-controlled, diagnostic investigations and has proven to be of major clinical importance. See Lord SM, Barnsley L, Wallis BJ, Bogduk N. Chronic cervical zygapophysial joint pain after whiplash. A placebo-controlled prevalence study. Spine. 1996 Aug 1;21(15):1737–44; discussion 1744–5.

An abundance of protein gene product (CGRP) 9.5 reactive nerve fibers indicates an extensive innervation of the cervical facet joint capsules. The presence of substance P (SP) and **calcitonin gene-related peptide reactive nerve fibers in a population of these lends credence to cervical facet joint capsules as a key source of neck pain**. Free nerve endings are also associated with SP. SP and CGRP have several peripheral effects that appear to be related to pain and inflammation. SP is involved in degranulation of mast cells and recruitment of inflammatory cells. The neuropeptides SP and CGRP in thin peripheral nerve fibers appear to have several functions related to nociception, inflammation, vasoactivity, and tissue repair. Kallakuri S, Singh A, Chen C, Cavanaugh JM. Demonstration of Substance P, Calcitonin Gene-Related Peptide, and Protein Gene Product 9.5 Containing Nerve Fibers in Human Cervical Facet Joint Capsules. Spine 2004;29:1182–1186.

§ 6:21 Facet joints—Capsular ligament stretching during whiplash

A study to examine the effectiveness of a new sensor that measures ligament length during motion testing of the right C6–C7 capsular ligament during flexibility tests and simulated whiplash found "The maximum C6–C7 capsular ligament elongation (7.2 mm) during the specimen flexibility testing occurred in the left lateral bending. During whiplash simulations, the maximum recorded ligament lengths were 7.2, 7.4, 7.8, and 8.2 mm, respectively, for 3, 4, 8, 10 G accelerations of the sled. These lengths exceeded the earlier-established ligament elongation during the flexibility testing." **These findings indicate that relatively minor collisions may result in excessive loading to the spinal ligaments. (A collision of**

just 6 mph can result in G forces of 6.5g.) From the preliminary findings of this current study, this low speed collision may result in ligament stretch. See Cholewicki J, Panjabi MM, Nibu K, Macias ME. Spinal ligament transducer based on a hall effect sensor. J Biomech. 1997 Mar;30(3):291–3.

Cervical zygapophysial joint pain was the most common source of chronic neck pain after whiplash. Painful joints were identified in 54% of the patients (95% confidence interval, 40% to 68%). Barnsley L, Lord SM, Wallis BJ, Bogduk N. The prevalence of chronic cervical zygapophysial joint pain after whiplash. Spine. 1995 Jan 1;20(1):20–5; *discussion 26.*

The presence of mechanoreceptors and nociceptive nerve endings in the cervical facet joint proves that these tissues are monitored by the central nervous system and implies that neural input from the facets is important to proprioception and pain sensation in the cervical spine. The small number of mechanoreceptor endings in the facet capsules suggests that these receptors have a large receptor field. **Damage to even a small part of the capsule might denervate that articular structure, which could have important implications for long-term joint function**. McLain RF. Mechanoreceptor endings in human cervical facet joints. Spine. 1994 Mar 1;19(5):495–501; McLain RF, Pickar JG. Mechanoreceptor endings in human thoracic and lumbar facet joints. Spine. 1998 Jan 15;23(2):168–73.

Peripheral inflammation results in an enlargement of the receptor fields of many neurons. Increases in neuronal activity in response to tissue injury lead to changes in gene expression and prolonged changes in the nervous system. The functional result is hyperalgesia and spontaneous pain associated with tissue injury. Dubner R, Ruda MA. Activity-dependent neuronal plasticity following tissue injury and inflammation. Trends Neurosci. 1992 Mar;15(3):96–103.

Peak facet joint compression and facet joint sliding exceeded the physiologic limits at **3.5** and **5 g**, respectively. Capsular ligament strains exceeded the physiologic strains at 6.5 g and were largest in the lower cervical spine. Peak facet joint compression occurred at maximum intervertebral extension, whereas peak capsular ligament strain occurred after the maximum intervertebral extension had been reached as the facet joint was returning to its neutral position. **Facet joint components are at risk for injury during whiplash due**

to facet joint compression and excessive capsular ligament strain. Pearson AM, Ivancic PC, Ito S. Panjabi MM. Facet Joint Kinematics and Injury Mechanisms During Simulated Whiplash. Spine 2004;29:390–397.

§ 6:22 Facet joints—Facet joint synovial folds

Not only can the facet capsule be a source of pain, the synovial folds, which are fibroadipose meniscoids attachments of the facet capsule, may be a source of pain. This injury may be caused by the jamming of the facet joint due to the change of the instanteous axis of rotation during the S-shape phase shift of the whiplash event. There are 3 types of synovial folds in the cervical facet joint. See Inami S, Kaneoka K, Hayashi K, Ochiai N. Types of synovial fold in the cervical facet joint. J Orthop Sci. 2000;5(5):475–80.

The presence of putative nociceptive fibers in the cervical synovial folds supports a possible role for these structures as a source of cervical facet joint pain. Inami S, Shiga T, Tsujino A, Yabuki T, Okado N, Ochiai N. Immunohistochemical demonstration of nerve fibers in the synovial fold of the human cervical facet joint. J Orthop Res. 2001 Jul;19(4):593–6.

The function of fibroadipose meniscoids seems to be to protect the articular cartilages in gliding joints that subluxate during normal movement. Arguments are raised that these structures may act as a nidus for intra-articular fibrosis, and that meniscus entrapment may be a mechanism for torticollis. Mercer S, Bogduk N. Intra-articular inclusions of the cervical synovial joints. Br J Rheumatol. 1993 Aug;32(8):705–10.

§ 6:23 Facet joints—Testing for joint pain

Comment:

Specific procedures must be followed by medical doctors in testing for facet joint pain. The facet joint is supplied by nerves from the medial branch of the dorsal primary rami.

In clinical testing of facet joint pain, a positive diagnosis was made only if both blocks relieved the patient's pain and bupivacaine provided longer relief. Painful joints were identified in 54% of the patients (95% confidence interval, 40% to 68%). **The cervical zygapophysial joint pain was the most common source of chronic neck pain after whiplash.** See Barnsley L, Lord SM, Wallis BJ, Bogduk N. The prevalence of chronic cervical zygapophysial joint pain after whiplash. Spine. 1995 Jan 1;20(1):20–5.

To further prove the facet joints are a source of pain, a double-blinded testing procedure was done. Among patients with dominant headache, comparative blocks revealed that the prevalence of C2–C3 zygapophysial joint pain was 50%. Among those without C2–C3 zygapophysial joint pain, placebo-controlled blocks revealed the prevalence of lower cervical zygapophysial joint pain to be 49%. Overall, the prevalence of cervical zygapophysial joint pain (C2–C3 or below) was 60% (95% confidence interval, 46%–73%). **Cervical zygapophysial joint pain is common among patients with chronic neck pain after whiplash. This entity (facet joint pain) has survived challenge with placebo-controlled, diagnostic investigations and has proven to be of major clinical importance.** Lord SM, Barnsley L, Wallis BJ, Bogduk N. Chronic cervical zygapophysial joint pain after whiplash. A placebo-controlled prevalence study. Spine. 1996 Aug 1;21(15):1737–44; discussion 1744–5.

On the basis of the current patient sample, this study demonstrates that although Pain Pressure Thresholds findings may generally be applied for monitoring change in chronic whiplash patients, the use of VAS scores should be limited to patients whose initial score is above 4. It is also suggested that if the PPT is to serve as an outcome measure, its measurement should be performed by the same tester. Prushansky T, Handelzalts S, Pevzner E. Reproducibility of Pressure Pain Threshold and Visual Analog Scale Findings in Chronic Whiplash Patients. Clin J Pain. 2007 May;23(4):339–345

§ 6:24 Facet joints—Multiple areas of pain

The investigation of neck pain by discography alone or by zagapophysial block alone constitutes an inadequate approach to neck pain that fails to identify the majority of patients whose symptoms stem from multiple elements in the 3-joint complexes of the neck.

Disc and Facet pain	41%
Facet pain	23%
Disc pain	20%

See Bogduk N, Aprill C. On the nature of neck pain, discography and cervical zygapophysial joint blocks. Pain. 1993 Aug;54(2):213–7.

§ 6:25 Facet joints—Manual palpation-facet joint pain

Manual palpation correctly identified all 15 patients with proven symptomatic zygapophysial joints, and specified correctly the segmental level of the symptomatic joint. None of the five patients with asymptomatic joints was misdiagnosed as having a symptomatic zygapophysial joint. Jull G, Bogduk N, Marsland A. The accuracy of manual diagnosis for cervical zygapophysial joint pain syndromes. Med J Aust. 1988 Mar 7;148(5):233–6.

§ 6:26 Spinal ganglion nerves

Comment:

Damage to muscles, tendons, or ligaments doesn't account for all whiplash injuries. Injuries from pathology of other structure can be serious and chronic. The symptoms may include tingling and numbness in the arms and legs and/or chronic pain that can last for months. Such symptoms appear to be caused by damage to the nerve tissue. The spinal ganglions (dorsal root ganglion) are a collection of nerve cell bodies that convey sensory information from the peripheral nervous system into the central nervous system (spinal cord).

The dorsal root ganglion demonstrates mechanical sensitivity in its normal state, with some discharges occurring spontaneously. This baseline excitability is heightened after peripheral nerve injury, contributing ectopic barrages above and beyond those generated by the region of nerve injury. See LaRocca H. A taxonomy of chronic pain syndromes. Spine. 1992 Oct;17(10 Suppl):S344–55.

With increasing age, there can be sprouting of sympathetic nerves in the dorsal root ganglion, which may be responsible for sympathetic pain generation or maintenance of pain. Ramer MS, Bisby MA. Normal and injury-induced sympathetic innervation of rat dorsal root ganglia increases with age. J Comp Neurol. 1998 Apr 27;394(1):38–47.

There is no blood brain barrier. **Endoneurial tissue pressure can develop easily when mechanical compression is applied to the ganglion, which is closely related to the onset of nerve cell dysfunction**. Kobayashi S, Yoshizawa H. Effect of mechanical compression on the vascular permeability of the dorsal root ganglion. J Orthop Res. 2002 Jul;20(4):730–9.

There are about 12,000 sensory fibers in the Dorsal Root and 6,000 motor fibers in the Ventral Root. Located between the sensory input and motor output are 375,000 cell bodies. Bland. Disorders of the Cervical Spine, 1994, pg 354.

Taylor et al. reported interstitial hemorrhage in cervical dorsal root ganglia in an autopsy study of victims who had sustained severe inertial neck loading during impacts to the torso or to the head. The structures around the ganglia were mostly uninjured. These findings correlate to experimental findings in pigs of nerve cell membrane dysfunction in cervical spinal root ganglia reported by (Ortengren, Svensson) and the pressure impulse in human cadavers (Eichberger). See Taylor JR, Twomey LT, Kakulas BA. Dorsal root ganglion injuries in 109 blunt trauma fatalities. Injury. 1998 Jun;29(5):335–9; Ortengren T, Hansson HA, Lovsund P, Svensson MY, Suneson A, Saljo A. Membrane leakage in spinal ganglion nerve cells induced by experimental whiplash extension motion: a study in pigs. J Neurotrauma. 1996 Mar;13(3):171–80; Svensson MY, Bostrom O, Davidsson J, Hansson HA, Haland Y, Lovsund P, Suneson A, Saljo A. Neck injuries in car collisions—a review covering a possible injury mechanism and the development of a new rear-impact dummy. Accid Anal Prev. 2000 Mar;32(2):167–75; Eichberger A, Darok M, Steffan H, Leinzinger PE, Bostrom O, Svensson MY. Pressure measurements in the spinal canal of post-mortem human subjects during rear-end impact and correlation of results to the neck injury criterion. Accid Anal Prev. 2000 Mar;32(2):251–60.

In an experiment to simulate the trauma to the neck in rear-end impacts, anesthetized pigs were exposed to a swift extension-flexion motion of the cervical spine. This motion also produced an S-shaped phase shift of the cervical spine. Fluid pressure in the spinal canal was monitored and nerve tissue was microscopically examined with findings of significant injuries in the lower cervical region. Injuries to the spinal ganglia were found, particularly in the lower cervical region. Ortengren T, Hansson HA, Lovsund P, Svensson MY, Suneson A, Saljo A. Membrane leakage in spinal ganglion nerve cells induced by experimental whiplash extension motion: a study in pigs. J Neurotrauma. 1996 Mar;13(3):171–80.

§ 6:27 Spinal ganglion nerves—Relationship between pressure pulse and Neck Injury Criterion (NIC)

The spinal ganglion nerves (dorsal root ganglion) contain the sensory neurons to the spinal structures (disc, dacet, ligaments).

Research at Chalmers University of Technology in Sweden

has shown that damage to the nerves entering the spinal column can occur with rapid changes in spinal column pressure. When the head moves back, relative to the torso, the shape of the neck changes. This increases or decreases the interior volume of the spinal column, but, because spinal fluid is incompressible, the changes in the spinal column volume result in pressure changes. Under normal circumstances—when you nod your head, for example—there's time for the fluid to move into or out of the spinal column to equalize the pressure. **In a rear impact, changes in the spinal column volume can be too rapid for normal fluid exchanges to occur, and the resulting pressure damages the nerve fibers where they enter the spinal column. This research indicates that a critical issue isn't the extent of the neck motion—it's the speed at which the motion occurs**. (See detailed citations in following paragraph.)

The Neck Injury Criterion (NIC) is a measure of neck injury risk that can be recorded on advanced crash test dummies. NIC doesn't measure spinal column pressure directly, but, as a surrogate, it compares the speed and acceleration of the head at the top of the neck with the speed and acceleration of the first thoracic vertebra at the bottom of the neck. This indicates how much the head motion is delayed behind the torso motion. Lower NIC values indicate shorter delays. The NIC is based on tests involving pigs. Researchers at Chalmers University of Technology in Sweden recorded significant spinal column pressure changes in tests that also caused nerve damage to pigs. The type of nerve damage the researchers observed could explain the kinds of symptoms suffered in human cases of whiplash injury with long-term symptoms. **Based on research with both pigs and humans, the Swedish researchers have proposed a value of 15 as the threshold below which the chances of whiplash injury with prolonged symptoms are very low.** See Ortengren T, Hansson HA, Lovsund P, Svensson MY, Suneson A, Saljo A. Membrane leakage in spinal ganglion nerve cells induced by experimental whiplash extension motion: a study in pigs. J Neurotrauma. 1996 Mar;13(3):171–80; Svensson MY, Bostrom O, Davidsson J, Hansson HA, Haland Y, Lovsund P, Suneson A, Saljo A. Neck injuries in car collisions—a review covering a possible injury mechanism and the development of a new rear-impact dummy. Accid Anal Prev. 2000 Mar;32(2):167–75; Eichberger A, Darok M, Steffan H, Leinzinger PE, Bostrom O, Svensson MY. Pressure measurements in the spinal canal of post-mortem human subjects during rear-end impact and correlation of results to the neck injury criterion. Accid Anal Prev. 2000 Mar;32(2):251–60.

It appears that the threshold for acute injury in the general population is likely to require a lowering of the originally proposed NIC value, and additional parameters, such as considering a forward rebound phase or neck extension criteria may be necessary. Croft AC, Herring P, Freeman MD, Haneline MT. The neck injury criterion: future considerations. Accid Anal Prev. 2002 Mar;34(2) :247–55.

In controlled human crash testing, a subject was injured with a NIC level of 10.9 with a crash pulse of 120 ms. Eichberger A, et al. Evaluation of the applicability of the neck injury criterion (NIC) in rear impacts on the basis of human subject tests. IRCOBI conference, September 1998, Goteborg, Sweeden, p. 331.

It was found that the commonly used change of velocity, Delta V, was not a good predictor for NIC, nor was the crash-pulse peak acceleration. **The change of velocity during the first 85ms of the impact correlated with the NIC**. Eriksson L, Bostrom O. Assessing the relevance of NIC and its correlation with crash-pulse parameters: using the mathematical bioRID 1 in rear impacts. Traffic Injury Prevention 2002;3:175–82.

The Intervertebral Neck Injury Criterion (IV-NIC) is based on the hypothesis that intervertebral motion beyond the physiological limit may injure spinal soft tissues during whiplash; while the Neck Injury Criterion (NIC) hypothesizes those sudden changes in spinal fluid pressure may cause neural injury. Average IV-NIC injury thresholds (95% confidence limits) varied among the intervertebral levels and ranged between 1.5 (1.1, 1.9) at C5–C6 and 3.4 (2.4, 4.4) at C7–T1. The NIC injury threshold was **8.7** (7.7, 9.7) m2/s2, substantially less than the proposed threshold of 15 m2/s2. Panjabi MM, Ito S, Ivancic PC, Rubin W. Evaluation of the intervertebral neck injury criterion using simulated rear impacts. J Biomech. 2005 Aug;38(8):1694–701.

Results indicated that the soft tissue injury occurred due to **flexion** mode of injury and its threshold was **8 g**. The average IV-NIC injury threshold (95% confidence interval) was 2.0 (1.2–2.8) at C4–C5 and 2.3 (1.6–3.0) at C6–C7, while the average NIC injury threshold was 18.4 (17.9–19.0) m2/s2. The NIC injury threshold was reached significantly earlier than all the IV-NIC injury thresholds, demonstrating that the **NIC may be**

unable to predict facet and soft tissue injury caused by non-physiologic inververtebral rotation. Ivancic PC, Ito S, Panjabi MM, Pearson AM, Tominaga Y, Wang JL, Gimenez SE. Intervertebral neck injury criterion for simulated frontal impacts. Traffic Inj Prev. 2005 Jun;6(2):175–84.

A correlation was found between duration of symptoms and crash severity measured as mean acceleration and change of velocity. The risk of WAD symptoms for more than one month was found to be **20%** at a change of velocity of approximately **8 km/h** and at a mean acceleration approximately 5 g. A correlation was found between grades of WAD according to Quebec Task Force and crash severity measured as mean acceleration and change of velocity. Out of all crashes with a recorded crash pulse only one out of 207 occupants sustained WAD symptoms for more than one month at mean acceleration below 3.0 g. Given the same crash severity, **females had a higher risk of initial WAD symptoms than males**. Kraft M, Kullgren A, Malm S, Adenius A. Influence of crash severity on various whiplash injury symptoms: a study based on real-life rear-end crashes with recorded crash pulses. ESV 2005; Paper Number: 05-0363

§ 6:28 Spinal ganglion nerves—Referred pain from deep tissues

The defense medical examiner may state that the patient's pain is "non-dermatomal." That is, the pain the person is complaining of does not correspond to the level of nerves of the skin coming from the spinal nerve root. No study has definitively demonstrated that the symptoms provoked by nerve root irritation will occur only within that nerve's dermatomal map. The results of the current study would either suggest that they may be referred in a dynatomal pattern or that the classic dermatomal maps are, to some extent, inaccurate. In either case, **the findings in this study may explain some patient's seemingly non-dermatomal pain complaints**. See Slipman CW, Plastaras CT, Palmitier RA, Huston CW, Sterenfeld EB. Symptom provocation of fluoroscopically guided cervical nerve root stimulation. Are dynatomal maps identical to dermatomal maps? Spine. 1998 Oct 15;23(20):2235–42.

Pain from the deep tissues, disc, facet, ligaments, is not dermatomal. It is a referred type of pain. **Referred pain of deep somatic structures may come from interspinous ligaments, paravertebral muscles, facets or discs**. Kellgren JH. On the distribution of pain arising from deep somatic structures with charts of segmental pain areas. Clin Sci 1939;4:35–46; Inman VT, Saunders JB, Abbott LC. Observations of the function of the shoulder joint. Clin Orthop. 1944 Sep;(330):3–12; Feinstein B, Langton JNK, Jameson RM, Schiller F. Experiments on pain referred from deep somatic tissues. J Bone Jt Surg 1954; 36-A(5):981–997; Cloward RB. Cervical discography. A contribution to the etiology and mechanism of neck, shoulder and arm pain. Ann Surg 1959;150:1052–1064; Cloward RB. The clinical significance of the sinu-vertebral nerve of the cervical spine in relation to the cervical disc syndrome. J Neurol Neurosurg Psychiatry 1960;23:321–326; Dwyer A, Aprill C, Bogduk N. Cervical zygapophyseal joint pain patterns. I: A study in normal volunteers. Spine. 1990 Jun;15(6):453–7; Aprill C, Dwyer A, Bogduk N. Cervical zygapophyseal joint pain patterns. II: A clinical evaluation. Spine. 1990 Jun;15(6):458–61.

§ 6:29 Low back complaints and whiplash

Lumbar spinal pain is defined as "pain perceived as arising from anywhere within a region bounded superiorly by an imaginary transverse line through the tip of the last thoracic spinous process, inferiorly by an imaginary transverse line through the tip of the first sacral spinous process, and laterally by vertical lines tangential to the lateral borders of the lumbar erectors spinae." Merskey H and Bogduk N (eds). Classification of chronic pain. 2nd ed. Seattle, USA: IASP Press;1994.

Sacral spinal pain is defined as "pain perceived as arising from anywhere within a region bounded superiorly by an imaginary transverse line through the tip of the first sacral spinous process, inferiorly by an imaginary transverse line through the sacrococcygeal joints, and laterally by imaginary lines passing through the posterior superior and posterior inferior iliac spines."

The spine consists of the bony vertebral column and cartilaginous discs that support ligaments, muscles, joints, soft tissues, and nerve tissue. The spine not only supports the weight of the head and torso, it also supports and protects the spinal cord, nerve roots, sensory and autonomic ganglia, and the peripheral nerves. Nearly all of the tissues of the spine have sensory innervation and are capable of producing pain and other sensations. There is great overlap in the patterns of pain that arise from injury to different structures and, thus, it is not hard to understand why identifying the anatomic cause of spine pain is so difficult. To understand the pathophysiology of back pain, practitioners must have a thorough knowledge of the different anatomic structures in the region, their nerve supplies, and the pain patterns that typically arise from abnormalities in each structure.

Terms to specify the source of the perceived pain.

- **Somatic pain** arises from the stimulation of the nerve endings in the skin and musculoskeletal components, such as the bone, ligament, joint, or muscle.
- **Referred pain** is pain perceived as arising or occurring in a region of the body supplied by nerves other than those that innervate the true source of the pain. Referred pain may be perceived in areas relatively distant from the actual source of pain, but when the true source of pain and area of referred pain are adjacent to each other, they seem to be confluent.
- **Radicular pain** is pain that is caused by the stimulation of the sensory dorsal root of a spinal nerve, or its dorsal root ganglion, and is not the same as radiculopathy. Radicular pain may resemble the distribution of classic dermatomal maps, but pain can be outside the distribution of the classic dermatomal maps.
- **Radiculopathy** is a pathological condition in which the function of the nerve root is impaired leading to numbness, motor loss, and pain, depending on which fibers of the nerve root are involved. Paresthesia, segmental numbness, weakness, and loss of reflexes are reliable and valid signs of radiculopathy that allow the diagnosis to be made clinically, without recourse to investigations.

Ahmed S. The Anatomic Basis of Low Back Pain. Pain Management Rounds, Massachusetts General Hospital. 2005;1(10).

Lower back pain is associated with cervical acceleration/deceleration (CAD) injury. Low back pain is a fairly common symptom following a whiplash trauma, as noted by the following tests:

Author	Year	% with Low Back Complaints
Cassidy et al	2003	61–64
Berglund et al	2001	20
Sqiures	1996	48
Sturzenegger	1995	46

Author	Year	% with Low Back Complaints
Radanov et al	1994	39
Magnusson	1994	47
Teasel	1993	40–60
Hildingson and Toolanen	1990	25
Hohl	1974	35

Radanov BP, Sturzenegger M, de Stefano G, Schnidrig A. Relationship between early somatic, radiological, cognitive and psychosocial findings and outcome during a one-year follow-up in 117 patients suffering from common whiplash. British Journal of Rheumatology 1994; 33:442–448; Cassidy JD, Carroll L, Cote P, Berglund A, Nygren Å. Low back pain after traffic collisions: A population based cohort study. Spine 2003; 28(10):1002–1009; Berglund A, Alfredsson L, Jensen I, Cassidy JD, Nygren Å. The association between exposure to a rear-end collision and future health complaints. J Clin Epidemiology 2001; 54:851–856; Hildingsson C, Toolanen G. Outcome after soft-tissue injury of the cervical spine. A prospective study of 93 car-accident victims. Acta Orthop Scand. 1990 Aug;61(4):357–9; Magnusson T. Extracervical symptoms after whiplash trauma. Cephalalgia. 1994 Jun;14(3):223–7; Hohl M, Hills B. Soft-Tissue Injuries of the Neck in Automobile Accidents. J Bone Joint Surg 1974; 56-A:1675–1682; Squires B, Gargan MF, Bannister GC. Soft-tissue injuries of the cervical spine. 15-year follow-up. J Bone Joint Surg (Br) 1996; 6:955–7; Sturzenegger M, Radanov BP, DiStefano G. The effect of accident mechanisms and initial findings on the long-term course of whiplash injury. J Neuro 1995; 242:443–449; Teasell RW. The clinical picture of whiplash injuries: An Overview. SPINE: State of the Art Reviews 1993; 7:373–389

§ 6:30 Low back complaints and whiplash—Neurological concerns—Low back pain from whiplash

Following a collision, multiple forces act upon the spine. Forces generated during simulated whiplash collision induce biphasic lumbar spinal motions (increased-decreased lordosis) of insufficient magnitude to cause bony injuries, but they may be sufficient to cause soft-

tissue injuries. The anterior shear strains had a biphasic shape. Spinal strains peaked at the T12 at approximately 120 and 370 msec, whereas in the L4 vertebra, it peaked at 200 and 380 msec. The anterior strain pattern of the L4 and T12 vertebrae were in diametrically opposite directions. See Fast A, Sosner J, Begeman P, Thomas MA, Chiu T. Lumbar Spinal Strains Associated with Whiplash Injury: A Cadaveric Study. Am J Phys Med Rehabil. 2002 Sep;81(9):645–650.

The forces act upon multiple tissues on the spine. In activating the nerve endings in the outer annulus fibrosus of the disc, in the capsule of the zygapophysial joints, and in the ligaments are most likely part of the proprioceptive system responsible for optimal recruitment of the paraspinal muscles. **Mechanical stimulation of the spinal viscoelastic tissues excites the muscles with higher excitation intensity when more than one tissue (e.g. ligaments and disc) is stimulated**. See Holm S, Indahl A, Solomonow M. Sensorimotor control of the spine. J Electromyogr Kinesiol. 2002 Jun;12(3):219–34.

There is coexistence of two different types of innervation: one originating directly from the spinal nerve segmentally, and one reaching vertebral structures via the sympathetic nerves nonsegmentally. **Therefore, sympathetic nerves are likely involved in the proprioception of the spinal column**. See Higuchi K, Sato T. Anatomical study of lumbar spine innervation. Folia Morphol (Warsz). 2002;61(2):71–9.

An injury may cause increased muscle tone. Hypertonicity of the lumbar soft supporting tissues and especially the lumbar erector muscles (caused by the over-excitement of the lumbar proprioceptors) can overload the nervous system. **Pain in the low back following whiplash may be a decrease in this propriceptive information from the low back.** Hinoki M, Hine S, Ushio N, Ishida Y, Koike S. Studies on ataxia of lumbar origin in cases of vertigo due to whiplash injury. Int J Equilib Res. 1973 Jun;3(1):141–52.

Pain is determined by the neurologic properties of receptor organs, neurons, and their interconnections. These may become supersensitive or hyperreactive following denervation (Cannon's Law). Gunn type 3 pain. (A neuropathic type of pain.) Gunn CC. "Prespondylosis" and some pain syndromes following denervation supersensitivity. Spine. 1980 Mar–Apr;5(2):185–92.

§ 6:31 Low back complaints and whiplash—Related soft tissue findings

Miniature endplate trauma may be responsible for low

back pain in patients with normal radiographic appearance. Yoganandan N, Larson SJ, Gallagher M, Pintar FA, Reinartz J, Droese K. Correlation of microtrauma in the lumbar spine with intraosseous pressures. Spine. 1994 Feb 15;19(4):435–40.

Injury in the form of microfractures of the endplate not detected on radiography, however, was observed under cryomicrotomy for structures loaded into the traumatic loading phase. Yoganandan N, Maiman DJ, Pintar F, Ray G, Myklebust JB, Sances A Jr, Larson SJ. Microtrauma in the lumbar spine: a cause of low back pain. Neurosurgery. 1988 Aug;23(2):162–8.

There is a strong theoretic basis to support the concept that the clinical features of many lumbar disc patients may be explained by inflammation caused by biochemical factors alone or combined with mechanical deformation of lumbar tissues, rather than mechanical factors alone. Saal JS. The role of inflammation in lumbar pain. Spine. 1995 Aug 15;20(16):1821–7.

The origin of pain is multi-factorial and that inflammation probably predominates over merely mechanical mechanisms. Leonardi M, Simonetti L, Agati R. Neuroradiology of spine degenerative diseases. Best Pract Res Clin Rheumatol. 2002 Jan;16(1):59–87.

Histological techniques and the scanning electron microscope were used to examine the different structures of the spine under conditions of tensile overload. Chief attention was paid to the structures most exposed to mechanical stress, such as the interface between the vertebral body and the intervertebral disc. **The authors found that the insertion of collagen fibers in cartilage or bone in the regions overloaded by tensile forces is identical to that found in epicondylitis in other locations. Such enthesopathies in the spinal region may form a major component of back pain states.** See Horn V, Vlach O, Messner P. Enthesopathy in the vertebral disc region. Arch Orthop Trauma Surg. 1991;110(4):187–9.

Note that those suffering from whiplash not only have a higher rate of long-term neck and shoulder pain, but also low back pain and other health complaints. (See following study.)

We conclude that rear-end collisions resulting in reported whiplash injuries seem to have a substantial impact on health complaints, even a long time after the collision (7-year follow-up). Berglund A, Alfredsson L, Jensen I, Cassidy JD, Nygren A. The association between exposure to a rear-end collision and future health complaints. J Clin Epidemiol. 2001 Aug;54(8):851–6.

The following chart flows from the above Berglund study:

Complaint	**Increase in Relative Risk (1.0 = same risk as control)**	
Headache	3.7	(370% increase)
Thoracic pain	3.1	
Low back pain	1.7	
Ill health	3.3	
Sleep disturbance	2.4	
Stomach ache	1.9	
Fatigue	1.6	
Depressive mode	1.6	

A dysfunction of a joint is defined as a reversible functional restriction of motion presenting with hypomobility, according to manual medicine terminology. The aim of our study was to evaluate the frequency and significance of sacroiliac joint (SIJ) dysfunction in patients with low back pain, sciatica and imaging-proven disc herniaiton. **We conclude that, in the presence of lumbar and ischiadic symptoms, our presented data suggest consideration of SIJ dysfunction, requiring manual medicine examination and, in the presence of SIJ dysfunction, appropriate therapy, regardless of intervertebral disc pathomorphology.** See Galm R, Frohling M, Rittmeister M, Schmitt E. Sacroiliac joint dysfunction in patients with imaging-proven lumbar disc herniation. Eur Spine J. 1998;7(6):450–3.

§ 6:32 Shoulder, arm and hand complaints

Comment:

Clinicians often think in terms of "syndromes." A syndrome is a pattern of symptoms (what the patient complains about) and signs (what the physician finds) that suggest the location of a disease process and occasionally its nature. The consequence of nerve root damage (from any cause) is known as a radiculopathy, whereas, the syndrome of "myelopathy" results from spinal cord damage.

§ 6:33 Shoulder, arm and hand complaints—Cervical radiculopathies

There are 7 cervical vertebrae and 8 cervical roots. The root number exiting between two vertebrae is always the number of the lower vertebra. For example, the C5 root exits between the C4–C5 vertebrae and would be affected by a C4/5 disc herniation; the C8 root exits between C7–T1 vertebrae and would be compressed by a C7/T1 disc.

Pain due to a C6 and C7 radiculopathy radiates from the neck and from around the shoulder into outer aspect of the arm and forearm. C6 radiculopathy may cause pain and numbness along the dorsal aspect of the thumb and index finger. C7 pain and paresthesia may radiate into the middle finger.

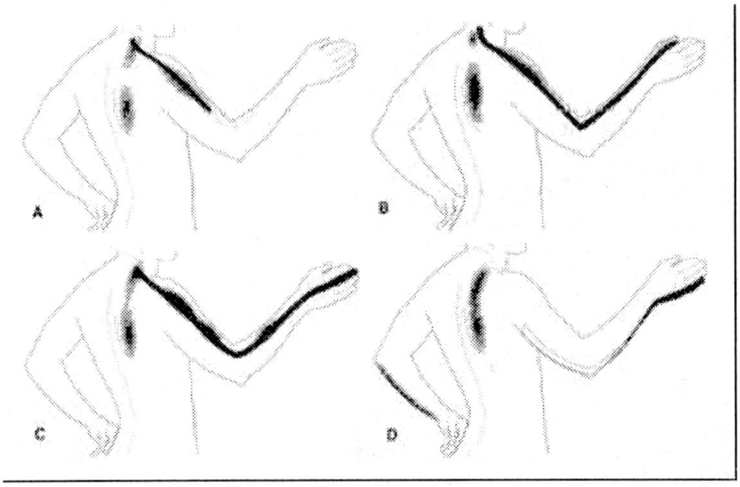

Above: Radicular signs/symptoms from lower cervical spine levels

§ 6:34 Shoulder, arm and hand complaints—Brachial plexus lesions

Physical signs included: decreased range of movement of the neck; paraesthesiae in the upper arm; forearm and/or hand weakness; coldness, discoloration and hyperhydrosis in the upper limb; upper limb swelling; positive Tinel sign over the scalene muscles or in the supraclavicular fossa, the cubital tunnel, the radial nerve at the elbow and/or the carpal tunnel; and discomfort with the maneuvers causing traction to the brachial plexus. A significant proportion of patients with irritation of the brachial plexus can have abnormal autonomic status, including neck and arm pain or numbness, headache, nausea, sleeplessness, general fatigue, hyperhydrosis and swelling of the hand. See Ide M, Ide J, Yamaga M, Takagi K. Symptoms and signs of irritation of the brachial plexus in whiplash injuries. J Bone Joint Surg Br. 2001 Mar;83(2):226–9.

Brachial plexus irritation diagnosis was determined by:(1) Persistent diffuse pain or paraesthesiae in the upper limb aggravated by carrying, lifting, overhead elevation or repetitive use of the arm. (2) A positive Tinel sign over the brachial plexus at the scalene muscles or supraclavicular fossa. (3) Reproduction of pain or paraesthesiae by maneuvers stressing the brachial plexus with the shoulder at 90° of abduction in external rotation, or with a traction maneuver. See Ide M, Ide J, Yamaga M, Takagi K. Symptoms and signs of irritation of the brachial plexus in whiplash injuries. J Bone Joint Surg Br. 2001 Mar;83(2):226–9.

Brachial plexus injury occurs often from whiplash. In this study it was found to be 37.8% of patients. Delay onset for brachial plexus symptoms is very common, with a mean of 6.7 days and some being delayed as long as 37 days. Brachial plexus injury is not related to patient age (range 16–69 years) or to mechanism of injury. Brachial plexus injury is significantly more likely to occur in women compared to men (nearly twice as common). The brachial plexus injury and its associated symptoms involve the sympathetic portion of the autonomic nervous system. Post-ganglionic sympathetic efferents are termed gray rami because they are non-myelinated, and problems in these non-myelinated sympathetic fibers are not assessed with nerve conduction studies. **This article gives evidence of support for the Double Crush Syndrome**. See Ide M, Ide J, Yamaga M, Takagi K. Symptoms and signs of irritation of the brachial plexus in whiplash injuries. J Bone Joint Surg Br. 2001 Mar;83(2):226–9.

§ 6:35 Shoulder, arm and hand complaints—Shoulder symptoms

The shoulder is affected by irritation of a cervical nerve root or referred pain. The anteroposterior diameter of the spinal canal at C5 and C6 in the painful-shoulder group was significantly narrower than in the control group. **It is well known that cervical radiculopathy sometimes causes shoulder pain. The cervical spine without obvious radiculopathy appears to be involved in patients with a painful shoulder. We speculate that the shoulder is affected by irritation of a cervical nerve root or referred pain.** See Mimori K, Muneta T, Komori H, Okawa A, Shinomiya K. Relation between the painful shoulder and the cervical spine with narrow canal in patients without obvious radiculopathy. J Shoulder Elbow Surg. 1999 Jul–Aug; 8(4):303–6.

This study emphasizes the need for a careful evaluation of patients with combined neck-shoulder pain syndrome in a systematic approach, allowing appropriate treatment. The complex problem of combined neck and shoulder pain was investigated in 26 operations in 13 patients who had a shoulder procedure (subacromial decompressions or rotator cuff repairs) and an anterior cervical spine fusion. Hawkins RJ, Bilco T, Bonutti P. Cervical spine and shoulder pain. Clin Orthop. 1990 Sep; (258):142–6.

52.6% of subjects with late whiplash syndrome had periarticular disorders of the shoulder joint and shoulder pain that was exaggerated by shoulder movement and tenderness in the tendons of the rotator cuff or the biceps tendon. Magnusson T. Extracervical symptoms after whiplash trauma. Cephalalgia. 1994 Jun; 14(3):223–7; discussion 181–2.

The risk for neck and shoulder pain 7 years after the collision is increased nearly three-fold compared to unexposed subjects. Berglund A, Alfredsson L, Cassidy JD, Jensen I, Nygren A. The association between exposure to a rear-end collision and future neck or shoulder pain: a cohort study. J Clin Epidemiol. 2000 Nov; 53(11):1089–94.

Our study showed an incidence of **22% of shoulder pain after whiplash injury** and is comparable with other studies. Of the 102 patients entered into the study, 59 did not fit the criteria for the impingement. Only 43 patients had positive signs of impingement and a positive Neer test on injection of lignocaine. Of these patients, 36 showed alteration of scapulohumeral rhythm. Chauhan SK, Peckham T, Turner R. Impingement syndrome associated with whiplash injury. J Bone Joint Surg Br. 2003 Apr;85(3):408–10.

After a neck injury a significant proportion of patients present with shoulder pain, some of whom have treatable shoulder pathology such as impingement syndrome. The diagnosis is, however, frequently overlooked and shoulder pain is attributed to pain radiating from the neck resulting in long delays before treatment. It is important that this is appreciated and patients are specifically examined for signs of subacromial impingement after whiplash injuries to the neck. Direct seatbelt trauma to the shoulder is one possible explanation for its etiology.

Abbassian A, Giddins GE. Subacromial Impingement in patients with whiplash injury to the cervical spine. J Orthop Surg. 2008 Jun 27;3(1):25.

§ 6:36 Shoulder, arm and hand complaints—Thoracic Outlet Syndrome (TOS)

Comment:

There are various names for thoracic outlet syndrome (TOS) including: cervical rib, scalenus anticus, costoclavicular, hyperabduction, pectoralis minor, bachiocephalic, and fractured clavicle-rib syndromes, nocturnal paresthetic brachialgia, and effort vein thrombosis. It is documented that whiplash trauma can cause TOS. Whiplash-caused TOS can cause long-term disabling symptoms. Whiplash injury patients occasionally do not respond to conventional treatment and become worse. Common whiplash TOS symptoms include: nausea, dizziness, numbness, aching pain, disorientation, neck stiffness, arm heaviness, incapacitating headache, easy fatigability of the arm, tingling and numbness in the ulnar aspect of the hand.

Arm pain and paresthesia following neck injury in motor vehicle accidents arise from irritable cervical neural tissues. Quintner JL. A study of upper limb pain and paraesthesiae following neck injury in motor vehicle accidents: assessment of the brachial plexus tension test of Elvey. Br J Rheumatol. 1989 Dec; 28(6):528–33.

In chronic whiplash patients, thoracic outlet syndrome was diagnosed in 31.6% of the cases. Magnusson T. Extracervical symptoms after whiplash trauma. Cephalalgia. 1994 Jun; 14(3):223–7; discussion 181–2.

In cases of Thoracic outlet syndrome (TOS), 32% had been involved in a rear-end accident and 25% had been in a side or head-on collision. Sanders RJ. Etiology. In:

Sanders RJ, Haug CE, eds. Thoracic Outlet Syndrome: A common sequelae of neck injuries. Philadelphia: Lippincott, 1991:21–31.

33% of whiplash injury patients reported arm symptoms, which author related to TOS. Moore M Jr. Thoracic outlet syndrome experience in a metropolitan hospital. Clin Orthop. 1986 Jun;(207):29–30.

The diagnosis of non-specific neurogenic thoracic outlet syndrome (TOS) is controversial, as there are no conclusive objective tests. This subset of TOS may represent over 85% of TOS patients. Ault J, Suutala K. Thoracic outlet syndrome. J Manual & Manipulative Therapy 1998; 6:118–29.

67% of the TOS symptoms were on the side of the driver's shoulder strap, suggesting that the force of the body against the shoulder restraint during whiplash may be responsible for some TOS problems. Lindgren KA, Oksala I. Long-term outcome of surgery for thoracic outlet syndrome. Am J Surg. 1995 Mar;169(3):358–60.

Patients with chronic cervicobrachialgia may have pain thresholds and pain tolerances lower than normal. In a normal person, A-beta afferent (large mylenated) fibers participate in transmitting low-threshold stimuli from mechanoreceptors, and A-delta/C fibers participate in transmitting high threshold stimuli, such as pain and thermal signals. Loss of input from A-beta afferent fibers may diminish the inhibition of the projecting neurons and give rise to "low-input" pain. **With a phenotype change in the spinal cord, A-beta afferent fibers that would normally evoke non-painful sensations (gate theory of pain) may elicit and maintain pain (allodynia).** See Voerman VF, van Egmond J, Crul BJ. Elevated detection thresholds for mechanical stimuli in chronic pain patients: support for a central mechanism. Arch Phys Med Rehabil. 2000 Apr; 81(4):430–5.

Posttraumatic **brachial plexus** entrapment in fibrotic scarring tissue is taken into consideration as the cause of complaints for patients who suffered a hyperextension-hyperflexion cervical injury. All 54 patients included in this analysis where symptom-free before the accident and subsequently complained for pain, paresthesia and slight weakness in the arm. In 14 neurological signs of brachial plexus entrapment were observed. Electroneurophysiological, summary index testing was positive for a brachial plexus involvement in all cases. Conservative measures, comprising physical therapy and vasoactive drugs were applied for a period of 6 to 12 (mean 8.4) months; surgical procedure of neurolysis was then proposed in 39 cases to solve the problem. Thirty-two patients were operated on. Twenty of these had a neat improvement on a 6-month to 1-year follow-up. Seven patients had refused surgery; of these 6 patients had clinical worsening at the same follow-up period while 1 remained unchanged. **All patients with clinical symptoms not reversed after some time post-injury should be investigated for a possible brachial plexus entrapment.** Alexandre A, Coro L, Azuelos A, Pellone M. Thoracic outlet syndrome due to hyperextension-hyperflexion cervical injury. Acta Neurochir Suppl. 2005;92:21–4.

§ 6:37 Shoulder, arm and hand complaints—Thoracic Outlet Syndrome (TOS)—Diagnostic tests for TOS

Comment:

Thoracic outlet syndrome may be identified by a positive Tinel's sign. For this test, pressure is applied to the brachial plexus for 10 to 60 seconds. If positive, the patient's symptoms may appear, including numbness in the hand. (Note that this test is similar to the Morley test.) Another useful test is the Roos test in which the patient hyperabducts and externally rotates the arms, while opening and closing his or her hands. If positive, the patient's symptoms will appear.

"Any injury causing a severe 'jerk' of the shoulder or neck may precipitate the outlet syndrome, including the so-called 'whiplash' auto injury. Arm symptoms may not develop for several days, weeks, or even months after the injury; however, they tend to be relentless and poorly responsive to physical therapy when they do develop." See Roos DB, Owens JC. Thoracic outlet syndrome. Arch Surg. 1966 Jul;93(1):71–4.

Neck-shoulder-arm symptoms represent the classic features of thoracic outlet syndrome (TOS). "Severe symptoms such as aching pain, arm 'heaviness,' easy fatigability of the arm, tingling and numbness in the ulnar aspect of the hand, and headache may appear in whiplash patients."

TOS symptoms can be neurogenic and/or vascular, and the vascular type occurs less frequently than the neurogenic type. Vascular type TOS is mainly due to the congenital anomalies of the scalenus muscle insertion to the first rib, or from osseous anomalies. Neurogenic type TOS may arise from edema or spasm of the anterior scalenus muscle or from postural abnormalities. Whiplash traumatic TOS can cause long-term disabling symptoms following rear-end auto accidents. "Neural irritation of the TOS elicited by cervical injuries has emerged as a principal cause of chronic shoulder-arm symptoms in these patients." "The Morley or Roos maneuver appears to have a significant value in the diagnosis, because the development of NTOS after cervical trauma may be caused solely by pressure on the brachial plexus by the overlying scalenus muscle."

The finding of cervical kyphosis will lead to total spinal malalignment or rounded shoulders. This malalignment will result in headache, neck pain, scapular pain, and low back pain with postural sway or continuous contraction of trunk muscles.

The authors also note that "the mainstays of nonoperative treatments that include the use of medication, the modification of activities, the use of a neck collar, and some injections," will not result in the needed changes in spinal alignment, noting: "Changes in the muscles and spinal alignment, standard treatments may be beneficial for short-term relief of painful symptoms, but will not be effective or essential for long-term relief."

Regarding the above citations, see Kai Y, Oyama M, Kurose S, Inadome T, Oketani Y, Masuda Y. Neurogenic thoracic outlet syndrome in whiplash injury. J Spinal Disord. 2001 Dec; 14(6):487–93.

§ 6:38 Shoulder, arm and hand complaints—Thoracic Outlet Syndrome (TOS)—Treatment for TOS

"Early mobilization after a whiplash injury may decrease neck-shoulder pain more than a standard program using a soft collar or initial rest." See Kai Y, Oyama M, Kurose S, Inadome T, Oketani Y, Masuda Y. Neurogenic thoracic outlet syndrome in whiplash injury. J Spinal Disord. 2001 Dec; 14(6):487–93.

A recent study has indicated that manipulative therapy for neurogenic cervicobrachial pain has been shown to help. Cowell IM, Phillips DR. Effectiveness of manipulative physiotherapy for the treatment of a neurogenic cervicobrachial pain syndrome: a single case study—experimental design. Man Ther. 2002 Feb; 7(1):31–8.

The relative mobility at levels C7–T1 and T1–T2 significantly predicted neck-shoulder pain and the symptom weakness in the hands. Manual therapy has shown to be effective in treating neck-shoulder pain and

mobility in the cervico-thoracic spine. Norlander S, Nordgren B. Clinical symptoms related to musculoskeletal neck-shoulder pain and mobility in the cervico-thoracic spine. Scand J Rehabil Med. 1998 Dec; 30(4):243–51.

§ 6:39 Shoulder, arm and hand complaints—Double crush syndrome

"Double crush" refers to the hypothesis that a single lesion along the course of a nerve predisposes that nerve to a second lesion further along its course. The reason for this is uncertain, and indeed the existence of the double crush syndrome is itself debated. **Cases with cervical root disease support the notion that the cervical radiculopathy may have predisposed the nerve to a second lesion along its course, resulting in the so-called double crush syndrome, and that this syndrome may therefore be a true entity.** See Raps SP, Rubin M. Proximal median neuropathy and cervical radiculopathy: double crush revisited. Electromyogr Clin Neurophysiol. 1994 Jun; 34(4):195–6.

The "double crush" syndrome has been proven in the laboratory. Dellon AL, Mackinnon SE. Chronic nerve compression model for the double crush hypothesis. Ann Plast Surg. 1991 Mar; 26(3):259–64.

Note that double crush syndrome may also occur in the lower extremities. See Golovchinsky V. Double crush syndrome in lower extremities. Electromyogr Clin Neurophysiol. 1998 Mar;38(2):115–20.

The association between thoracic outlet syndrome (TOS) and carpal tunnel syndrome (CTS) (40 cases), ulnar neuropathy (UN) (19 cases) and radial tunnel syndrome (29 cases) was investigated. **The possibility of a double crush syndrome is demonstrated that, in approximately half of all cases, the proximal neuropathy precedes the distal one.** Narakas AO. The role of thoracic outlet syndrome in the double crush syndrome. Ann Chir Main Memb Super. 1990; 9(5):331–40.

Cervical spondylosis and disc prolapse were more common in the patients than the controls at the C5–C6 and C6–C7 levels, and their locations were on the same side as the symptoms in the wrist(s) in 50% of cases. There was no difference in the size of the cervical canal between the two groups. **The higher incidence of narrowed cervical foramens in the patients and its concordance with affected nerve roots on the same side as the CTS symptoms support the hypothesis of a double-crush phenomenon**. Pierre-Jerome C, Bekkelund SI. Magnetic resonance assessment of the double-crush phenomenon in patients with carpal tunnel syndrome: a bilateral quantitative study. Scand J Plast Reconstr Surg Hand Surg. 2003;37(1):46–53.

It is evident that the arm and hand complaints have a cervical component. The following medical literature supports this idea:

Tinazzi M, Zanette G, Volpato D, Testoni R, Bonato C, Manganotti P, Miniussi C, Fiaschi A. Neurophysiological evidence of neuroplasticity at multiple levels of the somatosensory system in patients with carpal tunnel syndrome. Brain. 1998 Sep; 121 (Pt 9):1785–94.

Chang MH, Chiang HT, Ger LP, Yang DA, Lo YK. The cause of slowed forearm median conduction velocity in carpal tunnel syndrome. Clin Neurophysiol. 2000 Jun;111(6):1039–44.

Upton AR, McComas AJ. The double crush in nerve entrapment syndromes. Lancet. 1973 Aug 18; 2(7825):359–62; Hurst LC, Weissberg D, Carroll RE. The relationship of the double crush to carpal tunnel syndrome (an analysis of 1,000 cases of carpal tunnel syndrome). J Hand Surg [Br]. 1985 Jun; 10(2):202–4.

Wood VE, Biondi J. Double-crush nerve compression in thoracic-outlet syndrome. J Bone Joint Surg Am. 1990 Jan; 72(1):85–7.

Golovchinsky V. Relationship between damage of cervical nerve roots or brachial plexus and development of peripheral entrapment syndromes in the upper extremities (Double Crush Syndrome). J Neurol Orthop Med Surg 1995; 1:61–9.

Liu JE, Tahmoush AJ, Roos DB, Schwartzman RJ. Shoulder-arm pain from cervical bands and scalene muscle anomalies. J Neurol Sci. 1995 Feb;128(2):175–80.

Rydevik BL. The effects of compression on the physiology of nerve roots. J Manipulative Physiol Ther. 1992 Jan;15(1):62–6.

Rydevik B, Brown MD, Lundborg G. Pathoanatomy and pathophysiology of nerve root compression. Spine. 1984 Jan–Feb;9(1):7–15.

Epstein NE, Epstein JA, Carras R. Coexisting cervical spondylotic myelopathy and bilateral carpal tunnel syndromes. J Spinal Disord. 1989 Mar;2(1):36–42.

§ 6:40 Shoulder, arm and hand complaints—Temporomandibular joint disorders and whiplash

There seems to be a relationship between whiplash and

temporomandibular joint disorder (TMD), but the exact mechanism of injury has yet to be discovered.

The incidence of reduced and/or painful jaw movement was 14.9 percent (n = 1,158), and it was higher in subjects with WADs (15.8 percent) than in those without WADs (4.7 percent; relative risk = 3.36, 95 percent confidence interval, 2.36 to 4.78). Within the WAD injuries, multivariable logistic regression revealed that the onset of reduced and/or painful jaw movement was associated with female sex; age < 50 years; having hit one's head in the collision; and postinjury symptoms of difficulty swallowing, ringing in the ears, dizziness or unsteadiness, and more intense neck pain. Collision parameters, such as head position at the time of the crash and headrest use and type, were not associated with onset of jaw symptoms.

Reduced or painful jaw movement was more common in people with WADs than in those with other collision-related injuries. Among those with WADs, reduced or painful jaw movement was more common in women and younger people.

Reduced or painful jaw movement is an important aspect of WADs, and more studies are needed to determine how to best assess and treat this problem.

Carroll LJ, Ferrari R, Cassidy JD. Reduced or painful jaw movement after collision-related injuries: a population-based study. J Am Dent Assoc. 2007 Jan;138(1):86–93.

Sensory innervation of temporomandibular joint disk. Free nerve endings and sensory nerve end organs are present in the disk parenchyma of the human temporomandibular joint and are associated with sensation and proprioception, just as they are in the acetabular labrum, glenoid labrum, triangular fibrocartilage complex, and meniscus.

Asaki S, Sekikawa M, Kim YT. Sensory innervation of temporomandibular joint disk. J Orthop Surg (Hong Kong). 2006 Apr;14(1):3–8.

The higher prevalence of widespread pain and psychologic distress in patients with chronic whiplash-associated disorder suggests that the higher prevalence of temporomandibular disorder pain in these patients is part of a more widespread chronic pain disorder. In conclusion, **patients with chronic WAD showed higher prevalence of TMD pain**.

Visscher C, Hofman N, Mes C, Lousberg R, Naeije M. Is temporomandibular pain in chronic whiplash-associated disorders part of a more widespread pain syndrome? Clin J Pain. 2005 Jul-Aug;21(4):353–7.

The purpose of this study was to compare the prevalence of temporomandibular disorders (TMD) between individuals with chronic whiplash-associated disorders (WAD) and a group of age- and sex-stratified patients attending a Public Dental Service (PDS) clinic. Fifty-four individuals diagnosed with chronic WAD that were referred to a rehabilitation centre constituted the WAD group. The control group consisted of 66 patients at a PDS clinic (C group). Both groups underwent a standardised examination of the masticatory system comprising a questionnaire and a clinical examination. Eighty-nine per cent of the individuals in the WAD group had severe symptoms of TMD according to Helkimo's anamnestic index of dysfunction (A1) compared with 18% in the C group ($p < 0.001$). The individuals in the WAD group had also more signs of TMD. The maximum mouth opening capacity was 48 mm in the WAD group and 54 mm in the C group ($p < 0.001$). In the WAD group 17% had a mouth opening capacity < 40 mm compared with 2% in the C group ($p < 0.05$). Pain on palpation of the jaw muscles and on lateral palpation of the temporomandibular joints was more common in the WAD group ($p < 0.001$). Pain on mandibular mobility was reported by 30% in the WAD group and by 3% in the C group ($p < 0.001$). In conclusion, the prevalence of TMD was higher among individuals with chronic WAD compared with an age- and sex-stratified cohort of patients in a general dental practice. **The results indicate that trauma to the neck also affects temporomandibular function**.

Klobas L, Tegelberg A, Axelsson S. Symptoms and signs of temporomandibular disorders in individuals with chronic whiplash-associated disorders. Swed Dent J. 2004;28(1):29–36.

Symptoms of temporomandibular disorder (TMD) include the following:1) Pain emanating from the temporomandibular joints; 2) Facial pain; 3) Popping or cracking of the joints; 4) Grinding noises in the joint; 5) Closed lock phenomenon (28–33 mm mouth opening); 6) Headaches; 7) Neck pain and/or spasm; 8) A feeling of fullness in the ears; tinnitus (ringing in the ears); 9) Perceived hearing loss; 10) Deviation on jaw opening; 11) Lateral neck and trapezius pain. **It has been difficult to estimate the actual incidence of whiplash associated TMJ disorders primarily due to the common delay in onset of symptoms, which may be as long as several months**. See Steigerwald DP. Acceleration/deceleation injury as a precipitating cause of temporomandibular joint dysfunction. ACA J Chiro., 26(11):61–64, 1989; Steigerwald DP, Croft AC. Whiplash and TMJ Disorders: an Interdisciplinary Approach to Case Management. La Jolla, J.B. Media Int., 1992.

Some estimates have been as high as 37 percent of those who were involved in whiplash-type collision injuries. Frankel VH. Temporomandibular pain syndrome following deceleration injury to the cervical spine. Bull Hosp Joint Dis., 26:47, 1969.

Some have suggested referred TMD pain from damaged soft-tissues from the posterior neck. Christensen LV, McKay DC. Reflex jaw motions and jaw stiffness pertaining to whiplash injury of the neck. Cranio. 1997 Jul;15(3):242–60.

The medullary dorsal reticular nucleus (a structure in the brainstem) plays a pronociceptive role in both acute and tonic inflammatory pain, leading to amplification of the nociceptive signal. Almeida A, Storkson R, Lima D, Hole K, Tjolsen A. The medullary dorsal reticular nucleus facilitates pain behaviour induced by formalin in the rat. Eur J Neurosci. 1999 Jan;11(1):110–22.

It (the medullary dorsal reticular nucleus) may also underlie the noxious response to the temporomandibular joint. Tsai C. The caudal subnucleus caudalis (medullary dorsal horn) acts as an interneuronal relay site in craniofacial nociceptive reflex activity. Brain Res. 1999 May 1;826(2):293–7.

There does seem to be some kind of relationship between motor vehicle accidents with other studies that have reported objective tissue damage to the TMJ in patients with a history of whiplash injury. **Goldberg et al reported that post-traumatic TMD sufferers reported higher levels of pain in the jaw musculature and showed similarities to patients with mild traumatic brain injury**. (The brain is an active part of the descending pain inhibition system.) Goldberg MB, Mock D, Ichise M, Proulx G, Gordon A, Shandling M, Tsai S, Tenenbaum HC. Neuropsychologic deficits and clinical features of posttraumatic temporomandibular disorders. J Orofac Pain. 1996 Spring;10(2):126–40.

Garcia and Arrington found that whiplash patients were significantly more likely to have TMJ changes evident on MRI, and concluded that TMJ tissue damage should be evaluated in all whiplash patients. Segmental limitations (especially at the C0–C3 levels and tender points SCM, trapezius), are significantly more present with patient of temporomandibular disorders. Garcia R Jr, Arrington JA. The relationship between cervical whiplash and temporomandibular joint injuries: an MRI study. Cranio. 1996 Jul;14(3):233–9; De Laat A, Meuleman H, Stevens A, Verbeke G. Correlation between cervical spine and tempromandibular disorders. Clin Oral Invest 1998;2:54–7.

The TMJ, cervical spine and shoulder girdle should be evaluated in patients with complex or persistent symptoms in the head and neck region. de Wijer A, Steenks MH, de Leeuw JR, Bosman F, Helders PJ. Symptoms of the cervical spine in temporomandibular and cervical spine disorders. J Oral Rehabil. 1996 Nov;23(11):742–50.

The TMJ can refer pain to the neck. Hellstrom F, Thunberg J, Bergenheim M, Sjolander P, Djupsjobacka M, Johansson H. Increased intra-articular concentration of bradykinin in the temporomandibular joint changes the sensitivity of muscle spindles in dorsal neck muscles in the cat. Neurosci Res. 2002 Feb;42(2):91–9.

Our results suggest that neck injury, leading to whiplash associated disorders, is associated with **deranged control of mandibular and head-neckmovements during jaw opening-closing tasks**, and therefore might compromise natural jaw function. The present findings should be taken into account in assessment and management of patients in pain and dysfunction following neck injury, and in related research. Eriksson P-O, Zafar H, Ha"ggman-Henrikson B. Deranged jaw-neck motor control in whiplash-associated disorders. Eur J Oral Sci 2004; 112: 25–32.

The relationship between forward head posture and temporomandibular disorders. This study investigated the relationship between forward head posture and temporomandibular disorder symptoms. Thirty-three temporomandibular disorder patients with predominant complaints of masticatory muscle pain were compared with an age- and gender-matched control group. Head position was measured from photographs taken with a plumb line drawn from the ceiling to the lateral malleolus of the ankle and with a horizontal plane that was perpendicular to the plumb line and that passed through the spinous process of the seventh cervical vertebra. The distances from the plumb line to the ear, to the seventh vertebra, and to the shoulder were measured. Two angles were also measured: (1) ear-seventh cervical vertebra-horizontal plane; and (2) eye-ear-seventh cervical vertebra. The only measurement that revealed a statistically significant difference was angle ear-seventh cervical vertebra-horizontal plane. This angle was smaller in the patients with temporomandibular disorders than in the control subjects. In other words, **when evaluating the ear position with respect to the seventh cervical vertebra, the head was positioned more forward in the group with temporomandibular disorders than in the control group** ($P < .05$). Lee WY, Okeson JP, Lindroth J. The relationship between forward head posture and temporomandibular disorders. J Orofac Pain. 1995 Spring;9(2):161–7.

Temporomandibular disorders, headaches, and neck pain after motor vehicle accidents: a pilot investigation of persistence and litigation effects. There is a lack of long-term follow-up studies that involve post-motor vehicle accident temporomandibular disorders and compensation. The purposes of this retrospective pilot study were: (1) to assess patients who had previously been treated for temporomandibular disorders after motor vehicle accidents to determine the nature of their symptoms in terms of jaw, head, and neck pain and jaw dysfunction; and (2) to determine whether there was a difference in the pain and dysfunction between those who had settled and those who had not settled their insurance claims. Thirty previously treated patients with temporomandibular disorders after motor vehicle accidents were questioned by telephone regarding litigation status and current jaw, head, and neck pain and jaw dysfunction symptoms. **They did not differ substantially from a smaller group who were not able to be interviewed.** Descriptive statistics were calculated and statistical tests were performed. A total of 22 patients had their claims settled. Approximately 75% had persistent complaints of jaw pain, jaw dysfunction, and headache, and more than 80% reported persistent neck pain. No apparent differences were found between those who had and had not settled their insurance claims. **Jaw, head, and neck pain, and jaw dysfunction continued to be problems for the majority of this patient population, regardless of litigation status** in this retrospective study. Kolbinson DA, Epstein JB, Burgess JA, Senthilselvan A. Temporomandibular disorders, headaches, and neck pain after motor vehicle accidents: a pilot investigation of persistence and litigation effects. J Prosthet Dent. 1997 Jan;77(1):46–53.

Endurance during chewing in whiplash-associated disorders and TMD. An association was previously shown between neck injury and disturbed jaw function. This study tested the hypothesis of a relationship between neck injury and impaired endurance during chewing. Fifty patients with whiplash-associated disorders (WAD) were compared with 50 temporomandibular disorders (TMD) patients and 50 healthy subjects. Endurance was evaluated during unilateral chewing of gum for 5 minutes when participants reported fatigue and pain. Whereas all healthy subjects completed the task, 25% of the TMD and a majority of the WAD patients discontinued the task. **A majority of the WAD patients also reported fa-**

tigue and pain. These findings suggest an **association between neck injury and reduced functional capacity of the jaw motor system**. From the results, we propose that **routine examination of WAD patients should include jaw function** and that an endurance test as described in this study could also be a useful tool for non-dental professionals. Haggman-Henrikson B, Osterlund C, Eriksson PO. Endurance during chewing in whiplash-associated disorders and TMD. J Dent Res. 2004 Dec;83(12):946–50.

§ 6:41 Shoulder, arm and hand complaints—Temporomandibular joint disorders and whiplash—Imaging the TMJ

Researchers performed MRI scans on 87 whiplash patients (174 joints) with TMJ pain. These subjects had no direct trauma to the face in the accident and had no pre-accident TMJ symptoms. The study found that, "**Internal derangement was present in 143/164 (87%) of the TMJs. 118/164 (72%) demonstrated displacement with reduction (DDR), and 25/164 (15%) demonstrated disk displacement without reduction (DDNR); only 21/164 (13%) of the TMJs were found to be normal**." Garcia R Jr, Arrington JA. The relationship between cervical whiplash and temporomandibular joint injuries: an MRI study. Cranio. 1996 Jul;14(3):233–9.

One hundred patients with TMJ disorders (200 TMJs) were investigated by an experienced radiologist with HR-US (**high resolution ultrasound**) and **magnetic resonance imaging** (MRI). The MRI investigation showed degenerative changes in 190 joints (95%), while an effusion was found in 59 (29.5%) joints. At closed-mouth position a disc dislocation was found in 138 joints (69%) and in maximum-mouth-opening position disc dislocation was diagnosed in 76 joints (38%). In the determination of degenerative changes HR-US showed a sensitivity of 94%, a specificity of 100% and an accuracy of 94%. In the detection of effusion HR-US yielded a sensitivity of 81%, a specificity of 100% and an accuracy of 95%. In the determination of disk displacement at closed-mouth position HR-US showed a sensitivity, specificity and an accuracy of 92% each. At maximum-mouth-opening position HR-US reached a sensitivity of 86%, a specificity of 91% and an accuracy of 90%. **The results of the current study imply that HR-US is a valuable diagnostic imaging method of the TMJ** which can be used as an alternative method to a MRI-investigation, but is yet not able to replace it. Jank S, Emshoff R, Norer B, Missmann M, Nicasi A, Strobl H, Gassner R, Rudisch A,

Bodner G. Diagnostic quality of dynamic high-resolution ultrasonography of the TMJ—a pilot study. Int J Oral Maxillofac Surg. 2005 Mar;34(2):132–7.

MRI depicted intra-articular effusion in 41 of the 88 TMJs (46.5%) while no effusion was detected in the remaining 47 joints (53.5%). Ultrasonographic imaging revealed effusion in 42/88 joints (47.8%), while the remaining 46 joints (52.2%) showed no effusion. US showed a sensitivity of 75.6% and a specificity of 76.5%. The PPV and NPV were 73.8% and 78.2% respectively. US vs MRI agreement for the diagnosis of TMJ effusion was fairly good (pct. agreement 76.1%; K=0.521). Diagnostic ultrasound is a low-cost, easy-performing, non-invasive, rapidly-executing imaging technique whose possible employ in the study of the TMJ is very promising. Tognini F, Manfredini D, Melchiorre D, Zampa V, Bosco M. Ultrasonographic vs magnetic resonance imaging findings of temporomandibular joint effusion. Minerva Stomatol. 2003 Jul–Aug;52(7–8):365–70, 370–2.

§ 6:42 Shoulder, arm and hand complaints—Temporomandibular joint disorders and whiplash—Defense perspective on TMJ

A defense article on TMJ disorders, authored by Howard et al., asserted that forces at TMJ encountered during a CAD injury were no greater than those occurring during the simple act of chewing. As evidence for this, they provided a diagram illustrating the head-neck-jaw dynamics during a rear-impact collision. In their model, no motion occurs at the head-neck junction. Furthermore, no motion occurs in the cervical spine. There are two degrees of motion (flexion and extension) occurring at a pivot point at the cervicothoracic junction. Finally, as the head-neck moves into extension, the jaw does not open. See Howard RP, Benedict JV, Raddin JH Jr, Smith HL. Assessing neck extension-flexion as a basis for temporomandibular joint dysfunction. J Oral Maxillofac Surg. 1991 Nov;49(11):1210–3.

If one considers this a reliable model, the hypothesis might have some credibility. However, there is virtually no experimental evidence to verify or support such a simplistic model. **After the publication of the Howard paper, the American Academy of Head, Neck, Facial Pain & TMJ Orthopedics published a critical review of the paper, pointing out its numerous flaws and calling it "unfortunate."** See Rogal OJ, Haden J, Keropian B, et al. (representing the College of Trauma, American Academy of Head, Neck, Facial Pain and TMJ Orthopedics): Whiplash-TMD theory refuted. News J Am Acad Head Neck Facial Pain TMJ Orthop 4(1):3–4, 19.

§ 6:43 Vertebral artery injury and whiplash

The vertebral artery is the pipeline carrying blood and oxygen to the brain stem. After passing through the foramen transversarium of the atlas, the vertebral artery turns sharply medially, pierces the thick membrane between the atlas and the occiput, and enters the cranial cavity through the foramen magnum. "Very little slack exists in the vertebral artery and, during severe hyperextension and hyperflexion and especially during extreme lateral rotation, partial to complete obstruction of the vertebral artery has been demonstrated by arteriography." Angiography has shown constriction or occlusion of the vertebral artery in patients with persistent symptoms of vertigo, ataxia, headache, diplopia, and unsteadiness of gait. "The usual site of occlusion is at the second cervical level, which is the point of greatest rotation of the head on the neck." **"A great majority of symptoms that have been designated as psychoneurotic, namely, attacks of vertigo, ataxia, diplopia, severe attacks of migraine-like headache, hemicrania with nausea and vomiting, and, at times disturbances of speech and swallowing, are all due to disturbed circulation of the vertebral artery after neck sprain."** Seletze E. Whiplash injuries; neuro-physiological basis for pain and methods used for rehabilitation. J Am Med Assoc. 1958 Nov 29;168(13):1750–5.

With head-forward, "head extension occurred causing minimal VA elongation. In sharp contrast, rotated head posture at the time of rear impact caused dramatic effects on VA elongation peaks and timing." **Significant increases in dynamic vertebral artery elongation above physiological limits were observed due to head-turned rear impact beginning at 5 g, while no significant increases due to head-forward rear impact were observed.** "Dynamic VA elongation of up to 30.5 mm due to head-turned rear impact significantly exceeded physiological values beginning at 5 g, while VA elongation during head-forward rear impact remained within physiological limits." Chronic symptoms in whiplash patients include headaches, blurred vision, tinnitus, dizziness, and vertigo. Peak VA elongation occurred as early as 84.5 ms following head-turned rear impact. Cervical muscle activity can be achieved no earlier than 192 ms following head-turned rear impact. Thus, VA injury during head-turned rear impact occurs prior to neuromuscular protective mechanisms achieved via peak muscle tension. "In contrast, peak VA elongation during head-forward rear impact occurred significantly later. **Elongation-induced VA injury is more likely to occur in those with rotated head posture at the time of rear impact, as compared to head forward.**" Because the cadavers used in this study were between 70 – 80 years old, their spinal mechanical properties are stiffer than those of a younger population, which would reduce the stress on the vertebral artery. Therefore, the "peak dynamic VA elongation data of the present study are conservative, as compared to the younger population." "VA elongation causes a decrease in its diameter due to Poisson's effect and may lead to transient vascular compromise." While being elongated, the VA may be pinched and injured, potentially tearing the intimal layer, primarily at C1–C2. "Severe VA injury results in acute vascular compromise caused by arterial dissection with possible rupture or thrombosis leading to stroke." In the present study, head-turned rear impact caused highest peak elongation rate in the left VA, significantly greater (more than 6 times greater) than the corresponding head-forward peak rate. The high elongation rate observed due to head-turned rear impact may accentuate elongation-induced injury of the vertebral artery. Ivancic PC, Ito S, Tominaga Y, Carlson EJ, Rubin W, Panjabi MM. Effect of rotated head posture on dynamic vertebral artery elongation during simulated rear impact. Clin Biomech (Bristol, Avon). 2006 Mar;21(3):213–20.

Both neck manipulation and motor vehicle collision events apply loads to the spinal column rapidly. While neck manipulation loads are slower to develop and displacements smaller, they may reach peak amplitudes on maximum effort comparable to those seen in low-velocity collision experiments. In contrast to reports that the vertebral artery experiences elongations exceeding its physiological range by up to 9.0 mm during simulated whiplash, strains incurred during cervical manipulative therapy have been reported to be approximately one ninth of those required for mechanical failure, comparable to forces encountered in the course of diagnostic range of motion examination. Additionally, long-lasting abnormalities of blood flow velocity within the vertebral artery have been reported in patients following common whiplash injuries, whereas no significant changes in vertebral artery peak flow velocity were observed following cervical chiropractic manipulative therapy. Perceived causation of reported cases of cervical artery dissection is more frequently attributed to chiropractic manipulative therapy procedures than to motor vehicle collision related injuries, even though the comparative biomechanical evidence makes such causation unlikely. **The direct evidence suggests that the healthy vertebral artery is not at risk from properly performed chiropractic manipulative procedures.** Haneline M, Triano J. Cervical artery dissection. A comparison of highly dynamic mechanisms: manipulation versus motor vehicle collision. J Manipulative Physiol Ther. 2005 Jan;28(1):57–63.

The S-shaped phase shift of the spine in a whiplash injury may also have effects on vertebral artery. Nibu K, Cholewicki J, Panjabi MM, Babat LB, Grauer JN, Kothe R, Dvorak J. Dynamic elongation of the vertebral artery during an in vitro whiplash simulation. Eur Spine J. 1997;6(4):286–9; Seric V, Blazic-Cop N, Demarin V. Haemodynamic changes in patients with whiplash injury measured by transcranial Doppler sonography (TCD). Coll Antropol. 2000 Jun;24(1):197–204.

In a study by Chung et al, 29 patients with vertebrobasilar dissections (VBD) were evaluated to investigate the correlation between minor trauma and VBD and the clinical features of this trauma-related condition. Mean age was 43 years, with a male predominance (male/female ratio was 25/4). Seventeen patients presented with subarachnoid hemorrhage (SAH), and 12 with ischemic symptoms. Two patients presenting with ischemia had extracranial VBD (V3 segment). Seven patients had received minor or trivial head/cervical trauma, due to whiplash injury, minor fall, or during exercise, which were identified to precede with the lapse of some time (a few minutes or days) the onset of symptoms. **All of these patients presented with ischemic symptoms, and they were younger than the other ischemic or SAH patients. The site of vertebral artery dissection was intracranial in four cases, extracranial in one case, and combined in two cases. The clinicopathological findings of ischemia and angiographic narrowing/occlusion suggest that dissections were subintimal. Therefore, it is believed that this minor or trivial trauma may primarily cause subintimal dissection with luminal compromise, leading to ischemic symptoms, rather than subadventitial or transmural dissection with aneurysmal dilatation, leading to SAH.** This lesion may also occur in younger patients with a favorable outcome. Careful note should be made of patient for the early recognition of this disorder. See Chung YS, Han DH. Vertebrobasilar dissection: a possible role of whiplash injury in its pathogenesis. Neurol Res. 2002 Mar;24(2):129–38.

§ 6:44 Vertigo and dizziness

As discussed earlier, whiplash can produce non-painful conditions. The cause may be the over-excitation of the joint receptors that are injured or stimulated in a whiplash injury. This may produce a proprioceptive disturbance. Proprioception is the knowledge of where your body parts are. Proprioceptive receptors in the cervical spine play a key role in the Posture Control System (PCS)—the mechanism by which the body maintains balance and equilibrium.) See Hinoki studies below.

§ 6:45 Vertigo and dizziness—Input to cerebellum from spine

Cerebellar symptoms can be manifested by over-excitation of cervical and lumbar proprioceptors. Autonomic reflexes with, i.e. pupillo-constrictory reaction to light, are from over-excitation of the cervical proprioceptors. **Sympathetically induced hypertonicity of the deep neck muscles can cause disturbances of the oculomotor system (abnormal eye movement), particularly in the brain stem.** Hinoki M. Vertigo due to whiplash injury: a neurotological approach. Acta Otolaryngol Suppl. 1984;419:9–29; Hinoki M, Nakanishi K, Matsuura K, Ushio N. Proprio-vegetative reflexes in relation to bodily equilibrium: clinical observations on pupillary reactions in patients with neck and lumbar pain following whiplash injury. Agressologie. 1978;19(2):137–44.

Traumatic chronic cervical pain patients have shown impaired cervicocephalic kinesthetic sensibility. Non-traumatic neck pain patients show little evidence of impaired cervicocephalic kinesthetic sensibility. Rix GD, Bagust J. Cervicocephalic kinesthetic sensibility in patients with chronic, nontraumatic cervical spine pain. Arch Phys Med Rehabil. 2001 Jul;82(7):911–9.

Neck proprioceptive input is primarily by muscle spindles. Richmond FJ, Abrahams VC. Physiological properties of muscle spindles in dorsal neck muscles of the cat. J Neurophysiol. 1979 Mar;42(2):604–17; Richmond FJ, Bakker DA. Anatomical organization and sensory receptor content of soft tissues surrounding upper cervical vertebrae in the cat. J Neurophysiol. 1982 Jul;48(1):49–61; Mergner T, Anastasopoulos D, Becker W. Neuronal responses to horizontal neck deflection in the group X region of the cat's medullary brainstem. Exp Brain Res. 1982;45(1–2):196–206; Anastasopoulos D, Mergner T, Becker W, Deecke L. Sensitivity of external cuneate neurons to neck rotation in three-dimensional space. Exp Brain Res. 1991;85(3):565–76.

A study reported that whiplash patients showed a significantly reduced ability to determine head placement. "Patients with whiplash injury return to their reference position after an active movement with significantly less accuracy than healthy subjects. It has been suggested that neck kinesthetic sensibility is involved in this inaccuracy. The whiplash subjects also showed less accuracy in vertical plane repositioning movements, which might be explained by the hyperextension, hyperflexion trauma mechanism. They showed an overshooting tendency in vertical plane repositioning movements and even a tendency in the horizontal plane movements. This overshooting could indicate a lack of proprioceptive information and a search for additional proprioceptive information coming from stretched antagonist muscles . . . " Heikkila H, Astrom PG. Cervicocephalic kinesthetic sensibility in patients with whiplash injury. Scand J Rehabil Med. 1996 Sep;28(3):133–8.

Symptoms of vertigo, dizziness, and visual disturbance are common after whiplash injuries, which may be due to the proprioceptive functions of the cervical spine. There were significant differences between the two groups on reading behavior. **The whiplash patients showed reading behaviors similar to children in the first three years of elementary school, while the control subjects showed behaviors in the high school range. These reading problems were found to be closely linked to problems with smooth pursuit.** See Gimse R, Tjell C, Bjorgen IA, Saunte C. Disturbed eye movements after whiplash due to injuries to the posture control system. J Clin Exp Neuropsychol. 1996 Apr;18(2):178–86.

Three distinct pathological conditions, related to different means by which dense intralabyrinthine particles interfere with the function of a semicircular canal and cause nystagmus and vertigo, are amenable to treatment with repositioning maneuvers. Known as benign paroxysmal positional vertigo and variants, these conditions are better designated collectively by the term "vestibular lithiasis." Each form requires a different treatment strategy of head maneuvers and application of other modalities to restore normal semicircular function and thereby eliminate the positional nystagmus and vertigo. Real-time observation of the nystagmus induced by the particles during the maneuvers can greatly facilitate the repositioning process. See Epley JM. Human experience with canalith repositioning maneuvers. Ann N Y Acad Sci. 2001 Oct;942:179–91.

§ 6:46 Cervicogenic headache

The onset of headache is an important variable that should be controlled for when attempting to characterize the physical impairments associated with cervicogenic headache. Dumas JP, Arsenault AB, Boudreau G, Magnoux E, Lepage Y, Bellavance A, Loisel P. Physical impairments in cervicogenic headache: traumatic vs. nontraumatic onset. Cephalalgia. 2001 Nov;21(9):884–93.

Previous car accidents, pre-existing headache and neck pain were more frequent in chronic CEH (cervicogenic headache) individuals than in those in the cohort without CEH. Range of motion in the neck was reduced in 65% of chronic CEH individuals hours after the accident, compared with 41% in the cohort. Cybex inclinometer, at 6 weeks and 1 year, demonstrated reduced extension in the neck. CEH seems to be present after whiplash injury, particularly in the early phase. It seems similar to, but probably not identical to, non-whiplash CEH. Drottning M, Staff PH, Sjaastad O. Cervicogenic headache (CEH) after whiplash injury. Cephalalgia. 2002 Apr;22(3):165–71.

We conclude that the high degree of cytokine and NO (nitric oxide) production in CH may depend on the differing pathophysiological mechanisms at work in CEH than in other forms of headache. Martelletti P. Proinflammatory pathways in cervicogenic headache. Clin Exp Rheumatol. 2000 Mar–Apr;18(2 Suppl 19):S33–8.

Neck disorders implicated as causes of headache fall into two groups: a) those in which the cervical lesions are unequivocally demonstrable, and in which treatment of those lesions helps the headache; these are widely accepted as causes of headache, and include congenital and acquired craniovertebral junction disorders, rheumatoid arthritis and ankylosing spondylitis of the upper cervical spine, and dissection or trauma to the carotid or vertebral arteries; **b) those in which the neck disorder is either banal or not objectively demonstrable, and which seldom improves following treatment of the neck**; these are not widely accepted as causes of headache; they include whiplash syndrome, segmental hypomobility-hypermobility syndrome, the posterior cervical sympathetic syndrome, cervical migraine, third occipital nerve headache, and cervicogenic headache. **Features of a headache suggesting its cervical origin are: 1) abrupt onset following sudden excessive movement of the head; 2) persistent unilateral suboccipital or oc-**

cipital pain; 3) consistent reproduction by neck movements and by nothing else; 4) abnormal postures of head and neck; 5) significant painful limitation of movement of upper cervical spine; 6) abnormal mobility at craniovertebral junction; 7) C2 sensory abnormalities or lower medulla or upper cervical cord signs. See Edmeads J. [Headache of cervical origin] Rev Prat. 1990 Feb 11;40(5):399–402. French.

Interleukin-1 beta (IL-1 beta) and Tumour Necrosis Factor-alpha (TNF-alpha) exert their multifunctional biological effect by promoting and increasing the molecular events of cellular inflammation. **The aim of this study was to find out whether the cytokine pattern of cervicogenic headache (CH) patients tends, like that seen in cluster headache, toward an inflammatory status**. Fifteen CH patients, diagnosed according to the 1998 CHISG criteria, were analysed for serum IL-beta (ELISA) and TNF-alpha (bioassay and ELISA), both during the natural course of a painful attack and during a phase of mechanically worsened pain. The control groups consisted of 15 migraine without aura (MWA) patients and 15 historically healthy subjects. The MWA patients were studied both during (MWA-IN) and outside (MWA-OUT) a migraine attack. Higher levels of both IL-1 beta and TNF-alpha were detected in the sera of CH patients than in that of MWA-IN and MWA-OUT and C subjects. A difference also emerged in CH between spontaneous and mechanically worsened pain phases. **We conclude that the degree of cytokine production may depend on the different pathophysiological mechanisms at work in MWA and CH.** See Martelletti P, Stirparo G, Giacovazzo M. Proinflammatory cytokines in cervicogenic headache. Funct Neurol. 1999 Jul–Sep;14(3):159–62.

§ 6:47 Mild Traumatic Brain Injuries (MTBI)

Brain function can be disrupted by trauma. Some of the symptoms included, but not limited to, are excessive sleepiness, inattention, difficulty concentrating, impaired memory, faulty judgment, depression, irritability, emotional outbursts, disturbed sleep, diminished libido, difficulty switching between two tasks, and slowed thinking. A severe brain injury can be easily observable with symptoms, including partial or complete paralysis, speech problems, impaired cognitive functioning, disability from employment, long periods of coma, and CT, MRI, SPECT, PET brain-imaging changes. Mild traumatic brain injury may cause long-term residual problems with symptoms not apparent to the casual observer. These symptoms that can occur even without a loss of consciousness at the time of the traumatic event include: headaches, dizziness, lethargy, memory loss, irritability, personality changes, cognitive deficits, and/or perceptual changes. Clinically, cerebral concussion then represents a graded set of syndromes that occur with tissue disruption (mechanical and/or biochemical). Ommaya states that the loading of the brain mass initially provides for the development of shear strain distributions in the peripheral aspects of the cortex. Increasing load severities results in the development of damaging shear strain distributions in a centripetal manner. **Involvement of the cortical and the subcortical structures is, therefore, always significant in cases in which the shear strain distribution results in damage to the mesencephalic part of the brain stem.** (The brain stem is composed of the mesencephalon (midbrain), pons and medulla and is an upward extension from the spinal cord). **Cortical structures such as the temporal lobes, frontal lobes and the orbital cortex may be prone to damage**. See Ommaya AK. Head injury mechanisms and the concept of preventive management: a review and critical synthesis. J Neurotrauma. 1995 Aug; 12(4):527–46.

Motion of the head in three dimensions is represented by three rotational degrees of freedom and by three translational degrees of freedom. **Rotational forces are more important than translation forces in producing brain injury from whiplash**. See Ommaya, AK, FJ Fisch, RM Mahone, P Corrao and F Letcher. Comparative Tolerances for Cerebral Concussion by Head Impact and Whiplash Injury in Primates. Society of Automotive Engineers, New York, 1970; Ommaya, AK. Mechanisms and Preventive Management of Head Injuries: A Paradigm for Injury Control. 32nd Annual Proceedings, Association for the Advancement of Automotive Medicine, 1988; Gennarelli TA, Ommaya AK, Thibault LE. Comparison of translational and rotational head motions in experimental cerebral concussion. SAE 710882.

Scaling of data obtained through sub-human primate testing resulted in the development of the 50% probability level for onset of cerebral concussion given as being at head rotational velocities exceeding 50 radians/sec with head accelerations exceeding 1800 radians/sec2 and may be as low as 1600 radians/sec2. Ommaya AK, Hirsch AE. Tolerances for cerebral concussion from head impact and whiplash in primates. J Biomech. 1971 Jan;4(1) :13–21.

Animal studies have indicated that a side impact may have a lower threshold to cause concussion. Hodgson VR, Thomas LM, Khalil TB. The role of impact location in reversible cerebral concussion. SAE tech paper 831618;1983.

Qualitative (visual) and quantitative (strain) results illustrate clearly the deformation of brain matter due to occipital deceleration. Strains of 0.02–0.05 were typical during these events (0.05 strain corresponds roughly to a 5% change in the dimension of a local tissue element). Notably, **compression in frontal regions and stretching in posterior regions were observed**. The motion of the brain appears constrained by structures at the frontal base of the skull; it must pull away from such constraints before it can compress against the occipital bone. This mechanism is consistent with observations of contrecoup injury in occipital impact. Bayly PV, Cohen TS, Leister EP, Ajo D, Leuthardt EC, Genin GM. Deformation of the human brain induced by mild acceleration. J Neurotrauma. 2005 Aug;22(8):845–56.

The injury predictors and injury levels were analyzed based on resulting brain tissue responses and were correlated with the site and occurrence of mild traumatic brain injury (MTBI). Predictions indicated that the shear stress around the brainstem region could be an injury predictor for concussion. **The estimated HIC15** (head injury criterion) **threshold levels for 25%, 50%, and 80% of probability of MTBI were 151, 240, and 369.** Apparently, the threshold derived from this study was less than the regulatory limit for serious brain injury of 1,000, specified in FMVSS 208. Zhang L, Yang KH, King AI. A proposed injury threshold for mild traumatic brain injury. J Biomech Eng. 2004 Apr;126(2):226–36.

The group with MTBI scored significantly higher on the majority of primary symptom dimensions and global distress indices of the SCL-90-R, compared to both the diabetes and non-clinical control groups. Analysis of individual cases further revealed that 68.2% of the participants in the group with MTBI were classified as positive cases, a rate significantly higher than that of the diabetes and non-clinical control groups. The group with MTBI or the number of cases classified as positive did not differ significantly from the group of individuals with whiplash associated disorder with respect to elevation of primary symptom dimensions or global distress indices. The results of this study suggest that the **SCL-90-R has considerable utility as a general measure of psychological and symptomatic distress following MTBI**. Westcott MC, Alfano DP. The symptom checklist-90-revised and mild traumatic brain injury. Brain Inj. 2005 Dec;19(14):1261–7.

Translational and rotational accelerations from blunt head impact can induce excessive brain strain and cause traumatic brain injuries. However, it is not clear which acceleration plays a major role in the mechanism. The current study used the SIMon human finite element head model (FEHM) and delineated the contributions of these accelerations using postmortem human subject (PMHS) lateral head impact experimental data. Results indicated that rotational acceleration contributes more than 90% of total strain, and translational acceleration produces minimal strain. Therefore, **the rotational component is a more important biomechanical metric in this study**. Zhang J, Yoganandan N, Pintar FA, Gennarelli TA. Role of translational and rotational accelerations on brain strain in lateral head impact. Biomed Sci Instrum. 2006;42:501–6.

Intracranial hypotension following motor vehicle accident: an overlooked cause of post-traumatic head and neck pain?

Motor vehicle accidents result in many patients with chronic head and neck pain, some of which meet the criteria for a "whiplash syndrome." The cervical zygapophysial joint synovium, muscular, and ligamentous strains and other anatomical sites are often implicated in the pathophysiology of these cases. Some patients have a characteristic constellation of vague neurological symptoms, often including **headache, posterior neck discomfort, dizziness**, **nausea**, and **sometimes visual changes**. Recently presented research has noted that some patients who have a whiplash-associated disorder have imaging findings consistent with a **low-pressure cerebrospinal fluid leak**. Some of these patients respond favorably to high-volume epidural blood patch.

Huntoon MA, Watson JC. Intracranial hypotension following motor vehicle accident: an overlooked cause of post-traumatic head and neck pain? Pain Pract. 2007 Mar;7(1):47–52

Epidural blood patch therapy for chronic whiplash-associated disorder.

Patients with chronic whiplash-associated disorder (WAD) complain of symptoms such as **headache, dizziness, and nausea**.

These symptoms are also often experienced by patients with cerebrospinal fluid (CSF) leak. It was recently reported that radioisotope (RI) cisternography is useful in the diagnosis of intracranial hypotension due to CSF leak.

We investigated the relation between chronic WAD and CSF

leak by RI cisternography and evaluated whether epidural blood patch (EBP) administration is effective in the treatment of chronic WAD. We studied 66 patients with chronic WAD with symptoms lasting longer than 3 mo. All patients underwent RI cisternography to determine the presence of CSF leak. In patients in whom CSF leak was identified, EBP was administered. Symptoms were assessed before, 1 wk after, and 6 mo after EBP. Work status was also assessed and follow-up RI cisternography was performed.

Of the 66 patients, 37 showed CSF leak, and 36 of these patients received EBP 2.2 +/- 0.7 times. **The mean duration of symptoms was 33 mo.** One week after EBP, the percentage of patients with symptoms was decreased significantly compared with that before EBP; headache: **100%** vs 17%, respectively, **memory loss: 94%** vs 28%, **dizziness: 83%** vs 47%, **visual impairment: 81%** vs 25%, **nausea: 78%** vs 42% ($P < 0.01$). These effects were also observed at the 6 month follow-up examination ($P < 0.01$). Work status was also significantly improved at follow-up.

We conclude that CSF leak should be considered in some cases of chronic WAD and that EBP is an effective therapy for chronic WAD.

Ishikawa S, Yokoyama M, Mizobuchi S, Hashimoto H, Moriyama E, Morita K. Epidural blood patch therapy for chronic whiplash-associated disorder. Anesth Analg. 2007 Sep;105(3):809–14.

Chronic headache after cranio-cervical trauma—hypothetical pathomechanism based upon neuroanatomical considerations.

Chronic headache after whiplash injury is common, but the underlying mechanisms have not yet been elucidated. On the basis of human neuroanatomy, we hypothesize that rear-end collision can cause leakage of the cerebrospinal fluid (CSF) into the epidural space most frequently at the lumbosacral level, inducing chronic headache.

We considered that the following phenomena would be evident in patients with chronic headache after rear-end collision: (1) **orthostatic headache** with early onset and long duration, (2) low intracranial pressure (ICP =or< 60 mm H2O), (3) CSF leakage mainly in the lumbosacral region on radioisotope-myelocisternography, and (4) diffuse pachymeningeal enhancement (DPE) on gadolinium enhanced magnetic resonant image (Gd-MRI). The clinical signs and symptoms, ICP and neuroimaging findings were analyzed retrospectively in 20 patients who complained of chronic headache after rear-end collisions.

Headaches were orthostatic and started on the day of the accident in 14 patients. The headaches lasted more than 3 months in all patients. Mean ICP was 120 +/- 30 cm H2O. Only one patient showed low ICP. RI-myelocisternography revealed signs of CSF leakage at the lumbosacral level in 10 patients. Gd-MRI showed no abnormalities known to be characteristic of spontaneous intracranial hypotension (SIH). Chronic headache disappeared or was diminished in all patients by epidural blood patching in the lumbosacral region.

This clinical study partly supports the validity of our verifiable hypothetical mechanism. The ICP is not low and DPE is not observed on Gd-MRI. Therefore, CSF leakage into the epidural space may not occur, but spinal CSF absorption may be over-activated. This condition may represent a new clinical entity.

Takagi K, Bolke E, Peiper M, van Griensven M, Orth K, Son JH, Ueno T, Oshima M. Chronic headache after cranio-cervical trauma—hypothetical pathomechanism based upon neuroanatomical considerations. Eur J Med Res. 2007 Jun 27;12(6):249–54.

Both whiplash injury and concussion alter processing of the middle-latency SEP component N60 in the acute post traumatic period. The acute changes appear to normalize between three-six months post injury. The SEP similarities suggest that the overlapping clinical symptomatology post whiplash and concussion may reflect a similar underlying mechanism of rotational mild traumatic brain injury.

Zumsteg D, Wennberg R, Gutling E, Hess K. Whiplash and concussion: similar acute changes in middle-latency SEPs. Can J Neurol Sci. 2006 Nov;33(4):379–86.

This study addresses head responses causing concussion in National Football League players. Although efforts are underway to reduce impact acceleration through helmet padding, further study is needed of head kinematics after impact and their contribution to concussion, including rapid head displacement, z-axis rotation, and neck tension up to the time of maximum strain in the midbrain. **Neck strength influences head (DELTA) V** and head injury criterion and may help explain different concussion risks in professional and youth athletes, women, and children.

Viano D, Casson I, Pellman E. Concussion in professional football: Biomechanics of the struck player-Part 14. Neurosurgery. 2007 Aug;61(2):313–328.

§ 6:48 Mild Traumatic Brain Injuries (MTBI)—Defense perspective on MTBI

A common defense tactic is to assert that "primate studies show it takes 100 to 200 G forces to produce brain injury." This is based on a study that indicated 100 "G" forces produce concussion in 50% of tested rhesus monkeys. The definition of concussion in this study was a loss of responses to aversive stimuli and abolition of superficial reflexes. See Ommaya AK, Faas F, Yarnell P. Whiplash injury and brain damage: an experimental study. JAMA. 1968 Apr 22;204(4):285–9. *Based on this definition, these are not mild brain injuries.*

Another defense assertion is that "closed head injury does not occur at less than 70 Gs of acceleration." This was based on experimentally induced brain hemorrhage in ferrets. Viano DC, Lovsund P. Biomechanics of brain and spinal-cord injury: analysis of neuropathic and neurophysiologic experiments. J Crash Prevention and Injury Control 1999;1:35–43.

In Ommaya & Hirsch, tolerance for cerebral concussion in primates indicated the smaller the brain the better tolerance to concussion. Their criteria for concussion were:

Loss of coordinated responses to external stimuli

Apnea > 3 sec. followed by irregular slow respiration

Bradycardia (rate decreased by 20–30 beats/min)

Loss of corneal and palpebral reflexes

Loss of voluntary movements

Pupillary dilation > 15 sec.

This study extrapolates the 50% injury threshold for humans would be 1,800 radians/sec2 and may be as low as 1,600 radians. (This is a rotational rate of the head). **Again, this criterion is more than a mild brain injury.** Ommaya AK, Hirsch AE. Tolerances for cerebral concussion from head impact and whiplash in primates. J Biomech. 1971 Jan;4(1):13–21.

§ 6:49 Mild Traumatic Brain Injuries (MTBI)—Definition of MTBI

American Congress of Rehabilitation Medicine (1993) defines a mild traumatic brain injury as follows: **the criteria for a person to have sustained a mild traumatic brain injury**

is manifested by any loss of memory for events immediately before or after the accident; any alteration in mental state at the time of the accident (e.g., feeling dazed, disoriented, or confused); focal neurological deficit(s) that may or may not be transient. See Mild Traumatic Brain Injury Committee of the Head Injury Special Interest Group of the American Congress of Rehabilitation Medicine. Definition of mild traumatic brain injury. J Head Trauma Rehabil 1993; 8: 86–7.

Following concussion, cerebral patholophysiology can be adversely affected for days in animals and weeks in humans. **Significant changes in cerebral glucose metabolism can exist in brain injured patients with normal Glasgow Coma Scores. Cerebral concussion is an event followed by a complex cascade of ionic, metabolic, and physiological events**. Giza CC, Hovda DA. The neurometabolic cascade of concussion. J Athletic Training 2001;36:228–35.

In relatively mild brain injuries, an excessive release of excitatory neurotransmitters, such as acetylcholine and excitatory amino acids (glutamate, aspartate), can contribute to the pathobiologic reaction in the brain resulting in permanent deficits. This process may be mediated by a loss of calcium homeostasis. Endogenous opiates may mediate some of the neurologic damage. **Minor TBI can produce diffuse reductions in cerebral metabolic activity and disrupt the blood-brain-barrier**. See Hayes RL, Dixon CE. Neurochemical changes in mild head injury. Semin Neurol. 1994 Mar;14(1):25–31; Zwienenberg M, Gong QZ, Berman RF, Muizelaar JP, Lyeth BG. The effect of groups II and III metabotropic glutamate receptor activation on neuronal injury in a rodent model of traumatic brain injury. Neurosurgery. 2001 May;48(5):1119–26.

§ 6:50 Mild Traumatic Brain Injuries (MTBI)—Definition of MTBI—The neurophysiology of brain injury (Gaetz)

With mild forces, the sequence begins at the surface of the brain and progressively affects deeper structures as forces become more severe. A classification system was developed to identify the progressive grades of cerebral injury ranging from minor to severe disruptions of consciousness. Briefly, **grades I and II** involved cortical-subcortical disconnection, grades III and IV involved cortical-subcortical and diencephalic disconnection, with grades IV and V involving cortical-subcortical, diencephalic, and mesencephalic disconnection. According to their system, a **grade I to II concussion may involve memory disturbance without loss of motor control and partially impaired awareness**. In this case they suggested that significant mechanical strains did not reach the reticular system. On the other hand, severe cases typically demonstrated greater degrees of diffuse irreversible damage and when diffuse damage reached a critical point, a grade V coma occurred. Gaetz M. The neurophysiology of brain injury. Clinical Neurophysiology 2004;115:4–18.

Another point reinforced by the Ommaya-Gennarelli model was the notion of a continuum of injury. **Succinctly stated, mild, moderate, and severe brain injuries caused by A/D (acceleration/deceleration) forces are not discrete entities but occur on a continuum ranging from the surface of the brain inward with increasing amounts of damage occurring at each level of depth as forces increase.** This concept has been supported recently in an animal model where mild to moderate forces caused traumatic axonal injury (TAI) in corpus callosum, with animals exposed to the most impact energy showing the greatest number of abnormalities. In another study, mild forces produced no loss of delayed microtubule-associated protein-2 (MAP-2) within the ipsilateral dentate hilus, while moderately injured animals exhibited immunoreactive shrunken neurons and with MAP-2 changes observed in multiple areas of hippocampus. Id.

Numerous studies point to cellular injury that does not specifically involve brainstem, especially with injuries produced by mild to moderate forces. Others have shown that in subjects diagnosed with **mild TBI**, all lesions were located at the grey-white interface and associated white matter with none located in the brainstem or corpus callosum. Id.

Within 30 min of a mild traumatic insult, scattered axons showed focal increases of labeled 68kD neurofilament immunoreactivity and slight swelling, sometimes accompanied by blebbing (multiple axonal swellings) or infolding of the axolemma, or both. In this group, there was focal neurofilament disarray, misalignment of the axon with local axolemmal infolding, with no HRP entering the intracellular milieu. Therefore an early distinction between mild and moderate injury was that moderate injury produced a perturbation of the axolemma large enough for the HRP tracer to enter the cell, while mild injuries disrupted the axolemma enough to allow entry of small molecular ion species. Nonetheless, both mild and moderate injuries resulted in densely packed neurofilaments and subsequent cellular pathology. Id.

Ca++ (calcium) has long been considered a primary factor in axonal neurofilament compaction caused by damage to the associated sidearms. However, recent studies have shown that damage to neurofilaments depends on a variety of factors and may not occur as previously thought. First, the degree of neurofilament damage varies with the severity of force applied to the cell. For example, mild TBI is associated with misalignment of the cytoskeleton while severe injuries cause rapid neurofilament compaction. Id.

Ca2+ influx occurs during stretch. One of the more recent perspectives regarding how Ca2+ enters the cell following stretch was a process labeled "mechanoporation". Mechanoporation was defined as the "development of transient defects in the cell membrane that are due to its mechanical deformation". The mechanically induced pores were considered to be either transient or stable, the latter associated with long-term membrane leakage. According to Gennarelli, ions were driven by diffusion through the pores and into cells with Ca2+ entering due to the large extracellular gradient. Choi suggested that the influx of extracellular Ca2+, combined with any Ca2+ release triggered from intracellular stores, would elevate cytosolic free Ca2+ and would be cytotoxic if Ca2+ levels were sustained for at least 4 reasons. Id.

A form of cytotoxic edema occurs during hypoxic conditions where cells swell within a period of seconds after a hypoxic episode due to failure of the adenosine triphosphate (ATP) dependent Na K pump. As a result, Na2+ rapidly accumulates within cells, as does water due to osmotic pressure.Asecond cause of cytotoxic edema involves increased amounts of extracellular excitatory amino acid neurotransmitters such as glutamate and glycine that can cause acute swelling in dendrites and cell bodies. The presence of **high extracellular glutamate** levels causes membrane channels to open, which in turn leads to Na2+ influx, membrane depolarisation, and secondary influx of Cl- and water resulting in excitotoxic swelling. This type of pathology, and the Ca2+ dependent late degeneration induced by **glutamate**, can act in isolation to produce irreversible neuronal injury. Id.

Mild injuries typically result in axonal damage found within brain parenchyma showing no other signs of neuronal or vascular change. In this case, vascular disruption does not appear to influence the overall pathogenesis of axonal swelling and disconnection. Moderate to severe injuries on the other hand frequently result in vasculature damage. It is important for the neurophysiologist to understand the pathophysiology of

TBI, and to understand features of injury including the fact that impact is not required for significant damage to occur and that **mild A/D forces can cause injury to axons and dendrites in the presence of non-injured neural tissue and cerebrovasculature.** Gaetz M. The neurophysiology of brain injury. Clinical Neurophysiology 2004;115:4–18.

See also Kushner D. Mild traumatic brain injury: toward understanding manifestations and treatment. Arch Intern Med. 1998 Aug 10–24;158(15):1617–24.

§ 6:51 Mild Traumatic Brain Injuries (MTBI)—Definition of MTBI—Diagnostic grading scales of concussion

Severity of Grade			
Guidelines/ Source	**1**	**2**	**3**
Cantu	(1) No loss of consciousness (2) Post-traumatic amnesia last less than 30 min.	(1) Loss of consciousness less than 5 min. OR (2) Post-traumatic amnesia lasts longer than 30 min.	(1) Loss of consciousness lasts longer than 5 min. OR (2) Post-traumatic amnesia lasts longer than 24 hr.
Colorado	(1) Confusion without amnesia (2) No loss of consciousness	(1) Confusion with amnesia (2) No loss consciousness	(1) Loss of consciousness (of any duration)
Practice Parameter American Academy of Neurology	(1) Transient confusion (2) No loss of consciousness (3) Concussion symptom or mental status changes resolves in less than 15 min.	(1) Transient confusion (2) No loss of consciousness (3) Concussion symptoms or mental status change last longer than 15 min.	(1) Loss of consciousness (brief or prolonged)

Cantu RC. When to return to contact sports after a cerebral concussion. Sports Med Digest 1988;10:1–2.

Colorado Medical Society. Report of the Sports Medicine Committee. Guidelines for the management of concussion in sports. Denver: Colorado Medical Society; 1991.

Quality Standards Subcommittee, American Academy of Neurology. Practice Parameter. Neurology 1997;48:581–5.

§ 6:52 Mild Traumatic Brain Injuries (MTBI)—Serious and severe brain injury

Head accelerations as low as 30 g produce neuropsychological evidence of significant brain injury. **It must be concluded that accelerations in excess of 34 g can cause apparently irreversible brain injury.** Varney NR, Roberts RJ. Forces and accelerations in car accidents and resultant brain injuries. Chapter 3, pp:39–47. *The evaluation and treatment of mild traumatic brain injury.* Varney NR, Roberts RJ, eds. Lawrence Erlbaum Associates, Mahwah, New Jersey, 1999.

§ 6:53 Mild Traumatic Brain Injuries (MTBI)—Recovery and MTBI

Comment:

Most cases of mild brain injury are limited; the literature suggests that between **70–80% of patients with minor head trauma will recover quickly and without complications. The problem lies with the 20–30% of those with MTBI who have long-term problems**.

This study examined 70 patients with MTBI—35 at 6 months and 35 at 12 months or more. Each patient was given the Behavior Change Inventory (BCI). The BCI is a list of 68 behavior changes that are common after brain injury. The patient and the patient's spouse or close family member completed the survey. Only those behaviors that were marked by both individuals were recorded as a real behavior change. The results for these patients were compared with those from 40 non-injured control patients. **The authors state that many patients continue to have behavioral changes, even 12 months after the injury: "While most behavioral problems showed improvement, 21% tended to show significant behavioral impairment compared to controls at 12 or more months post-injury."** Treatment seemed to help:

"Neurobehavioral changes symptoms were considerably less severe among treated patients and, in fact, showed progressive lessening over time." See Hartlage LC, Durant-Wilson D, Patch PC. Persistent neurobehavioral problems following mild traumatic brain injury. Archives of Clinical Neuropsychology 2001;16:561–570.

§ 6:54 Mild Traumatic Brain Injuries (MTBI)—Lab tests and MTBI

Patients with high levels of **S-100B** at initial assessment (>2.5 µg/L) may represent a high risk group for disability after head trauma.

Townend W, Ingebrigtsen T. Head injury outcome prediction: A role for protein S-100B? Injury. 2006 Dec;37(12):1098–108.

Middle-latency somatosensory evoked potentials (SEPs) following median nerve stimulation can provide a sensitive measure of cortical function.

Both whiplash injury and concussion alter processing of the middle-latency SEP component N60 in the acute post traumatic period. The acute changes appear to normalize between three-six months post injury. The SEP similarities suggest that the overlapping clinical symptomatology **post whiplash and concussion** may reflect a similar underlying mechanism of **rotational mild traumatic brain injury.**

Zumsteg D, Wennberg R, Gutling E, Hess K. Whiplash and concussion: similar acute changes in middle-latency SEPs. Can J Neurol Sci. 2006 Nov;33(4):379–86.

S-100 is a protein synthesized by astroglial cells (supporting cells) in all parts of the central nervous system (CNS). Although not normally detectable in serum, following MTBI, it has been shown to be frequently elevated. It is also elevated in multiple sclerosis exacerbations, intracranial tumors, encephalomyelitis, and spinal cord compression. A recently conducted controlled study indicated that S-100 may be an important marker for persistent neurocognitive dysfunction after MTBI. **There appears to be a direct relationship between the concentration of serum S-100 and severity of brain injury. However, not all cases of MTBI will show an elevated protein level. The test must be conducted very soon after injury (peak levels occur at about two hours post-injury) because values decline steadily**. *See* Waterloo K, Ingebrigtsen T, Romner B. Neuropsychological function in patients with increased serum levels of protein S-100 after minor head injury. Acta Neurochir (Wien). 1997;139(1):26–31; discussion 31–2; Ingebrigtsen T, Romner B. Serial S-100 protein serum measurements related to early magnetic resonance imaging after minor head injury. J Neurosurg. 1996 Nov;85(5):945–8.

Determination of S-100 protein may be more related to post-concussion symptoms caused by mild traumatic brain injury than to symptoms of psychological origin. Ingebrigtsen T, Romner B, Marup-Jensen S, Dons M, Lundqvist C, Bellner J, Alling C, Borgesen SE. The clinical value of serum S-100 protein measurements in minor head injury: a Scandinavian multicentre study. Brain Inj. 2000 Dec;14(12):1047–55.

Undetectable serum levels of S-100 protein predict normal intracranial findings on CT scan, indicating serum S-100 protein may be used to select patients for CT scanning. Romner B, Ingebrigtsen T, Kongstad P, Borgesen SE. Traumatic brain damage: serum S-100 protein measurements related to neuroradiological findings. J Neurotrauma. 2000 Aug;17(8):641–7.

Evidence of changes in brain function in individual with persistent post-concussion symptoms is consistent with the position that the post-concussion syndrome has a substantial biological, as opposed to a psychological, basis. Gaetz M, Weinberg H. Electrophysiological indices of persistent post-concussion symptoms. Brain Inj. 2000 Sep;14(9):815–32.

Quantitative electroencephalography may help provide support for an organic basis for the subjective and objective cognitive dysfunction. Henry GK, Gross HS, Herndon CA, Furst CJ. Nonimpact brain injury: neuropsychological and behavioral correlates with consideration of physiological findings. Appl Neuropsychol. 2000;7(2):65–75.

The P300 recording is an electrophysiological marker of cognitive ability. The P300 amplitude indicates the amount of stimulus information that is processed, and the P300 latency denotes the speed of this processing. "The P300 event-related potential is a stimulus-independent wave related to cognitive processing of an unexpected stimulus. It is either delayed, absent, or of lower amplitude in a variety of confusional states or dementing disorders and in multiple sclerosis, but normal in depressive disorders." SPECT perfusion **abnormalities in patients with chronic whiplash syndrome correlate well with P300 recording (an electrophysiologic marker for**

cognitive ability). See Lorberboym M, Gilad R, Gorin V, Sadeh M, Lampl Y. Late whiplash syndrome: correlation of brain SPECT with neuropsychological tests and P300 event-related potential. J Trauma. 2002 Mar;52(3):521–6.

"None of the new brain imaging techniques nor quantitative EEG analyses have proved useful enough in the assessment of mild head injured, as well as whiplash, patients. The present study suggests an objective neurophysiological parameter, the P300 wave, as a possible diagnostic tool for the situation." Granovsky Y, Sprecher E, Hemli J, Yarnitsky D. P300 and stress in mild head injury patients. Electroencephalogr Clin Neurophysiol. 1998 Nov;108(6):554–9.

§ 6:55 Mild Traumatic Brain Injuries (MTBI)—Symptoms of MTBI after whiplash

In this study, **33 patients with mild traumatic brain injury (TBI) from whiplash accidents were given intensive interviews to observe the range of patient reactions to their injuries. The following reactions were observed:**Persistent altered consciousness: feelings of discomfort in one's body, dissociation, and being in a "fog." Cerebral personality disorder: a reduced intensity of feelings, apathy, depression, indifference. Aprosodia, or a lack of "expressive movements which serve communications and regulate social relationships" (i.e. facial responses, prosody of speech (e.g. deficits of pitch, loudness, timbre, tempo, stress, accent)). Irritability, violence, anger, anxiety. Personality changes. See Parker RS. The spectrum of emotional distress and personality changes after minor head injury incurred in a motor vehicle accident. Brain Inj. 1996 Apr;10(4):287–302.

Traumatic brain injury has been associated with many physical and neurobehavioral consequences, including pain problems. Documented most has been the presence of post-traumatic headaches that are associated with the postconcussion syndrome. This study therefore examined types and rates of chronic pain problems in patients seen in an outpatient brain injury rehabilitation program. A total of 104 patients were evaluated, 66 of whom were male and 38 female, and the average time postinjury was 26 months. Headaches were the most frequent chronic pain problem across both mild and the moderate/severe groups, although in the former, a significantly higher frequency was noted (89%) when compared against the latter group. The same relative rates were seen for chronic neck/shoulder, back, and other pain problems. **The mild group also showed a higher frequency of concurrent pain problems**, whereas in the moderate/severe group only one patient had more than one chronic pain problem. Results also showed that in the mild group neck/shoulder accompanied headaches 47% of the time, and back pain coexisted with headaches 44% of the time. These results underscore the high frequency of chronic pain problems in the mild head injury population and implicate the need for avoiding the mislabeling of symptoms such attentional deficits or psychological distress as attributable only to head injury sequelae in those with coexisting chronic pain.

Uomoto JM, Esselman PC. Traumatic brain injury and chronic pain: differential types and rates by head injury severity. Arch Phys Med Rehabil. 1993 Jan;74(1):61–4.

Chronic pain was reported by 58% of mild TBI and 52% of moderate/severe TBI patients. Headaches were the most commonly reported pain problem. Chronic headaches were reported by 47% of mild TBI patients and 34% of moderate/ severe TBI patients. Neck/shoulder, back, upper limb, and lower limb pain were reported similarly by mild and moderate/severe TBI patients.

Findings indicate that chronic pain is a significant problem in mild and moderate/severe TBI patients.

Lahz S, Bryant RA. Incidence of chronic pain following traumatic brain injury. Arch Phys Med Rehabil. 1996 Sep;77(9) :889–91.

Painful regions also exhibited very high rates of allodynia, hyperpathia and exaggerated wind-up. The characteristics of the chronic pain resembled those of other central pain patients although TBIP displayed several unique features. **Neuronal hyperexcitability** may be a contributing factor to the chronic pain.

Ofek H, Defrin R. The characteristics of chronic central pain after traumatic brain injury. Pain. 2007 Oct;131(3):330–40.

Pain in patients with mild TBI

Ten studies [1–10] reported the prevalence of pain in patients with mild traumatic brain injury (TBI). Of the 1046 patients included in these studies, 788 reported pain, producing a prevalence rate of 75.3% (95% CI, 72.7%–77.9%).

Nine studies [3,9. 10 11. 12–15,] furnished data on the prevalence of pain in patients with severe traumatic brain injury TBI. Of the 1063 patients included in these studies, 341 reported chronic pain, producing a prevalence rate of 32.1% (95% CI, 29.3%–34.9%).

Although this review confirmed the clinical perception that patients with **mild TBI have a higher prevalence of chronic pain syndromes than those with moderate to severe TBI** (*P*<.001).

1. Alfano DP, Asmundson GJG, Larsen DK, et al. MTBI and chronic pain: preliminary findings [abstract]. Arch Clin Neuropsychol. 2000;15:831–832.

2. Alfano DP. Emotional and pain-related factors in neuropsychological assessment following mTBI. BrainCogn. 2006;60(2):193–217.

3. Beetar JT, Guilmette TJ, Sparadeo FR. Sleep and pain complaints in symptomatic TBI and neurologic populations. Arch Phys Med Rehabil. 1996;77(12):1298–1302.

4. Jensen OK, Nielsen FF. The influence of sex and pre-traumatic HA on the incidence and severity of HA after head injury. Cephalalgia. 1990;10(6):285–293.

5. Lahz S, Bryant RA. Incidence of chronic pain following TBI. Arch Phys Med Rehabil. 1996;77(9):889–891.

6. Mooney G, Speed J, Sheppard S. Factors related to recovery after mTBI. Brain Inj. 2005;19(12):975–987.

7. Rimel RW, Giordani B, Barth JT, et al. Disability caused by minor head injury. Neurosurgery. 1981; 9(3):221–228.

8. Smith-Seemiller L, Fow NR, Kant R, et al. Presence of post-concussion syndrome symptoms in patients with chronic pain vs. mTBI. Brain Inj. 2003;17(3):199–206.

9. Uomoto JM, Esselman PC. TBI and chronic pain:differential types and rates by head injury severity. Arch Phys Med Rehabil. 1993;74(1):61–64.

10. Yamaguchi M. Incidence of headache and severity of head injury. Headache. 1992;32(9):427–431.

11. Bryant RA, Marosszeky JE, Crooks J, et al. Interaction of posttraumatic stress disorder and chronic pain following TBI. J Head Trauma Rehabil. 1999;14(6):588–594.

12. Cosgrove JL, Vargo M, Reidy ME. A prospective study of peripheral nerve lesions occurring in traumatic brain-injured patients. Am J Phys Med Rehabil.1989;68(1):15–17.

13. Garland DE, Blum CE, Waters RL. Periarticular heterotopic ossification in head-injured adults: incidence and location. J Bone Joint Surg Am. 1980;62(7):1143–1146.

14. Gellman H, Keenan ME, Stone L, et al. Reflex sympathetic dystrophy in brain-injured patients. Pain. 1992;51(3) :307–311.

15. Hoffman JM, Pagulayan KF, Zawaideh N, et al.

Understanding pain after TBI: impact on community participation. Am J Phys Med Rehabil. 2007;86(12):962–969.

§ 6:56 Forces on head from low speed whiplash

During a low speed whiplash injury (7 mph) the head may be accelerated to 9–18 *g*. West DH, Gough JP, Harper TK: Low speed collision testing using human subjects. Accid Reconstr J 1993;5(3):22–26.

Since the brain is a soft structure, shear strains are created as the outer part of the brain moves at a different pace than the inner part of the brain. This is intensified as the momentum of the head changes rapidly in a sagittal direction during a whiplash trauma. **Controlled low speed crash studies have produced angular accelerations of volunteers' heads of up to 1000 rad/sec, in one study, to as high as 1260 rad/sec2 in another.** See van den Kroonenberg A, Philippens H, Cappon J, Wismans J, Hell W, Langweider K: Human head-neck response during low-speed rear end impacts. Proceedings of the 42nd Stapp Car Crash Conference, SAE 983157, 207–221, 1998; Siegmund GP, King DJ, Lawrence JM, Wheeler JB, Brault JR, Smith TA: Head/neck kinematic response of human subjects in low-speed rear-end collisions. SAE Technical Paper 973341, 357–385, 1997.

This is close to the 1,600 to 1,800 rad/sec as a proposed 50% threshold level. Ommaya AK, Hirsch AE. Tolerances for cerebral concussion from head impact and whiplash in primates. J Biomech. 1971 Jan;4(1):13–21.

The most important factors in whiplash-induced concussion are rotational acceleration, flexion/extension tensions in the neck, and intracranial pressure gradients. The whiplash mechanism in cerebral concussion is by the flexion-extension-tension distortion mechanism. Ommaya AK, Hirsch AE, Martinez JL. The role of whiplash in cerebral concussion. SAE Technical Paper 660804 197–203, 1966.

Rotation of the head is more likely to produce cerebral concussion than translation. Gennarelli TA, Ommaya AK, Thibault LE. Comparison of translational and rotational head motions in experimental cerebral concussion. SAE 710882.

§ 6:57 Forces on head from low speed whiplash—Structural neuroimaging—Post-concussion syndrome

Structural neuroimaging is not sensitive in detecting brain

pathology; quantitative electroencephalography was abnormal in all the subjects evaluated in this study. Frontocentral and increased spike wave activity was seen. **Whiplash injury can produce wide-ranging circuitry dysfunction, and that test selection is critical for identifying cognitive deficits.** Henry GK, Gross HS, Herndon CA, Furst CJ. Nonimpact brain injury: neuropsychological and behavioral correlates with consideration of physiological findings. Appl Neuropsychol. 2000;7(2):65–75.

Damages of the orbital surface on the frontotemporal lobes impair the gating mechanism that normally limits sensory input to the brain and further promotes central sensitization. Mamelak M. The motor vehicle collision injury syndrome. Neuropsychiatry Neuropsychol Behav Neurol. 2000 Apr;13(2):125–35.

Single photon emission computed tomography (SPECT) and positron emission tomography (PET) studies indicate brain activation patterns of nociceptive afferent nerves from the upper cervical spine in whiplash patients. Otte A, Ettlin TM, Nitzsche EU, Wachter K, Hoegerle S, Simon GH, Fierz L, Moser E, Mueller-Brand J. PET and SPECT in whiplash syndrome: a new approach to a forgotten brain? J Neurol Neurosurg Psychiatry. 1997 Sep;63(3):368–72; Radanov BP, Bicik I, Dvorak J, Antinnes J, von Schulthess GK, Buck A. Relation between neuropsychological and neuroimaging findings in patients with late whiplash syndrome. J Neurol Neurosurg Psychiatry. 1999 Apr;66(4):485–9.

The late whiplash syndrome shows slight abnormalities when examined with SPECT scans. The researchers concluded that the changes in brain structure were not due to direct head trauma, but "it may be that the perfusion deficits are caused by . . . a mechanism in the upper cervical spine." **The researchers speculate that these changes may be responsible for attentional dysfunction that is commonly found in whiplash patients.** See Otte A, Mueller-Brand J, Fierz L. Brain SPECT findings in late whiplash syndrome. Lancet. 1995 Jun 10;345(8963):1513.

A study indicates that PET and SPECT should not be routinely used. A **PET scan** generally **costs** anywhere from $3000 to $6000). Note: the control group of "normals" were cancer patients with melanoma. Bicik I, Radanov BP, Schafer N, Dvorak J, Blum B, Weber B, Burger C, von Schulthess GK, Buck A. PET with 18fluorodeoxyglucose and hexamethylpropylene amine oxime SPECT in late whiplash syndrome. Neurology. 1998 Aug;51(2):345–50.

§ 6:58 Cognitive performance & cervical spine dysfunction

Comment:

Not only can cerebral brain injury cause cognitive disturbances, a dysfunction of input to the nervous system may also cause cognitive disturbances.

The cervicoenchephalic syndrome is characterized by headache, fatigue, dizziness, poor concentration, disturbed accommodation (eye movements), and impaired adaptation to light sensitivity. See Radanov BP, Dvorak J, Valach L. Cognitive deficits in patients after soft tissue injury of the cervical spine. Spine. 1992 Feb;17(2):127–31.

Headache due to cervical pathology is likely to be responsible from impaired attention functioning whiplash patients. Radanov BP, Hirlinger I, Di Stefano G, Valach L. Attentional processing in cervical spine syndromes. Acta Neurol Scand. 1992 May;85(5):358–62.

Cognitive disturbances (i.e., deficient attentional functioning and impairment of memory) are frequent complaints in patients after whiplash injury. However, few prospective studies of non-selected patients have been performed. **These studies indicate that impaired cognitive functioning relates either to trauma-induced somatic symptoms (i.e., pain) or psychologic symptoms resulting from problems adjusting to trauma-related somatic symptoms. Accordingly, cognitive disturbances after whiplash show a fair rate of recovery, which parallels recovery from trauma-related somatic symptoms. Current research does not indicate disturbances in higher cognitive functions after whiplash.** See Radanov BP, Dvorak J. Spine update. Impaired cognitive functioning after whiplash injury of the cervical spine. Spine. 1996 Feb 1;21(3):392–7.

A mechanism that may have an influence on cognitive performance is by the dysfunction of the cerebellum. **The cerebellum has a contribution to cognition.** Schmahmann JD, Sherman JC. The cerebellar cognitive affective syndrome. Brain. 1998 Apr;121 (Pt 4):561–79.

Cognitive and emotional changes might be prominent or even principal manifestations of cerebellar lesions. **This realization supports evidence suggesting that the cerebellum is an important part of a set of distributed neural circuits that subserve higher-order processing.** Schmahmann JD. Dysmetria of thought: clinical consequences of cerebellar dysfunction on cognition and affect. TICS: Trends in Cognitive Sciences 1998; 2(9):362–71.

Positron emission tomography (PET) activations were observed in the right lateral cerebellum, left medial dorsal thalamus, medial and left orbital frontal cortex, anterior cingulate, and a left parietal region. These activations confirm **a cognitive role for the cerebellum, which may participate in an interactive cortical-cerebellar network that initiates and monitors the conscious retrieval of episodic memory.** Andreasen NC, O'Leary DS, Paradiso S, Cizadlo T, Arndt S, Watkins GL, Ponto LL, Hichwa RD. The cerebellum plays a role in conscious episodic memory retrieval. Hum Brain Mapp. 1999;8(4):226–34.

Cerebellar symptoms can be manifested by over-excitation of cervical and lumbar proprioceptors. Autonomic reflexes with, i.e. pupillo-constrictory reaction to light, are from over-excitation of the cervical proprioceptors. **Sympathetically induced hypertonicity of the deep neck muscles can cause disturbances of the oculomotor system (abnormal eye movement, particularly in the brain stem.)** Hinoki M. Vertigo due to whiplash injury: a neurotological approach. Acta Otolaryngol Suppl. 1984;419:9–29.

After attempting to rule out other ways of interpreting these differences (such as pain, depression, medication, and premorbid health problems), these data were interpreted as lending support to the notion of a causal connection between the disturbed posture control system and some cognitive malfunctions. Gimse R, Bjorgen IA, Tjell C, Tyssedal JS, Bo K. Reduced cognitive functions in a group of whiplash patients with demonstrated disturbances in the posture control system. J Clin Exp Neuropsychol. 1997 Dec;19(6):838–49.

There will be patients who claim no symptoms after trauma and demonstrate occulomotor dysfunction and repositioning dysfunction. Neck pain measure with cervicobrachial visual analog pain scale did not correlate significantly with occulomotor (eye muscle) performance and kinesthesthetic sensibility. **A proproceptive dysfunction might be one of the most important factors for understanding the morbidity after non-contact whiplash injury to the neck.** Heikkila HV, Wenngren BI. Cervicocephalic kinesthetic sensibility, active range of cervical motion, and oculomotor function in patients with whiplash injury. Arch Phys Med Rehabil. 1998 Sep;79(9):1089–94.

Dysfunction related to whiplash trauma may be seen with dysfunction of the smallest muscles (muscles of the eye). This is dysfunction in the frontal cortex. Mosimann UP, Muri RM, Felblinger J, Radanov BP. Saccadic eye movement disturbances in whiplash patients with persistent complaints. Brain. 2000 Apr;123:828–35.

Whiplash injury can produce wide ranging circuitry dysfunction and that test selection is critical for identifying cognitive deficits. Henry GK, Gross HS, Herndon CA, Furst CJ. Nonimpact brain injury: neuropsychological and behavioral correlates with consideration of physiological findings. Appl Neuropsychol. 2000;7(2):65–75.

§ 6:59 The immune system and whiplash

The possible involvement of the immune system during the disease process in Whiplash Associated Disorders (WAD) indicates that effector molecules, including chemokines and their receptors could play a role in WAD. These chemokines attract neutrophils, monocytes/macrophages [Innate Immune Response], eosinophils, basophils, and T cells [which are part of the body's Adaptive Immune Response]. WAD is associated with a systemic but transient dysregulation in percentages of RANTES and CCR-5 expressing MNC and T cells. "RANTES is a chemotactic cytokine (also called a chemokine) and attracts mainly monocytes/macrophages [which are part of the Innate immune response] and T cells [are part of the Adaptive immune response]."

Chemokines (chemotactic cytokines) are the key molecules involved in the activation and recruitment of immune system cells. Cytokines are proteins, which means they exist as an expression of one's DNA. These chemokines physiologically direct leukocyte recruitment trafficking in inflammatory conditions or in different disease processes.

Altered RANTES expression might be important in development of signs and symptoms associated with WAD. CCR-5 is chemokines receptor associated with Th1 cells. These were elevated in patients 3 days after whiplash injury.

Higher percentages of RANTES-expressing blood MNC and T cells were observed in patients with WAD examined within 3 days compared to 14 days after the whiplash injury and, likewise, compared with healthy controls.

"All 29 patients with WAD examined within 3 days after the accident had higher percentages" of chemokines expression associated with both the innate and adaptive immune responses as "compared with the healthy controls."

Some chemokines expression (CXCR-3 and CCR-5) is associated with Th1 cells.

Other chemokines expression (CCR-3 and CCR-4) is associated with Th2 cells.

"Therefore our data suggest that the elevated CCR-5-expressing levels may reflect Th1-type immune responses early in WAD."

"In conclusion, we show that WAD patients examined within 3 days after the accident have a systemic increase" in chemokine profile that is associated primarily with the Th1 [which is associated with immunogloblium G (IgG)] immune system response.

"These alterations are normalized 14 days after the whiplash trauma."

"These findings thus indicate that even a minor soft tissue trauma like WAD is associated with upregulated chemokine and chemokine-receptor expression." "Whether patients with permanent clinical symptoms after WAD, making up 5–10% of all patients with WAD, will develop long-standing changes in chemokine and chemokine receptors remains to be established." Kivioja J, Rinaldi L, Ozenci V, Kouwenhoven M, Kostulas N, Lindgren U, Link H. Chemokines and their receptors in whiplash injury: elevated RANTES and CCR-5. J Clin Immunol. 2001 Jul;21(4):272–7.

§ 6:60 The immune system and whiplash—Disc and immune system

Immunoglobins (Igs) are produced by plasma cells, which are also found in the central nervous system (CNS). Igs in the cerebral spinal fluid are normally derived by diffusion from plasma. Changes in serum Igs concentrations may occur in both brain tumors and lumbar disc disease. **Patients with lumbar disc disease showed a significantly decline in post-operative serum IgA and IgM levels.** See Yuceer N, Arasil E, Temiz C. Serum immunoglobulins in brain tumours and lumbar disc diseases. Neuroreport. 2000 Feb 7;11(2):279–81.

§ 6:61 The immune system and whiplash—Multiple sclerosis and whiplash

"In susceptible individuals, these effects might unleash critical changes in the levels of pro-inflammatory cytokines and nitric oxide, thus triggering MS symptoms ab initio or aggravating symptoms of pre-existing latent disease."

Possible mechanisms as to how specific focal trauma can aggravate multiple sclerosis:

(1) Increased permeability of blood-brain-barrier (BBB)
(2) Increased production of pro-inflammatory cytokines
(3) Increased production of nitric oxide synthetase
(4) Synergistic effect of psychological stress
(5) Direct axonal injury

See Chaudhuri A, Behan PO. Acute cervical hyperextension-hyperflexion injury may precipitate and/or exacerbate symptomatic multiple sclerosis. Eur J Neurol. 2001 Nov;8(6):659–64.

Inflammatory T Cells in the central nervous system play an important role in the pathogenesis of multiple sclerosis. A significantly increased migratory rate toward RANTES and MIP-1a, but not other chemokines, was found in T cells in multiple sclerosis patients and not in health individuals. **This study demonstrated that aberrant migration of multiple sclerosis derived T cells toward RANTES and MIP-1a resulted from over expression of their receptors (CCR5).** Zang YC, Samanta AK, Halder JB, Hong J, Tejada-Simon MV, Rivera VM, Zhang JZ. Aberrant T cell migration toward RANTES and MIP-1 alpha in patients with multiple sclerosis. Overexpression of chemokine receptor CCR5. Brain. 2000 Sep;123 (Pt 9):1874–82.

§ 6:62 The immune system and whiplash—Multiple sclerosis and whiplash—Blood-brain-barrier

Whiplash and other spinal trauma can initiate MS signs and symptoms in asymptomatic, perfectly healthy individuals. Of those with MS, 25% have asymptomatic "silent" MS. Whiplash and other trauma can adversely affect the course of benign MS. The initiation of MS symptoms following trauma may manifest within hours, peak within days to weeks, and is rare after 3 months. **Breakdown in the blood-brain barrier (BBB) is an essential event in the development of MS. Breaching of the BBB results in a pro-inflammatory cytokines immune system response. The whiplash trauma involved may be minor.** Chaudhuri A, Behan PO. Acute cervical hyperextension-hyperflexion injury may precipitate and/or exacerbate symptomatic multiple sclerosis. Eur J Neurol. 2001 Nov;8(6):659–64.

Inflammatory-mediated pain alters both the functional and

molecular properties of the blood-brain-barrier. **Inflammatory-induced changes may significantly alter delivery of therapeutic agents to the brain.** See Huber JD, Witt KA, Hom S, Egleton RD, Mark KS, Davis TP. Inflammatory pain alters blood-brain barrier permeability and tight junctional protein expression. Am J Physiol Heart Circ Physiol. 2001 Mar;280(3):H1241–8.

An alteration in the blood-brain-barrier (BBB) is a necessary step in the pathogenesis of the Multiple Sclerosis lesion, and trauma to the central nervous system (CNS) can result in a breach of the BBB. Poser CM. Trauma to the central nervous system may result in formation or enlargement of multiple sclerosis plaques. Arch Neurol. 2000 Jul;57(7):1074–7, discussion 1078.

Chapter 7

Tissue Healing

§ 7:1 Overview

Comment:

There are multiple phases of healing. Healing of ligaments and soft tissues has been shown to occur mainly by fibrous repair (scar tissue) and not by regeneration of the damaged tissue. The healing response of muscle, tendon, ligament, and disc results in weaker, stiffer and more sensitive tissue.

Activation of an innate immune response is among the first lines of defense after tissue injury. Restoring blood flow to the site of injured tissue is often a necessary prerequisite for mounting an initial immune response to pathogens and for subsequent initiation of a successful repair of wounded tissue.

Scarring occurs after trauma, injury or surgery to any tissue or organ in the body. Such scars are a consequence of a repair mechanism that replaces the missing normal tissue with an extracellular matrix consisting predominantly of fibronectin and collagen types I and III, as such scarring represents a failure of tissue regeneration.

Scar, our body's "glue" is formed through a highly organized sequence of physiologic events. The ability of one type of collagenous tissue to weld various tissues, adapt to their structural integrity, impart tensile strength, and permit return of function is reviewed.

The ultimate goal in collagen research may be the discovery of healing without scar formation.

Until then, to prevent scar formation is to prevent healing. It is an inferior method compared with regeneration, but it is the primary means of repair for all vertebrates.

Special cells in our body respond to injury by forming a collagenous glue." This body glue is called granulation scar tissue. The response to injury, either surgically or traumatically induced, is immediate.

The wound then passes through three phases toward final repair:

1.) the inflammatory phase,

2.) the fibroplastic phase,

3.) the remodeling phase.

The **inflammatory** phase prepares the area for healing,

The **fibroplastic** phase rebuilds the structure,

The **remodeling** phase provides the final form.

Hardy MA. The biology of Scar Formation. Physical Therapy 1989;69(12):1014–24.

Numerous articles discuss soft tissue trauma and healing time. Although published in different references, numerous similarities exist on the topic of healing of injured soft tissues. See, e.g., Oakes BW. Acute soft tissue injuries: nature and management. Aust Fam Physician. 1981 Jul;10(7 Suppl):3–16; Van Der Meulin JHC. Present state of knowledge on processes of healing collagen structures. Internatl J Sports Med (Suppl) 3:4–8, 1982; Frank C, Woo SL, Amiel D, Harwood F, Gomez M, Akeson W. Medial collateral ligament healing. A multidisciplinary assessment in rabbits. Am J Sports Med. 1983 Nov–Dec;11(6):379–89; Muckle DS. Injuries in sport. R Soc Health J. 1982 Jun;102(3):93–4; Noyes FR, Keller CS, Grood ES, Butler DL. Advances in the understanding of knee ligament injury, repair, and rehabilitation. Med Sci Sports Exerc. 1984 Oct;16(5):427–43; Kloth LC, McCullouch JM, Feedar JA. Wound Healing: Alternatives in Management. Philadelphia: FA Davis, 1990.

Healing has been demonstrated to occur in phases that can require one year for completion, and occasionally longer.

In the acute inflammatory phase, there is progressive bleeding from the damaged tissues, and subsequently an increase in pain for a period of approximately three days.

After the acute inflammatory phase begins, the body attempts to mend the damaged tissues. The body's attempt at mending the damaged tissues is called the phase of regeneration. During this phase, small cells called fibrocytes create protein glues called collagen that mend the gap in the torn tissues. This phase of regeneration takes approximately six to eight weeks to complete.

The third phase of healing is termed remodeling. It is during this phase that motion put into the healed tissues will induce them to line up along the direction of stress and strain, thereby improving the tissues' functional capabilities and minimizing the chances for future reoccurrence of pain and/or spasms that tend to occur at times of increased use or stress on the once damaged tissues. This phase of remodeling takes an average of twelve months to complete. In the healing process, numerous authors state that injured and healed tissues are frequently histologically different from the original tissues. This difference is classified as fibrosis, since there is a persistent disorganization in the tissues, giving the tissues a long-term dysfunctional residual. The fibrosis of repair noted that this fibrotic tissue subsequent to trauma and healing has a residual weakness and a residual stiffness or inelasticity. These mechanical residuals tend to cause exacerbations of pain and/or spasms at times of increased use or stress on these once damaged, but now fibrotically healed tissues.

Regarding the above, see, generally, Oakes BW. Acute soft tissue injuries: nature and management. Aust Fam Physician. 1981 Jul;10(7 Suppl):3–16; Van Der Meulin JHC. Present state of knowledge on processes of healing collagen structures. Internatl J Sports Med (Suppl) 3:4–8, 1982; Frank C, Woo SL, Amiel D, Harwood F, Gomez M, Akeson W. Medial collateral ligament healing. A multidisciplinary assessment in rabbits. Am J Sports Med. 1983 Nov–Dec;11(6):379–89; Muckle DS. Injuries in sport. R Soc Health J. 1982 Jun;102(3):93–4; Noyes FR, Keller CS, Grood ES, Butler DL. Advances in the understanding of knee ligament injury, repair, and rehabilitation. Med Sci Sports Exerc. 1984 Oct;16(5):427–43; Kloth LC, McCullouch JM, Feedar JA. Wound Healing: Alternatives in Management. Philadelphia: FA Davis, 1990.

§ 7:2 Healing process is a continuum

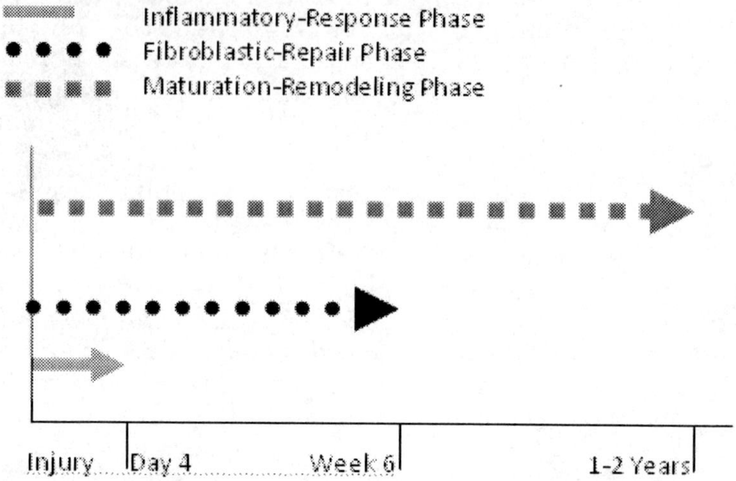

§ 7:3 Common sequence of healing

Phase 1: Acute inflammation
Phase 2: Repair or regeneration
Phase 3: Remodeling

Phase 1 is the acute phase, which lasts for about 72 hours, depending on the severity of the injury. In this phase, prostaglandins are released and are involved with pain production and increased capillary permeability.

Phase 2 may last from 48 hours up to 6 weeks. The repair of the tissue is when collagen fiber synthesis lays down new collagen. But, the new collagen is not fully oriented in the direction of stress.

Phase 3 may last from 3 weeks to 12 months or more. This is the phase in which collagen is remodeled to increase in functional capacity to withstand the stresses imposed on it. The tensile strength of the collagen is quite specific to the forces imposed on it during the remodeling phase. The distinction between phases 2 and 3 is one of increasing the quantity of collagen during the repair phase and improvement in the quality (orientation and strength) in the remodeling phase.

Normal ligaments are composed of type I collagen. Damaged and healed ligaments contain a large portion of type III collagen, which is deficient in the number cross-links and is weaker. At 40 weeks the new, healed collagen is deficient in content and quality.

Regarding the above, see Kellett J. Acute soft tissue injuries—a review of the literature. Med Sci Sports Exerc. 1986 Oct;18(5):489–500.

§ 7:4 Healing as described by American Academy of Orthopedic Surgeons

Woo et al. indicates that there are additional phases in the healing process: remodeling, which can take up to 12 months or longer, followed by the maturation phase, as follows:

Phase I: (acute inflammation) occurs during the first 72 hours.

Phase II (repair and regeneration) lasts from 48 to 72 hours after the injury, until approximately 6 weeks after the injury. It is characterized by the subsidence of inflammation and the beginning of healing.

Phase III (remodeling and maturation) requires 12 months or more to become maximal. Maximum ligament scar maturation is not achieved before 12 months. The original tensile strength is not regained (50–70% is the probable range).

See Woo S, Buckwalter JA. Injury and repair of the musculoskeletal soft tissues. American Academy of Orthopedic Surgeons. 1988. Pg. 106.

§ 7:5 Disc healing

The anular fibers have very little capacity to repair themselves, and the deep layers do not heal. Hampton D, Laros G, McCarron R, Franks D. Healing potential of the anulus fibrosus. Spine. 1989 Apr;14(4):398–401.

§ 7:6 Additional studies on healing

Injuries to ligaments induce a healing response that is characterized by the formation of a scar. The scar tissue is weaker, larger, creeps more than normal ligaments, and is associated with an increased amount of minor collagens (types III, V and VI), decreased collagen cross-links and an increased amount of glycosaminoglycans. Collagen constitutes 70 percent of the dry weight of ligament, the majority being type I collagen, which is also found in tendon, skin and bone. Collagen has a relatively long turnover rate, its average half-life being 300 and 500 days, which is slightly longer than that of bone. **Therefore, several months may be required for a ligament to alter its structure to meet changes in physical loading conditions or to repair itself after injury.** Hildebrand KA, Frank CB. Scar formation and ligament healing. Can J Surg. 1998 Dec; 41(6):425–9.

Repair is by the scar formation process, which may be influenced by environmental factors as well as by the severity of the lesion. See Oakes BW. Acute soft tissue injuries: nature and management. Aust Fam Physician. 1981 Jul;10(7 Suppl):3–16; van der Meulen JC. Present state of knowledge on processes of healing in collagen structures. Int J Sports Med. 1982 Feb;3 Suppl 1:4–8.

The statement that all sprains heal within 6 weeks is incorrect. This is a misstatement of a study that was done on rabbit knees. At 6 weeks, the increase in cells that laid down collagen peaked. This is the end of the cellular proliferation stage, but not in the stages of healing. Frank C, Woo SL, Amiel D, Harwood F, Gomez M, Akeson W. Medial collateral ligament healing. A multidisciplinary assessment in rabbits. Am J Sports Med. 1983 Nov–Dec; 11(6):379–89.

Even ankle sprains can become chronic. In a long-term follow up of inversion trauma of the ankle, 1012 patients with grade I–III lateral ankle ligament sprain were followed for 9 months and 6.5 years. Residual complaints of pain, fear of giving way, swelling, and actual instability were 30% at 9 months and 39% at 6.5 years. Verhagen RA, de Keizer G, van Dijk CN. Long-term follow-up of inversion trauma of the ankle. Arch Orthop Trauma Surg. 1995; 114(2):92–6.

Chapter 8

Pain From Whiplash Injuries

René Descartes, a philosopher and scientist, can be credited with the first documented attempt to understand pain. The origin of the theory that the transmission of pain is through a single channel from the skin to the brain can be traced to Descartes. This simplified scheme of the reflex, published in 1664 in the Treatise of Man, was the beginning of the development of the modern doctrine of reflexes. Descartes gives a purely mechanical view of the involuntary withdrawal of a foot that comes in contact with a noxious stimulus: "the small rapidly moving particle of fire moves the skin of the affected spot causing a thin thread to be pulled. This opens a small valve in the brain and through it animal spirits are sent down to the muscles which withdraw the foot. Just as by pulling at one end of a rope one makes to strike at the same instant a bell which hangs at the other end." Unfortunately, Descartes' reflex theory directed both the study and treatment of pain for more than 330 years. It is still described in physiology and neuroscience textbooks as fact rather than theory. This specificity theory proposes that a specific pain pathway carries the messages from a pain receptor in the skin to a pain center in the brain, implying that the simple cutting of this pathway should alleviate all pain.

Melzack and Wall intensely disputed Descartes' theory. Their gate control theory, proposed in 1965, rejuvenated the field of pain study and led to further investigation into the phenomena of spinal sensitization and central nervous system plasticity, which are the potential pathophysiologic correlates of chronic pain. At a conference in 1995, Wall commented that the classic picture of a single pain mechanism is being swept away in favor of a dynamic interlocking series of biological reactive mechanisms. Wall stated that the model that purports that a hard-wired, line-labeled, modality-specific, single pathway exists that leads from stimulus to sensation is pure fantasy and that the next few years (in understanding pain) are going to be revolutionary. The phenomenon of pain takes place in an integrated matrix throughout the neuroaxis and occurs on at least three levels—at peripheral, spinal, and supraspinal sites.

The basic strategy of pain control monopolize on this concept of integration by attenuation or blockade of pain through intervention at the periphery, by activation of inhibitory processes that gate pain at the spinal cord and brain, and by interference with the perception of pain.

Melzack R, Wall PD. Pain mechanisms: a new theory. Science. 1965 Nov 19;150(699):971–9.

DeLeo JA. Basic science of pain. J Bone Joint Surg Am. 2006 Apr; 88 Suppl 2:58–62.

§ 8:1 "Pain" defined

Pain is defined as "an unpleasant sensory and emotional experience associated with actual or potential tissue damage or described in terms of such damage." Nociceptive pain is the pain that results from activation of nociceptors, nerve fibers and pathways associated with tissue damage. Pain has subjective elements and does not necessarily require tissue damage. There are technical differences between pain and nociception. See Merskey H, Bogduk N. editors. Classification of Chronic Pain, 2nd ed. IASP Press, Seattle 1994.

As discussed in prior chapters, common areas of pain from whiplash injuries are the facet, disc, ligaments, spinal ganglion, and pain may be manifested in the muscle. The pains from whiplash injuries are most likely a referred type of pain. The pain is not a "classical dermatome" pattern.

Referred pain from muscle is manifested in somatic structures (skin, muscles, joints, and tendons). And visceral pain may be referred to somatic as well as visceral structures. See Arendt-Nielsen L, Laursen RJ, Drewes AM. Referred pain as an indicator for neural plasticity. Prog Brain Res. 2000;129:343–56.

The classic paper on pain is from Melzach & Wall, and it explains their "Gate Theory of Pain." This was published in the journal Science in 1965. The gate theory is based on larger diameter afferent nerves (coming from mechanoreceptors) inhibiting the information from small diameter afferent nerves (nociceptive-pain impulses). If there is a decrease in mechanoreceptive (proprioceptive) information from large diameter afferents, the nociceptive (painful) information then may become prominent. This is part of the gate theory of pain. Melzack R, Wall PD. Pain mechanisms: a new theory. Science. 1965 Nov 19;150(699):971–9.

Since Melzach & Wall's publication, other factors have been found to be involved, as referenced below, but this mechanism is still part of the pain experience.

§ 8:2 "Pain" defined—General classification of pain types

Comment:

Pain is classified as **nocicpetive** (from the injured tissue), inflammatory (sensitization of tissue and nerves) **and neurogenic/neuropathic** (from the nervous system itself). Tissue injury triggers an increase in the excitability of the neurons in the spinal cord. (This is known as central sensitization). Central sensitization is generated by C-afferent fibers. The changes in the nervous system can decrease the threshold of pain and increase the receptive field. Central sensitization has been documented in a large number of laboratories in a wide variety of species, including humans. It is now accepted as a major contributor to post-injury pain hypersensitivity.

Two simultaneous processes may be occurring to produce and maintain a central component of inflammatory hypersensitivity. The first is ongoing generation of central sensitization by nociceptors and sensitized by the inflammation. The second is a change in the phenotype of sensory neurons innervating the inflamed area.

§ 8:3 "Pain" defined—Facet joint as site of injury for causing chronic pain following whiplash injury

Overall, the prevalence of cervical zygapophysial joint pain (C2–C3 or below) was 60% (95% confidence interval, 46% — 73%). Cervical zygapophysial joint pain is common among patients with chronic neck pain after whiplash. **This entity (facet joint pain) has survived challenge with placebo-controlled, diagnostic investigations and has proven to be of major clinical importance.** Lord SM, Barnsley L, Wallis BJ, Bogduk N. Chronic cervical zygapophysial joint pain after whiplash. A placebo-controlled prevalence study. Spine. 1996 Aug 1;21(15):1737–44; discussion 1744–5.

When compared to the reported strains that facet joint capsules experienced in whiplash (35–60%) and the reported capsule subfailure strains (35–67%), the low strain thresholds are substantially lower whereas the high thresholds and afterdischarge strains are within that range. Thus, low threshold units appear to signal proprioception within the physiologic range. High threshold units likely signal nociception (pain sensation) while afterdischarge may signal **capsule strain injury** and contribute to persistent pain. Lu Y, Chen C, Kallakuri S, Patwardhan A, Cavanaugh JM. Neural response of cervical facet joint capsule to stretch: a study of whiplash pain mechanism. Stapp Car Crash J. 2005 Nov;49:49–65.

§ 8:4 "Pain" defined—Multiple-area source of pain

The investigation of neck pain by discography alone, or by zagapophysial block alone, constitutes an inadequate approach to neck pain that fails to identify the majority of patients whose symptoms stem from multiple elements in the 3-joint complexes of the neck.

Disc and Facet pain	**41%**
Facet pain only	**41%**
Disc pain only	**20%**

See Bogduk N, Aprill C. On the nature of neck pain, discography and cervical zygapophysial joint blocks. Pain. 1993 Aug; 54(2):213–7.

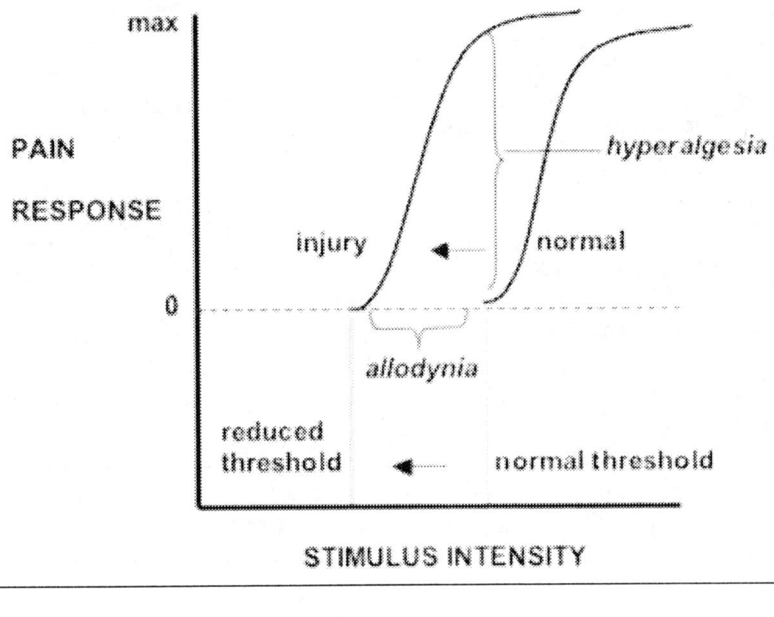

Alloydynia = reduced threshold for pain
Hyperalgesia = increase in pain level

§ 8:5 "Pain" defined—Nociception

The perception of pain involves activation of nociceptors in the periphery, which then activate second-order neurons in the spinal cord. At the cord level, pain signals can be transmitted and modulated. Areas of the brain, thalamus, and brainstem receive the nociceptive information and can originate descending inhibition. Nociceptors are primary afferent neurons that respond to noxious or potentially tissue-damaging stimuli and can be sensitized. Acute pain can induce long-term neuronal remodeling and sensitization. After joint or muscle injury, the spinal cord processes nociceptive information and controls peripheral inflammation. The dorsal horn neurons can be sensitized by peripheral injury with activation of N-methyl-D-aspartate (NMDA), non-NMDA excitatory amino acid, and neurokinin 1 (NK1) receptors. A non-NMDA receptor, a-amino-3-hydroxy-5-methyl-4-isoxazolepropionate (AMPA), appears to set the baseline level of nociception and faithfully transmits the intensity and duration of the stimulus. NMDA receptors enhance noxious information. Davis C. Chronic pain/dysfunction in whiplash-associated disorders. J Manipulative Physiol Ther. 2001 Jan;24(1):44–51.

After tissue damage, the substances released include potassium (from damaged cells), serotonin (platelets), bradykinin (plasma), histamine (mast cells), prostaglandins (PGE2; damaged cells), leukotrienes (damaged cells), and substance P (SP; primary afferent fibers). Davis C. Chronic pain/dysfunction in whiplash-associated disorders. J Manipulative Physiol Ther. 2001 Jan;24(1):44–51.

Tetrodotoxin sodium current receptors, nerve growth factor (NGF), NK1 receptors (for SP), d-μ—opioid receptors, glutamate, NMDA and AMPA receptors, nitric oxide (NO), cyclooxygenase, and other neurotrophic factors and neurotransmitters can also affect nociception. Glutamate is the main excitatory neurotransmitter in the central nervous system and has been implicated in neurodevelopment and synaptogenesis, neurodegenerative disorders, neurotoxicity, and synaptic plasticity, as in **long-term potentiation (LTP)** and **long-term depression (LTD)**. Adenosine 5′-triphosphate, which may also evoke nociceptor activation, is known to depolarize sensory neurons and may play a role in nociceptor activation when released from damaged tissue through primary afferent neurotransmission. Davis C. Chronic pain/dysfunction in whiplash-associated disorders. J Manipulative Physiol Ther. 2001 Jan;24(1):44–51.

§ 8:6 Facet joint

Comment:

In the facet joint, there are mechanoreceptors (proprioceptors) and nociceptive (pain) nerve endings.

The presence of mechanoreceptors and nociceptive nerve endings in the cervical facet joint proves that these tissues are monitored by the central nervous system and implies that neural input from the facets is important to proprioception and pain sensation in the cervical spine. The small number of mechanoreceptor endings in the facet capsules suggests that these receptors have a large receptor field. **Damage to even a small part of the capsule might denervate that articular structure, which could have important implications for long-term joint function.** See McLain RF. Mechanoreceptor endings in human cervical facet joints. Spine. 1994 Mar 1;19(5):495–501.

If there is a decrease in mechanoreceptive (proprioceptive) information from large diameter afferents, the nociceptive (painful) information then may become prominent. This is part of the gate theory of pain. Melzack R, Wall PD. Pain mechanisms: a new theory. Science. 1965 Nov 19;150(699):971–9.

Pain may be evoked by a 1) loss of low-threshold mechanoreceptive neurons, such that nociceptive neuronal output is now prominent, 2) reduced tonic inhibition of thalamic or cortical neurons, and/or 3) unmasking or strengthening of nociceptive pathways. Davis KD, Kiss ZH, Tasker RR, Dostrovsky JO. Thalamic stimulation-evoked sensations in chronic pain patients and in nonpain (movement disorder) patients. J Neurophysiol. 1996 Mar;75(3):1026–37.

40% of nerves in a joint show a low mechanical threshold during passive movements, a proprioceptive function. 60% of the joint innervation may be classified as nociceptive and is normally inactive. Pathological conditions like joint inflammation and severe stretching activate these receptors. Heppelmann B. Anatomy and histology of joint innervation. J Peripher Nerv Syst. 1997;2(1):5–16.

Summation of simultaneous nociceptive and non-nociceptive inputs plays an important role in the modulation of nociception. Romaniello A, Svensson P, Cruccu G, Arendt-Nielsen L. Modulation of exteroceptive suppression periods in human jaw-closing muscles induced by summation of nociceptive and non-nociceptive inputs. Exp Brain Res. 2000 Jun;132(3):306–13.

The process of summation of simultaneous nociceptive and non-nociceptive input into the nervous system may also apply to patients with chronic cervicobrachialgia. These patients have pain thresholds and pain tolerances lower than normal. In a normal person, A-beta afferent (large mylenated) fibers participate in transmitting low-threshold stimuli from mechanoreceptors and A-delta/C fibers participate in transmitting high threshold stimuli, such as pain and thermal signals. Loss of input from A-beta afferent fibers may diminish the inhibition of the projecting neurons and give rise to "low-input" pain. With a phenotype change in the spinal cord, A-beta afferent fibers that would normally evoke non-painful sensations may elicit and maintain pain (allodynia). Voerman VF, van Egmond J, Crul BJ. Elevated detection thresholds for mechanical stimuli in chronic pain patients: support for a central mechanism. Arch Phys Med Rehabil. 2000 Apr;81(4):430–5.

The phenotype change in the spinal cord, A-beta afferent fibers that would normally evoke non-painful sensations is a type of spinal neuronal plasticity shown to be a key contributor to pathologic pain hypersensitivity. These A-beta impulses, which would normally "gate out' the pain signals, now contribute to the pain process. This is a form of adverse neuronal plasticity. Mannion RJ, Woolf CJ. Pain mechanisms and management: a central perspective. Clin J Pain. 2000 Sep;16(3 Suppl):S144–56

§ 8:7 Facet joint cervical facet joint-synovial folds

Not only can there be an injury to the facet capsule, the facet joint has synovial folds. The synovial fibroadipose folds are connected to the capsule.

There are 3 types of synovial folds in the cervical facet joint. Inami S, Kaneoka K, Hayashi K, Ochiai N. Types of synovial fold in the cervical facet joint. J Orthop Sci. 2000;5(5):475–80.

Nociceptive (pain) fibers are found in the cervical synovial folds. Inami S, Shiga T, Tsujino A, Yabuki T, Okado N, Ochiai N. Immunohistochemical demonstration of nerve fibers in the synovial fold of the human cervical facet joint. J Orthop Res. 2001 Jul;19(4):593–6.

The presence of mechanoreceptors (for proprioception — joint position sense) and nociceptive nerve endings (for pain) in the cervical facet joint proves that

these tissues are monitored by the central nervous system and implies that neural input from the facets is important to proprioception and pain sensation in the cervical spine. McLain RF. Mechanoreceptor endings in human cervical facet joints. Spine. 1994 Mar 1;19(5):495–501.

The lack of proprioceptive inhibition of nociceptors at the dorsal horn of the spinal cord would result in chronic pain. Nussbaum EL, Downes L. Reliability of clinical pressure-pain algometric measurements obtained on consecutive days. Phys Ther. 1998 Feb;78(2):160–9.

Multifidus muscle insertions were found to cover 22.4 ± 9.6% of the capsule area. The forces acting on the facet capsular ligament, due to vertebral motions and eccentric muscle contractions, can be as high as 66 N. **These anatomical data provide quantitative evidence of substantial muscle insertions into the cervical facet capsular ligament and provide a possible mechanism for injury to this ligament and the facet joint as a whole.** Winkelstein BA, McLendon RE, Barbir A, Myers BS. An anatomical investigation of the human cervical facet capsule, quantifying muscle insertion area. J Anat. 2001 Apr;198(Pt 4):455–61.

§ 8:8 Disc pain

Pain travels mainly from nerve fibers that have small diameters. This study demonstrates an extensive distribution of small nerve fibers in the size range of C and A-delta fibers throughout the peripheral anulus and provides an illustration of this distribution. These findings support a role for the **disc as a source of low back pain**. Cavanaugh JM, Kallakuri S, Ozaktay AC. Innervation of the rabbit lumbar intervertebral disc and posterior longitudinal ligament. Spine. 1995 Oct 1;20(19):2080–5.

The lumbar intervertebral discs are innervated posteriorly by the **sinuvertebral nerves**, but laterally by branches of the **ventral rami and grey rami communicantes (the grey rami comes from the sympathetic nervous system)**. The posterior longitudinal ligament is innervated by the sinuvertebral nerves and the anterior longitudinal ligament by branches of the grey rami. Lateral and intermediate branches of the lumbar dorsal rami supply the iliocostalis lumborum and longissimus thoracis, respectively. Medial branches supply the multifidus, intertransversarii mediales, interspinales, interspinous ligament, and the lumbar zygapophysial joints. The distribution of the intrinsic nerves of the lumbar vertebral column systematically identifies those structures that are potential sources of **primary low-back pain**. Bogduk N. The innervation of the lumbar spine. Spine. 1983 Apr;8(3):286–93.

Microdissection and histologic studies were undertaken to determine the innervation of the cervical intervertebral discs. The **cervical sinuvertebral nerves** were found to have an upward course in the vertebral canal, supplying the disc at their level of entry and the disc above. Branches of the vertebral nerve supplied the lateral aspects of the cervical discs. Histologic studies of discs obtained at operation showed the presence of nerve fibers as deeply as the outer third of the anulus fibrosus. These anatomic findings provide the hitherto missing substrate for **primary disc pain and the pain of provocation discography**. Bogduk N, Windsor M, Inglis A. The innervation of the cervical intervertebral discs. Spine. 1988 Jan;13(1):2–8.

MRI is essential in the evaluation of patients with chronic neck pain who have failed conservative treatment and present with axial, rather than appendicular, complaints. Small central cervical disc ruptures can cause chronic, disabling neck pain. Metzger CS, Schlitt M, Quindlen EA, White RL. Small central cervical disc syndrome: evaluation and treatment of chronic disabling neck pain. J Spinal Disord. 1989 Dec;2(4):234–7.

Nerve ingrowth into the damaged intervertebral discs is a factor in the pathogenesis of chronic low back pain. Freemont AJ, Peacock TE, Goupille P, Hoyland JA, O'Brien J, Jayson MI. Nerve ingrowth into diseased intervertebral disc in chronic back pain. Lancet. 1997 Jul 19;350(9072):178–81.

Production of proinflammaory mediators within the disc may be a major factor in the genesis of a painful disc. Burke JG, Watson RW, McCormack D, Dowling FE, Walsh MG, Fitzpatrick JM. Intervertebral discs which cause low back pain secrete high levels of proinflammatory mediators. J Bone Joint Surg Br. 2002 Mar;84(2):196–201.

Glutamate originating from degenerated disc tissue (proteoglycan) may diffuse to the dorsal root ganglion and effect glutamate receptors causing pain. Harrington JF, Messier AA, Bereiter D, Barnes B, Epstein MH. Herniated lumbar disc material as a source of free glutamate available to affect pain signals through the dorsal root ganglion. Spine. 2000 Apr 15;25(8):929–36.

IL-1beta appeared to "sensitize" annulus cells to mechanical load. This increased responsiveness to

mechanical load in the face of inflammatory cytokines may imply the sensitivity of annulus cells to shear increases during inflammation and may affect initiation and progression of disc degeneration. Elfervig MK, Minchew JT, Francke E, Tsuzaki M, Banes AJ. IL-1beta sensitizes intervertebral disc annulus cells to fluid-induced shear stress. J Cell Biochem. 2001;82(2):290–8.

Tumor necrosis factor-alpha is involved in mechanisms of neuropathic pain. TNF-a is primarily responsible for the histological and behavioral manifestations of experimental sciatica associated with herniated lumbar discs. Igarashi T, Kikuchi S, Shubayev V, Myers RR. 2000 Volvo Award winner in basic science studies: Exogenous tumor necrosis factor-alpha mimics nucleus pulposus-induced neuropathology. Molecular, histologic, and behavioral comparisons in rats. Spine. 2000 Dec 1;25(23):2975–80.

Immunoglobins (Igs) are produced by plasma cells, which are also found in the central nervous system (CNS). Igs in the cerebral spinal fluid are normally derived by diffusion from plasma. Changes in serum Igs concentrations may occur in both brain tumors and lumbar disc disease. **Patients with lumbar disc disease showed a significant decline in post-operative serum IgA and IgM levels**. See Yuceer N, Arasil E, Temiz C. Serum immunoglobulins in brain tumours and lumbar disc diseases. Neuroreport. 2000 Feb 7;11(2):279–81.

§ 8:9 Disc pain—Referred pain from the cervical disc

Predominantly unilateral symptoms were provoked just as often as bilateral symptoms. The C2–C3 disc **referred pain** to the neck, subocciput and face. The C3–C4 **disc referred pain** to the neck, subocciput, trapezius, anterior neck, face, shoulder, interscapular and limb. The C4–C5 **disc referred pain** to the neck, shoulder, interscapular, trapezius, extremity, face, chest and subocciput. The C5–C6 **disc referred pain** to the neck, trapezius, interscapular, suboccipital, anterior neck, chest and face. The C6–C7 **disc referred pain** to the neck, interscapular, trapezius, shoulder, extremity and subocciput. At C7–T1 we produced neck and interscapular pain. Slipman CW, Plastaras C, Patel R, Isaac Z, Chow D, Garvan C, Pauza K, Furman M. Provocative cervical discography symptom mapping. Spine J. 2005 Jul–Aug;5(4):381–8.

These findings suggest the coexistence of **two different types of innervation**: one originating directly from the spinal nerve segmentally, and one reaching vertebral structures via the sympathetic nerves non-segmentally. Therefore, sympathetic nerves are likely involved in the proprioception of the spinal column. Higuchi K, Sato T. Anatomical study of lumbar spine innervation. Folia Morphol (Warsz). 2002;61(2):71–9.

Two kinds of innervation are present in the lumbar spine: one depends on the **somatic nervous system** and the other on the **sympathetic nervous system**. The sympathetic nerves are the sinu-vertebral nerves and the rami communicantes which innervate the intervertebral disc, the ventral surface of the dura mater, the longitudinal dorsal ligament and the longitudinal ventral ligament. The sinu-vertebral nerve was described first by Luschka in 1850. This nerve is implicated in diffuse low back pain because of its pathway and its sympathetic component. This nerve cannot directly reach a somatic element at each level of the lumbar spine, so must first reach the L2 spinal ganglion. Thus, there is a "hole" in the somatic innervation between L3 and L5 because the dorsal nerves do not reach the skin at these levels. The pain therefore takes another route through the sympathetic system. **Discogenic pain** is mediated by the sinu-vertebral nerves, and through the rami communicantes reaches the L2 spinal ganglion. Anatomical and clinical features reinforce this hypothesis. Raoul S, Faure A, Robert R, Rogez JM, Hamel O, Cuillere P, Le Borgne J. Role of the sinu-vertebral nerve in low back pain and anatomical basis of therapeutic implications. Surg Radiol Anat. 2003 Feb;24(6):366–71.

The distinct histological characteristic of the painful disc was the formation of a zone of vascularised granulation tissue from the nucleus pulposus to the outer part of the annulus fibrosus along the edges of the fissures. SP-, NF- and VIP-immunoreactive nerve fibres in the painful discs were more extensive than in the control discs. **Growth of nerves deep into the annulus fibrosus and nucleus pulposus was observed mainly along the zone of granulation tissue in the painful discs.** This suggests that the zone of granulation tissue with extensive innervation along the tears in the posterior part of the painful disc may be responsible for causing the pain of discography and of discogenic low back pain. Peng B, Wu W, Hou S, Li P, Zhang C, Yang Y. The pathogenesis of discogenic low back pain. J Bone Joint Surg Br. 2005 Jan;87(1):62–7.

§ 8:10 Disc pain—Disc injury causing changes in the nervous system

TSG-6 is induced by **pro-inflammatory cytokines** such as

TNFa (tissue necrosis factor) and IL-1 (interleukin). Staining for TSG-6 was greatest in herniated discs, particularly close to blood vessels. IaI immunostaining was frequently widespread throughout the disc but there was little in the cartilage endplate. It has been proposed that these molecules have widespread effects, including extracellular matrix stabilization, down regulation of the protease network and reduction of inflammation. Roberts S, Evans H, Menage J, Urban JP, Bayliss MT, Eisenstein SM, Rugg MS, Milner CM, Griffin S, Day AJ. TNFalpha-stimulated gene product (TSG-6) and its binding protein, IalphaI, in the human intervertebral disc: new molecules for the disc. Eur Spine J. 2005 Feb;14(1):36–42.

The local application of nucleus pulposus may induce a characteristic "inflammatory crescent" reaction when applied to the surface of the DRG **(dorsal root ganglion)**. ¶ There was a disintegration of the elastic fiber layer in the DRG 24 and 72 hours after disc incision. The disintegrated capsule showed an **increased permeability** even for a large molecule as albumin, which indicates a possible entrance route for various substances (i.e., tumor necrosis factor, nitric oxide, interleukin-1, interleukin-6, interleukin-10, and prostaglandin E2), induced by locally applied nucleus pulposus. Murata Y, Rydevik B, Takahashi K, Larsson K, Olmarker K. Incision of the intervertebral disc induces disintegration and increases permeability of the dorsal root ganglion capsule. Spine. 2005 Aug 1;30(15):1712–6.

Disc injury causing dorsal horn neuronal windup: The current finding of enhanced dorsal horn neuronal windup after exposure of the DRG to NP (nucleus pulposus) may partially explain the clinical manifestations of lumbar disc herniation-induced radiculopathy. ¶ Due to an enhanced dorsal horn neuronal excitability and windup response at low frequencies that do not normally elicit windup, the normally nonnoxious stimulus is inducing **dorsal horn neuronal windup** that is interpreted as **pain** . . . Cuellar JM, Montesano PX, Antognini JF, Carstens E. Application of nucleus pulposus to L5 dorsal root ganglion in rats enhances nociceptive dorsal horn neuronal windup. J Neurophysiol. 2005 Jul;94(1):35–48.

Wind-up is therefore triggered by temporal summation of C-fiber impulses and also by spatial summation of impulses arriving in the larger population of C-fibers recruited by wider pulses. Furthermore, an important parameter for the generation of wind-up is the previous level of excitability of spinal cord neurons. Accordingly, wind-up is generated at lower frequencies or pulse widths in situations of spinal cord hyperexcitability. Wind-up is not observed at frequencies below about 0.2–0.3 Hz is maximal around 1–2 Hz, and declines up to 20 Hz. Herrero JF, Laird JM, Lopez-Garcia JA. Wind-up of spinal cord neurones and pain sensation: much ado about something? Prog Neurobiol. 2000 Jun;61(2):169–203.

Both **wind-up** and temporal summation appear to be dependent on NMDA receptor activation. The results of clinical trials in patients with chronic pain suggest that the NMDA receptor may represent a new target for modulation of abnormal temporal summation of pain, as well as other characteristics of chronic pain. Eide PK. Wind-up and the NMDA receptor complex from a clinical perspective. Eur J Pain. 2000;4(1):5–15.

Wind-up is a process that is a different type of pain than the regular type of pain which is nociceptive type of pain. With wind-up pain, it is a neuropathic type of pain that is more difficult to treat.

§ 8:11 Deep tissue pain—Referred pain

Many times you will hear that the pain is non-dermatomal in origin. This statement may suggest that the patient is making it up. But, research has shown that injuries in vehicle collisions cause damage to the deeper structures than the skin.

Deep tissue pain is different from superficial pain, as deep pain lasts longer than superficial pain and does not follow dermatomal patterns. See Woolf CJ, Wall PD. Relative effectiveness of C primary afferent fibers of different origins in evoking a prolonged facilitation of the flexor reflex in the rat. J Neurosci. 1986 May;6(5):1433–42; Kellgren JH. On the distribution of pain arising from deep somatic structures with charts of segmental pain areas. Clin Sci 1939;4:35–46; Feinstein B, Langton JNK, Jameson RM, Schiller F. Experiments on pain referred from deep somatic tissues. J Bone Joint Surg (Am) 1954;36:981–97.

Referred pain of deep, somatic structures may come from interspinous ligaments, paravertebral muscles, facets or discs. See generally, Kellgren JH. On the distribution of pain arising from deep somatic structures with charts of segmental pain areas. Clin Sci 1939;4:35–46; Feinstein B, Langton JNK, Jameson RM, Schiller F. Experiments on pain referred from deep somatic tissues. J Bone Jt Surg 1954; 36-A(5):981–997; Cloward RB. Cervical discography. A contribution to the etiology and mechanism of neck, shoulder and arm pain. Ann Surg 1959;150:1052–1064; Cloward RB. The clinical significance of the sinu-vertebral nerve of the cervical spine in relation to the cervical disc syndrome. J Neurol Neurosurg Psychiatry 1960;23:321–326; Dwyer A, Aprill C, Bogduk N. Cervical zygapophyseal joint pain patterns. I: A study in normal volunteers. Spine. 1990 Jun;15(6):453–7; Aprill C, Dwyer A, Bogduk N. Cervical zygapophyseal joint pain patterns. II: A clinical evaluation. Spine. 1990 Jun;15(6):458–61.

§ 8:12 Deep tissue pain-referred pain Referred pain from facets

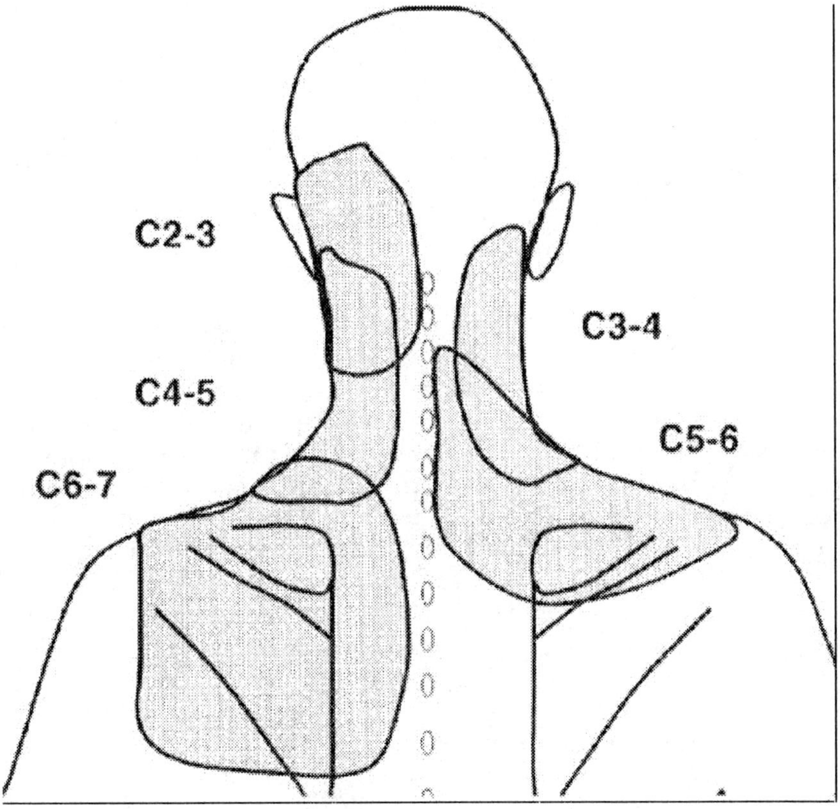

Above: Referred pain from the cervical facets. (Adapted from April C, Dwyer A, Bogduk N. Cervical zygopophyseal joint pain patterns II: A clinical evaluation. Spine 1990;15:458–61.) *See* Aprill C, Dwyer A, Bogduk N. Cervical zygapophyseal joint pain patterns. II: A clinical evaluation. Spine. 1990 Jun;15(6):458–61.

§ 8:13 Dorsal root ganglion (DRG)

The dorsal root ganglion is where the nerve cell bodies that go to the facet and spinal tissue are located.

The DRG is the most common site for ectopic discharge generation after spinal nerve injury, and separate mechanisms seem to be involved in the development of ectopic discharges and adrenergic sensitivity. A-beta (Aβ) and A-delta (Ad) primary afferent fibers start to produce ectopic discharges 13 hours after injury to the spinal nerve. These ectopic discharges originate most commonly from the DRG. **This may play an important role in the development of neuropathic pain** after peripheral nerve injury. Liu X, Chung K, Chung JM. Ectopic discharges and adrenergic sensitivity of sensory neurons after spinal nerve injury. Brain Res. 1999 Dec 4;849(1–2):244–7.

Compression of the dorsal root ganglion may lead to a neuropathic pain state. Abe M, Kurihara T, Han W, Shinomiya K, Tanabe T. Changes in Expression of Voltage-Dependent Ion Channel Subunits in Dorsal Root Ganglia of Rats with Radicular Injury and Pain. Spine. 2002 Jul 15;27(14):1517–1524.

After compression of the dorsal root ganglion at 122.4 mmHg or more, leakage of tracer into the endoneurial space was markedly increased compared with the sham-operated group, and severe edema was noted. **It was proven that the increased vascular permeability occurred as well as in leakage of dye within the dorsal root ganglion after a single hour of compression of the dorsal root ganglion.** Kobayashi S, Yoshizawa H. Effect of mechanical compression on the vascular permeability of the dorsal root ganglion. J Orthop Res. 2002 Jul;20(4):730–9.

These results suggest the possibility that TNF-a produced in the vicinity of nerve roots, due to disc herniation, might cause ectopic discharges in primary afferent fibers and thereby induce the prolonged excitation in pain-processing neurons responsible for radicular pain. Onda A, Hamba M, Yabuki S, Kikuchi S. Exogenous Tumor Necrosis Factor-alpha Induces Abnormal Discharges in Rat Dorsal Horn Neurons. Spine. 2002 Aug 1;27(15):1618–24.

An exaggerated and more prolonged response (hyperalgesia) bilaterally after reinjury suggests central sensitization after initial injury. **Neuroinflammatory activation in the spinal cord further supports the hypothesis that central neuroinflammation plays an important role in chronic**

radicular pain. Hunt JL, Winkelstein BA, Rutkowski MD, Weinstein JN, DeLeo JA. Repeated injury to the lumbar nerve roots produces enhanced mechanical allodynia and persistent spinal neuroinflammation. Spine. 2001 Oct 1;26(19):2073–9.

§ 8:14 Chronic pain

There is increasing interest about the possible involvement of the **sympathetic nervous system** (SNS) in initiation and **maintenance of chronic muscle pain syndromes** of different aetiology. Epidemiological data show that stresses of different nature, e.g. work-related, psychosocial, etc., typically characterised by SNS activation, may be a co-factor in the development of the pain syndrome and/or negatively affect its time course. In spite of their clear traumatic origin, whiplash associated disorders (WAD) appear to share many common features with other chronic pain syndromes affecting the musculo-skeletal system. These features do not only include symptoms, like type of pain or sensory and motor dysfunctions, but possibly also some of the pathophysiological mechanisms that may concur to establish the chronic pain syndrome. This review focuses on WAD, particular emphasis being devoted to sensorimotor symptoms, and on the actions exerted by the sympathetic system at muscle level. Besides its well-known action on muscle blood flow, the SNS is able to affect the contractility of muscle fibresfibers, to modulate the proprioceptive information arising from the muscle spindle receptors and, under certain conditions, to modulate nociceptive information. Furthermore, the activity of the SNS itself is in turn affected by muscle conditions, such as its current state of activity, fatigue and pain signals originating in the muscle. The possible involvement of the SNS in the development of WAD is discussed in light of the several positive feedback loops in which it is implicated.

Passatore M, Roatta S. Influence of sympathetic nervous system on sensorimotor function: whiplash associated disorders (WAD) as a model. Eur J Appl Physiol. 2006 Nov;98(5):423–49.

The hypothalamus-pituitary-adrenal (HPA) axis can act as the body's own anti-inflammatory system.

Reduced reactivity and enhanced negative feedback sensitivity of the hypothalamus-pituitary-adrenal axis in chronic whiplash-associated disorder. Dysregulations of the hypothalamus-pituitary-adrenal (HPA) axis have been discussed as a physiological substrate of chronic pain and fatigue. The aim of the study was to investigate possible dysregulations of the HPA axis in chronic whiplash-associated disorder (WAD). In 20 patients with chronic WAD and 20 healthy controls, awakening cortisol responses as well as a short circadian free cortisol profile were assessed before and after administration of 0.5mg dexamethasone. In comparison to the controls, chronic WAD patients had attenuated cortisol responses to awakening and normal cortisol levels during the day and showed enhanced and prolonged suppression of cortisol after the administration of 0.5mg dexamethasone. **Dysregulations of the HPA axis in terms of reduced reactivity and enhanced negative feedback suppression exist in chronic WAD.** The observed endocrine abnormalities could serve as a systemic mechanism of symptoms experienced by chronic WAD patients. Gaab J, Baumann S, Budnoik A, Gmunder H, Hottinger N, Ehlert U. Reduced reactivity and enhanced negative feedback sensitivity of the hypothalamus-pituitary-adrenal axis in chronic whiplash-associated disorder. Pain. 2005 Dec 15;119(1–3):219–24.

Acute hyperalgesia and some types of chronic pain result from continuous generation of pain mediators by damaged tissue. Ferreira SH, Lorenzetti BB, De Campos DI. Induction, blockade and restoration of a persistent hypersensitive state. Pain. 1990 Sep;42(3):365–71.

Small, persistent input of nociceptors can lead to chronic pain. See Greening J, Lynn B. Minor peripheral nerve injuries: an underestimated source of pain? Manual Ther 1998;3:187–94; Arendt-Nielsen L, Sonnenborg FA, Andersen OK. Facilitation of the withdrawal reflex by repeated transcutaneous electrical stimulation: an experimental study on central integration in humans. Eur J Appl Physiol. 2000 Feb;81(3):165–73; Yaksh TL, Hua XY, Kalcheva I, Nozaki-Taguchi N, Marsala M. The spinal biology in humans and animals of pain states generated by persistent small afferent input. Proc Natl Acad Sci U S A. 1999 Jul 6;96(14):7680–6.

Painful osteoarthritis can cause muscle hyperalgesia and extended pain due to central sensitization. Bajaj P, Bajaj P, Graven-Nielsen T, Arendt-Nielsen L. Osteoarthritis and its association with muscle hyperalgesia: an experimental controlled study. Pain. 2001 Aug;93(2):107–14.

Spinal neuronal plasticity has shown to be a key contributor to pathologic pain hypersensitivity. Mannion RJ, Woolf CJ. Pain mechanisms and management: a central perspective. Clin J Pain. 2000 Sep;16(3 Suppl):S144–56.

Using treatments that are for acute pain may not be effective for treating chronic pain.

Chronic pain cannot be treated by blocking pain pathways, which is effective against acute pain. Chronic pain may require a multidisciplinary approach. Kumazawa T. Primitivism and plasticity of pain—implication of polymodal receptors. Neurosci Res. 1998 Sep;32(1):9–31.

A synopsis of these most recent experimental data and results from previous electrophysiological in vivo and in vitro studies suggests that dorsal horn neurons, and most likely other neurons in pain-related structures, become spontaneously active and can maintain their activity without further noxious peripheral input. Schadrack J, Zieglgansberger W. Activity-dependent changes in the pain matrix. Scand J Rheumatol Suppl. 2000;113:19–23.

§ 8:15 Chronic pain—Chronic symptoms

Patients with chronic whiplash syndrome may have a generalized central hyperexcitability from a loss of tonic inhibitory input (disinhibition) and/or ongoing excitatory input. Dysfunction of the motor system may also occur, with or without pain. Davis C. Chronic pain/dysfunction in whiplash-associated disorders. J Manipulative Physiol Ther. 2001 Jan;24(1):44–51.

Studies on experimentally produced central hypersensitivity support three mechanisms; (1) maintenance of central hypersensitivity by ongoing peripheral nociceptive input, (2) persistence of central hypersensitivity after resolution of primary peripheral event, and (3) imbalance of the descending modulation system. Curatolo M, Petersen-Felix S, Arendt-Nielsen L, Giani C, Zbinden AM, Radanov BP. Central hypersensitivity in chronic pain after whiplash injury. Clin J Pain. 2001 Dec;17(4):306–15.

At equal levels of pressure, patients with CLBP **(chronic low back pain)** or **fibromyalgia** experienced significantly more pain and showed more extensive, common patterns of **neuronal activation in pain-related cortical areas.** When stimuli that elicited equally painful responses were applied (requiring significantly lower pressure in both patient groups as compared with the control group), neuronal activations were similar among the 3 groups. These findings are consistent with the occurrence of **augmented central pain processing** in patients with idiopathic CLBP. Giesecke T, Gracely RH, Grant MA, Nachemson A, Petzke F, Williams DA, Clauw DJ. Evidence of augmented central pain processing in idiopathic chronic low back pain. Arthritis Rheum. 2004 Feb;50(2):613–23.

Gray matter density was reduced in bilateral dorsolateral prefrontal cortex and right thalamus and was strongly related to pain characteristics in a pattern distinct for neuropathic and non-neuropathic chronic back pain (CBP). Our results imply that CBP is accompanied by **brain atrophy** and suggest that the pathophysiology of chronic pain includes thalamocortical processes. Apkarian AV, Sosa Y, Sonty S, Levy RM, Harden RN, Parrish TB, Gitelman DR. Chronic back pain is associated with decreased prefrontal and thalamic gray matter density. J Neurosci. 2004 Nov 17;24(46):10410–5.

In chronic back pain, the interrelationship between chemicals within and across **brain regions was abnormal**, and there was a specific relationship between regional chemicals and perceptual measures of pain and anxiety. Grachev ID, Fredrickson BE, Apkarian AV. Abnormal brain chemistry in chronic back pain: an in vivo proton magnetic resonance spectroscopy study. Pain. 2000 Dec 15;89(1):7–18.

Those with persistent moderate/severe symptoms at 6 months display, soon after injury, generalized hypersensitivity suggestive of changes in central pain processing mechanisms. This phenomenon did not occur in those who recover or those with persistent mild symptoms. Sterling M, Jull G, Vicenzino B, Kenardy J. Sensory hypersensitivity occurs soon after whiplash injury and is associated with poor recovery. Pain 2003;104:509–517.

Non-recovery after whiplash was associated with initially reduced cold pressor pain endurance and increased peak pain, suggesting that dysfunction of central pain modulating control systems plays a role in chronic pain after acute whiplash injury. Kasch H, Qerama E, Bach FW, Jensen TS. Reduced cold pressor pain tolerance in non-recovered whiplash patients: a 1-year prospective study. Eur J Pain. 2005 Oct;9(5):561–9.

§ 8:16 Chronic pain—Spinal cord, dorsal horn, and the brain

Brain Blood Flow and Chronic Whiplash Pain. WAD patients had no alterations in cerebral blood-flow pattern, as measured by rCBF-SPECT and SPM analysis, compared to healthy controls. This contrasts with the non-traumatic group with chronic neck pain, which showed marked blood-flow changes. The blood-flow changes in the non-traumatic group were similar to those described earlier in pain patients but,remarkably enough, were different from those in the WAD group. **Chronic neck pain of whiplash and non-traumatic**

origin appears to be unique in some respects. A better understanding of the underlying pathological mechanisms is a prerequisite for prevention of the development of such chronic pain syndromes and for improvement of the treatment of patients with severe symptoms. Guez M. Chronic neck pain. An epidemiological, psychological and SPECT study with emphasis on whiplash-associated disorders. Acta Orthop Suppl. 2006 Feb;77(320):preceding 1, 3–33.

The rCBF was monitored in 45 patients with chronic neck pain: 27 cases with chronic whiplash syndrome and 18 age- and gender-matched cases with non-traumatic chronic neck pain. The rCBF was estimated with single-photon emission computed tomography (SPECT) using technetium-99m hexamethylpropylene amine oxime (HMPAO). The non-traumatic patients displayed rCBF changes in comparison with the whiplash group and the healthy control group. These changes included rCBF decreases in a right temporal region close to hippocampus, and increased rCBF in left insula. The whiplash group displayed no significant differences in rCBF in comparison with the healthy controls. **The present study suggests different pain mechanisms in patients with chronic neck pain of non-traumatic origin compared to those with chronic neck pain due to a whiplash trauma.** Sundstrom T, Guez M, Hildingsson C, Toolanen G, Nyberg L, Riklund K. Altered cerebral blood flow in chronic neck pain patients but not in whiplash patients: a (99m)Tc-HMPAO rCBF study. Eur Spine J. 2006 Aug;15(8):1189–95.

Intervertebral disc disease is a common cause of radiculopathy, which can result in severe pain and suffering. In addition, disc pathologies may be an important generator of low back pain, a major source of disability that requires considerable health care resources. **Inflammatory agents released** from (or recruited by) NP affect the dorsal root ganglion (and/or are transported to cord) to enhance primary afferent excitation of nociceptive dorsal horn neurons.

The current finding of enhanced dorsal horn neuronal windup after exposure of the DRG to NP may partially explain the clinical manifestations of lumbar disc herniation-induced radiculopathy. It is possible that, due to an enhanced dorsal horn neuronal excitability and windup response at low frequencies that do not normally elicit windup, the normally non-noxious stimulus is inducing dorsal horn **neuronal windup** that is interpreted as pain and further enhances the dorsal spinal neuronal excitability to subsequent sensory input. Cuellar JM, Montesano PX, Antognini JF, Carstens E. Application of nucleus pulposus to L5 dorsal root ganglion in rats enhances nociceptive dorsal horn neuronal windup. J Neurophysiol. 2005 Jul;94(1):35–48.

Patients with chronic low back pain (CLBP) have **augmented central pain processing**. Giesecke T, Gracely RH, Grant MA, Nachemson A, Petzke F, Williams DA, Clauw DJ. Evidence of augmented central pain processing in idiopathic chronic low back pain. Arthritis Rheum. 2004 Feb;50(2):613–23.

Altered sensory processing is probably involved in the determination of pain and disability in patients with chronic pain after whiplash injury. This mechanism can explain symptoms in the absence of evident tissue damage. Petersen-Felix S, Lars Arendt-Nielsen L, Curatolo M. Chronic Pain After Whiplash Injury-Evidence for Altered Central Sensory Processing. Journal of Whiplash & Related Disorders, Vol. 2(1) 2003.

Chronic pain is accompanied by **cortical reorganization** and may serve an important function in the persistence of the pain experience. The enlarged cortical representation of chronic pain observed in this study might contribute to and maintain the continuing experience of pain in chronic pain patients. Flor H, Braun C, Elbert T, Birbaumer N. Extensive reorganization of primary somatosensory cortex in chronic back pain patients. Neurosci Lett. 1997 Mar 7;224(1):5–8.

The findings suggest a **generalized central hyperexcitability** in patients suffering from chronic whiplash syndrome. This indicates that the pain might be considered as a neurogenic type of pain. Koelbaek Johansen M, Graven-Nielsen T, Schou Olesen A, Arendt-Nielsen L. Generalised muscular hyperalgesia in chronic whiplash syndrome. Pain. 1999 Nov;83(2):229–34.

Chronic back pain alters the human brain chemistry. In chronic back pain, the interrelationship between chemicals within and across brain regions was abnormal. These findings provide direct evidence of abnormal brain chemistry in chronic back pain. Grachev ID, Fredrickson BE, Apkarian AV. Abnormal brain chemistry in chronic back pain: an in vivo proton magnetic resonance spectroscopy study. Pain. 2000 Dec 15;89(1):7–18.

Abnormality of the trigeminal inhibitory temporalis reflex is based on a transient **dysfunction of the brainstem-mediated reflex circuit** mainly of the late polysynaptic pathways. The reflex abnormalities are considered as a neurophysiological correlate of the posttraumatic (cervico)-

cephalic pain syndrome. They point to an **altered central pain control in acute post traumatic headache due to whiplash injury**. Keidel M, Rieschke P, Stude P, Eisentraut R, van Schayck R, Diener H. Antinociceptive reflex alteration in acute posttraumatic headache following whiplash injury. Pain. 2001 Jun;92(3):319–26.

Chronic back pain was defined as back pain in excess of 6 months. Neocortical gray matter volume was compared in both groups. **Patients with chronic back pain showed 5–11% less neocortical gray matter volume than control subjects.** The magnitude of this decrease in neocortical grey matter is equivalent to the gray matter volume lost in 10–20 years of normal aging. The authors showed that the longer the pain, the greater the brain grey matter loss. The chronic back pain patients lost an average of 1.3 cm3 loss of gray matter for every year of chronic pain. The authors referred to this loss of grey matter from chronic back pain as "brain atrophy." Apkarian AV, Sosa Y, Sonty S, Levy RM, Harden RN, Parrish TB, Gitelman DR. Chronic back pain is associated with decreased prefrontal and thalamic gray matter density. J Neurosci. 2004 Nov 17;24(46):10410–5.

Comment:

The authors in the above study further quantify that "normal whole-brain gray matter atrophy is 0.5% per year of aging" and that atrophy caused by chronic back pain is 5–11% per year, which means that the "brain gray matter atrophy caused by chronic back pain is equivalent to 10–20 years of aging" per year of chronic back pain. They also note that 10% of adults suffer from severe chronic pain, back problems constitute 25% of all disabling occupational injuries, and that in 85% of those with back pain, "no definitive diagnosis can be made." They note that chronic pain greatly diminishes quality of life and increases anxiety and depression. Apparently, the authors claim that if the chronic back pain is treated successfully and quickly, the gray matter shrinkage is reversible, but with more prolonged pain the atrophy may not be reversible because it is attributable to neurodegeneration. The authors further find that the cause of chronic back pain is excitotoxicity [i.e. exposure to glutamate and aspartate, which are commonly added to foods as taste enhancers] and inflammatory agents [such as the omega-6 arachidonic acid cascade to the pro-inflammatory eicosanoid prostaglandin E2]. These results imply that Chronic Back Pain is accompanied by brain atrophy and suggest that the pathophysiology of chronic pain includes thalamocortical processes.

Those with persistent moderate/severe symptoms at 6 months display, soon after injury, generalized hypersensitivity suggestive of changes in **central pain processing** mechanisms. Sterling M, Jull G, Vicenzino B, Kenardy J. Sensory hypersensitivity occurs soon after whiplash injury and is associated with poor recovery. Pain. 2003 Aug;104(3):509–17.

We provide evidence for spinal cord hyperexcitability in patients with chronic pain after whiplash injury and in fibromyalgia patients. This can cause exaggerated pain following low intensity nociceptive or innocuous peripheral stimulation. **Spinal hypersensitivity may explain, at least in part, pain in the absence of detectable tissue damage**. Banic B, Petersen-Felix S, Andersen OK, Radanov BP, Villiger PM, Arendt-Nielsen L, Curatolo M. Evidence for spinal cord hypersensitivity in chronic pain after whiplash injury and in fibromyalgia. Pain. 2004 Jan;107(1–2):7–15.

Tissue damage, detected or not by the available diagnostic methods, is probably the main determinant of central hypersensitivity. **Central hypersensitivity may explain exaggerated pain in the presence of minimal nociceptive input arising from minimally damaged tissues. This could account for pain and disability in the absence of objective signs of tissue damage in patients with whiplash.** Central hypersensitivity may provide a common neurobiological framework for the integration of peripheral and supraspinal mechanisms in the pathophysiology of chronic pain after whiplash. Curatolo M, Arendt-Nielsen L, Petersen-Felix S. Evidence, mechanisms, and clinical implications of central hypersensitivity in chronic pain after whiplash injury. Clin J Pain. 2004 Nov–Dec;20(6):469–76.

Accurate reproducible maps of cortical responses can be used to measure the neurological consequences of spinal joint manipulation. Cervical manipulation activates specific neurological pathways. **Manipulation of the cervical spine may be associated with an increase or a decrease in brain function depending upon the side of the manipulation and the cortical hemisphericity of a patient.** Carrick FR. Changes in brain function after manipulation of the cervical spine. J Manipulative Physiol Ther. 1997 Oct;20(8):529–45.

The **cerebral cortex is able to control the nociceptive processing in different pain syndromes (somatic, visceral or neuropathic pain).** Opioidergic and serotonergic systems play the key role in this control. The effect over the cortical descending control is likely to be one of the components of the analgetic effect exerted by opioids and some other central analgesics. Kharkevich DA, Churukanov VV. Pharmacological regulation of descending cortical control of the nociceptive processing. Eur J Pharmacol. 1999 Jun 30;375(1–3):121–31.

The correlations between the sensory and affective dimensions of pain were non-significant, which indicates that they are two independent constructs that describe various dimensions of whiplash-related pain. High pain intensity and pain affect, greater widespread pain, and high fear of movement/(re)injury corresponded to low self-efficacy. Multiple regression analyses showed that **self-efficacy was the most important predictor of persistent disability** contributing to 42% of the variation in the PDI score. The treatment approach for patients with subacute WAD should incorporate the multidimensional nature of pain, and special effort should be made to enhance the patient's self-efficacy beliefs to prevent disability. Bunketorp L, Lindh M, Carlsson J, Stener-Victorin E. The perception of pain and pain-related cognitions in subacute whiplash-associated disorders: Its influence on prolonged disability. Disabil Rehabil. 2006 Mar;28(5):271–9.

Significant correlation was identified with a high pain score and an increasing age of patient and high NDI scores. No correlation was found between the impact speed, speed of vehicle struck, or time since incident with the NDI. **Two-thirds of patients had some disability at 4–6 weeks after injury;** 91 patients (54.5%) saw their GP in the intervening period between attending the department and telephone follow up, and 87/170 patients had no idea about their prognosis. This study identifies that **there is significant disability associated with whiplash associated disorder**. Crouch R, Whitewick R, Clancy M, Wright P, Thomas P. Whiplash associated disorder: incidence and natural history over the first month for patients presenting to a UK emergency department. Emerg Med J. 2006 Feb;23(2):114–8.

To investigate differences in sensory and sympathetic nervous system (SNS) function between whiplash-injured persons with and without a posttraumatic stress reaction (PTSR) and explore associations between sensory, SNS function, and persistent PTSR at 6 months post-injury. Seventy-six acutely (<1 month) whiplash-injured persons (10 with PTSR persisting to 6 months post-injury, 14 with early PTSR that resolved, and 52 with no PTSR) were prospectively investigated. Those with persistent PTSR showed sensory hypersensitivity and impaired peripheral vasoconstriction, compared to those whose PTSR resolved and those without PTSR (P<.05). The early presence of sensory hypersensitivity was associated with PTSR at 6 months, but this relationship was mediated by pain and disability levels. Impaired vasoconstriction and higher pain and disability levels were associated with PTSR at 6 months. **Sensory disturbances following whiplash injury are associated with persistent PTSR but may be mediated by levels of pain and disability.** Sterling M, Kenardy J. The relationship between sensory and sympathetic nervous system changes and posttraumatic stress reaction following whiplash injury-a prospective study. J Psychosom Res. 2006 Apr;60(4):387–93.

§ 8:17 Chronic pain—Chronic myofascial pain

Chronic myofascial pain is more than just the muscle.

The nociceptive processes are qualitatively altered in patients with chronic myofascial pain and suggest that myofascial pain may be mediated by low-threshold mechanosensitive afferents projecting to **sensitized dorsal horn neurons (sensory neurons in the spinal cord)**. Bendtsen L, Jensen R, Olesen J. Qualitatively altered nociception in chronic myofascial pain. Pain. 1996 May–Jun;65(2–3):259–64.

The results of the review showed that the reported proportion of patients who **still experienced pain after 12 months was 62%** on average (range 42–75%), the percentage of patients sick-listed 6 months after inclusion into the study was 16% (range 3–40%), the percentage who experienced relapses of pain was 60% (range 44–78%), and the percentage who had relapses of work absence was 33% (range 26–37%). ¶ The mean reported prevalence of LBP in cases with previous episodes was 56% (range 14–93%), which compared with 22% (range 7–39%) for those without a prior history of LBP. The risk of LBP was consistently about twice as high for those with a history of LBP. The results of the review show that, despite the methodological variations and the lack of comparable definitions, the overall picture is that LBP does not resolve itself when ignored.

There is no evidence supporting the claim that 80–90% of LBP patients become pain free within 1 month. Hestbaek L, Leboeuf-Yde C, Manniche C. Low back pain: what is the long-term course? A review of studies of general patient populations. Eur Spine J. 2003 Apr;12(2):149–65.

75% with continue to have problems. At 3 and **12 months**

follow up, only 39/188 (21%) and 42/170 (25%) respectively **had completely recovered** in terms of pain and disability. The original article to which the statement of "90% recovery" can be traced to a record review in one general practice (Dixon ASJ. Progress and problems in back pain research. Rheumatol Rehabil 1973;12(4):165–75). If no further consultation within an episode is taken as the measure of "recovery" then record review is a valid measure of this. However, the inference that the patients have completely recovered is clearly not supported by our data. General practice records cannot be used to draw such conclusions. Croft PR, Macfarlane GJ, Papageorgiou AC, Thomas E, Silman AJ. Outcome of low back pain in general practice: a prospective study. BMJ 1998;316:1356–9.

55% had residual disorders referable to the original accident. Neck pain, radiating pain and headache were the most common symptoms. One-third of the patients with residual symptoms suffered from work disability, compared to 6% in the group of patients without residual disorders. All 25 patients who had reached a final claim settlement (42%) had a poor outcome. Patients with WAD reported a significantly higher score on the NDI than those without residual disorders. The results of the study show that approximately half of the patients with neck complaints following motor vehicle accidents in Gothenburg in 1983 suffered frequent residual symptoms 17 years after the accident, mostly comprising neck pain, radiating pain, and headache. The residual disorders contributed to the patients' overall disability. Bunketorp L, Nordholm L, Carlsson J. A descriptive analysis of disorders in patients 17 years following motor vehicle accidents. Eur Spine J. 2002 Jun;11(3):227–34.

§ 8:18 Chronic pain—Recurring pain

The clinical significance of nociceptor 'activity'-dependent spinal cord & supraspinal LTP to manipulative therapy is fairly obvious. It would constitute **not only a molecular mechanism for acute pain and its consequences, but also a potentially lasting physiologically and structurally mediated 'memory' basis for chronic continuous, or relapsing, pain and associated disability. Relapsing pain** and its consequences may, therefore, be seen as a periodic breakthrough (for a variety of reasons) of the less desirable of these 'memories'. Zusman M. Mechanisms of musculoskeletal physiotherapy. Phys Ther Rev. 2004;9:39–49.

To summarize, sensory input — nociceptive and proprioceptive — produced as a result of peripheral tissue insult leads to physiological and anatomical changes at synapses in the central nervous system, a form of LTP. As well as for pain, these synaptic events are a learned mechanism for the expression of maladaptive changes in motor function — muscle tone, and postures and movements collectively known as 'behavior'. **Unless and until movement can be carried out in the relative/total absence of pain, both the synaptic 'memory' and its behavioral consequences are likely to be self-reinforcing. Indeed, they have the potential to become chronic. This is generally averted by a combination of natural history and delivery of appropriate therapeutic interventions**. An important neurological consequence of the latter is to drastically change — that is 'normalize' — the pattern of sensory input. Zusman M. Mechanisms of musculoskeletal physiotherapy. Phys Ther Rev. 2004;9:39–49.

Research indicates that manipulative therapy is not a placebo therapy. Placebo analgesia uses endogenous opioids. Manual therapy is not opioid based, does not induce tolerance. (manipulative uses different pain inhibition processes) Paungmali A, O'Leary S, Souvlis T, Vicenzino B. Naloxone fails to antagonize initial hypoalgesic effect of a manual therapy treatment for lateral epicondylalgia.J Manipulative Physiol Ther. 2004 Mar–Apr;27(3):180–5; Paungmali A, Vicenzino B, Smith M. Hypoalgesia induced by elbow manipulation in lateral epicondylalgia does not exhibit tolerance. J Pain. 2003 Oct;4(8) :448–54.

Clinical and basic science literature suggests that the analgesic effects of manipulation are segmentally organized and probably result from large-diameter afferent stimulation. Further, this **analgesic effect is nonopioid but involves spinal activation of serotoneric and noradrenergic-receptors,** implicating descending inhibitory pathways from the RVM and the noradrenergic cells in the brainstem. Sluka KA, Hoeger MK, Skyba DA. Basic Science Mechanisms of Nonpharmacological Treatments for Pain. Pain 2002-An Updated Review: ISAP Press 2002.

§ 8:19 Muscle pain

Released by trauma or inflammatory injury, serotonin sensitizes muscle nociceptors to chemical and mechanical stimuli. Seratonin combined with bradykinin induces muscle hyperalgesia to pressure. **These are peripheral mechanisms for muscle tenderness and hyperalgesia**. Graven-Nielsen

T, Mense S. The peripheral apparatus of muscle pain: evidence from animal and human studies. Clin J Pain. 2001 Mar;17(1):2–10.

Outcome following whiplash injury of the cervical spine is variable, and the pathology of those with prolonged symptoms is uncertain. This was a prospective study in 25 patients to identify whether those with prolonged symptoms following whiplash injury exhibit a rise in serum creatine kinase consistent with significant muscle damage at the time of injury. Transient rise in creatine kinase level was seen in only 2 of 25 patients, neither of whom complained of prolonged symptoms. Of the 8 patients who developed chronic symptoms following whiplash injury, none demonstrated a serum creatine kinase rise. **Prolonged symptoms following whiplash injury cannot be explained by biochemically measurable muscle damage.** See Scott S, Sanderson PL. Whiplash: a biochemical study of muscle injury. Eur Spine J. 2002 Aug;11(4):389–92.

Chronic muscle pain lasting more for months would be caused by neurogenic type of pain and not continued nociception from the muscle. Koelbaek Johansen M, Graven-Nielsen T, Schou Olesen A, Arendt-Nielsen L. Generalised muscular hyperalgesia in chronic whiplash syndrome. Pain. 1999 Nov;83(2):229–34.

Chronic muscle pain is maintained by the central nervous system. Sluka KA, Kalra A, Moore SA. Unilateral intramuscular injections of acidic saline produce a bilateral, long-lasting hyperalgesia. Muscle Nerve. 2001 Jan;24(1):37–46.

This can be caused by a long-term increase of the excitability of wide dynamic neurons in the spinal cord. Rygh LJ, Svendsen F, Hole K, Tjolsen A. Natural noxious stimulation can induce long-term increase of spinal nociceptive responses. Pain. 1999 Sep;82(3):305–10.

This can also be caused by a decrease in cortical brain function. (The cerebral cortex activates descending pain inhibition). Kharkevich DA, Churukanov VV. Pharmacological regulation of descending cortical control of the nociceptive processing. Eur J Pharmacol. 1999 Jun 30;375(1–3):121–31.

§ 8:20 Muscle pain—Inflammation

Inflammation increases the sensitivity of the receptors in the periphery and in the central nervous system by altering membrane properties of nociceptors, permitting a higher discharge frequency and contributing to hyperalgesia, and by activating synapses that are usually inactive. Inflammatory pain and the sensitization of peripheral nociceptors can be very rapid and involve non-neuronal cells such as mast cells, neutrophils, fibroblasts, and macrophages. Inflammation increases the sensitivity in the peripheral terminals of A-d and C fibers. Davis C. Chronic pain/dysfunction in whiplash-associated disorders. J Manipulative Physiol Ther. 2001 Jan;24(1):44–51.

Inflammation causes A-β fibers, which normally inhibit nociception, to sprout into lamina II in the dorsal horn and express SP as C fibers. Inflammation elevates the neurotrophin NGF, increases levels of PGE2, activates cholecystokinin-B receptors, alters the sensory processing in the substantia gelatinosa, increases nociceptin (also known as *orphanin* FQ), sensitizes tetrodotoxin sodium current receptors that are present in peripheral terminals of primary afferent nociceptors, increases NO that is involved in the maintenance of mechanical allodynia, induces central sensitization in the spinal cord, and increases the number of sensory axons containing ionotropic glutamate receptors that contribute to peripheral sensitization. The medullary dorsal reticular nucleus plays a pronociceptive role in both acute and tonic inflammatory pain, leading to amplification of the nociceptive signal, and it may also underlie the noxious response to the temporomandibular joint. Davis C. Chronic pain/dysfunction in whiplash-associated disorders. J Manipulative Physiol Ther. 2001 Jan;24(1):44–51.

Cytokines released from an injury may be proinflammatory or anti-inflammatory, Cytokines are small proteins that are essential for healing of connective tissue after injury and play roles in cell-to-cell signaling. The interaction between a cytokine and its receptor is highly specific. The response of a cell to its own cytokine is known as an autocrine response; the response of a cell to cytokines produced by adjacent cells is known as a paracrine response. Cytokines can also act as endocrine signals. Evidence points to tumor necrosis factor-a (a proinflammatory cytokine) having a role in inducing the hyperalgesic response to inflammation; this is likely to be the consequence of its induction of later-acting intermediaries, particularly interleukin-1-β and NGF. Cytokines may act as a link between the nervous and immune systems. Davis C. Chronic pain/dysfunction in whiplash-associated disorders. J Manipulative Physiol Ther. 2001 Jan;24(1):44–51.

§ 8:21 Muscle pain—Chronic pain HPA axis

Hypothalamic-pituitary-adrenal stress axis function

and the relationship with chronic widespread pain and its antecedents. In clinic studies, altered hypothalamic-pituitary-adrenal (HPA) axis function has been associated with fibromyalgia, a syndrome characterized by chronic widespread body pain. These results may be explained by the associated high rates of psychological distress and somatisation. A hypothesis has been asserted that the latter, rather than the pain, might explain the HPA results. A population study ascertained pain and psychological status in subjects aged 25 to 65 years. Random samples were selected from the following three groups: satisfying criteria for chronic widespread pain; free of chronic widespread pain but with strong evidence of somatisation ("at risk"); and a reference group. HPA axis function was assessed from measuring early morning and evening salivary cortisol levels, and serum cortisol after physical (pain pressure threshold exam) and chemical (overnight 0.25 mg dexamethasone suppression test) stressors. The relationship between HPA function with pain and the various psychosocial scales assessed was modeled using appropriate regression analyses, adjusted for age and gender. In all 131 persons with chronic widespread pain (participation rate 74%), 267 "at risk" (58%) and 56 controls (70%) were studied. Those in the chronic widespread pain and "at risk" groups were, respectively, 3.1 (95% CI (1.3, 7.3)) and 1.8 (0.8, 4.0) times more likely to have a saliva cortisol score in the lowest third. **None of the psychosocial factors measured were, however, associated with saliva cortisol scores.** Further, those in the chronic widespread pain (1.9 (0.8, 4.7)) and "at risk" (1.6 (0.7, 3.6)) groups were also more likely to have the highest serum cortisol scores. High post-stress serum cortisol was related to high levels of psychological distress ($p = 0.05$, 95% CI (0.02, 0.08)). After adjusting for levels of psychological distress, the association between chronic widespread pain and post-stress cortisol scores remained, albeit slightly attenuated. **This is the first population study to demonstrate that those with established, and those psychologically at risk of, chronic widespread pain demonstrate abnormalities of HPA axis function,** which are more marked in the former group. Although some aspects of the altered function are related to the psychosocial factors measured, the occurrence of HPA abnormality in persons with chronic widespread pain is not fully explained by the accompanying psychological stress. McBeth J, Chiu YH, Silman AJ, Ray D, Morriss R, Dickens C, Gupta A, Macfarlane GJ. Hypothalamic-pituitary-adrenal stress axis function and the relationship with chronic widespread pain and its antecedents. Arthritis Res Ther. 2005;7(5):R992–R1000.

Dysregulations of the HPA (hypothalamus-pituitary-adrenal) axis in terms of reduced reactivity and enhanced negative feedback suppression exist in chronic WAD. This causes dysregulation of the neuroendrocrine mechanisms leading to continued pain. The observed endocrine abnormalities could serve as a systemic mechanism of symptoms experienced by chronic WAD patients. Gaab J, Baumann S, Budnoik A, Gmunder H, Hottinger N, Ehlert U. Reduced reactivity and enhanced negative feedback sensitivity of the hypothalamus-pituitary-adrenal axis in chronic whiplash-associated disorder. Pain. 2005 Dec 15;119(1–3):219–24.

At 8 weeks post-lesion, there was a dramatic increase in the density of peptidergic fibers in the upper dermis. Quantification revealed that densities of peptidergic fibers 8 weeks post-lesion were significantly above levels in sham animals. The ectopic sympathetic fibers did not innervate blood vessels but formed a novel association and wrapped around sprouted peptidergic nociceptive fibers. Data show a long-term sympathetic and sensory innervation change in the rat hind paw skin after the chronic constriction injury. **This novel fiber arrangement after nerve lesion may play an important role in the development and persistence of sympathetically maintained neuropathic pain after partial nerve lesions.** Yen LD, Bennett GJ, Ribeiro-da-Silva A. Sympathetic sprouting and changes in nociceptive sensory innervation in the glabrous skin of the rat hind paw following partial peripheral nerve injury. J Comp Neurol. 2006 Feb 27;495(6):679–690.

Autonomic (sympathetic and parasympathetic) fiber sprouting was first observed 1 week post-injury, with a peak in the number of sprouted fibers occurring at 4 and 6 weeks post-CCI. CGRP-IR fibers almost disappeared at 2 weeks post-CCI, but quickly sprouted, leading to a significant peak above sham levels 4 weeks post-injury. trkA receptor expression was found to be up-regulated in small cutaneous nerves 4 weeks post-CCI, returning to sham levels by 8 weeks post-CCI. There was no sympathetic fiber sprouting in the trigeminal ganglion following CCI. At 4 weeks post-CCI, rats displayed spontaneous, directed grooming to the area innervated by the MN that was not seen in sham animals, which we interpreted as a sign of spontaneous pain or dysesthesiae. Collectively, our findings indicate that as a result of **autonomic sprouting due to CCI of the MN, remaining intact nociceptive fibres may potentially develop sensitivity to sympathetic and parasympathetic stimulation, which may have a role in the generation of abnormal pain following nerve injury**.

Grelik C, Bennett GJ, Ribeiro-da-Silva A. Autonomic fibre sprouting and changes in nociceptive sensory innervation in the rat lower lip skin following chronic constriction injury. Eur J Neurosci. 2005 May;21(9):2475–87.

Glially-driven pain can also occur under pathological conditions, such as occurs following peripheral nerve inflammation or trauma. Here, **immune- and trauma-induced alterations in peripheral nerve function lead to the release of substances within the spinal cord that trigger the activation of glia**. Evidence is reviewed that such pathologically-driven glial activation is associated with enhanced pain states of diverse etiologies and that such pain facilitation is driven by **glial release of proinflammatory cytokines and other neuroexcitatory substances**. This recently recognized role of spinal cord glia and glially derived proinflammatory cytokines as powerful modulators of pain is exciting as it may provide novel approaches for controlling human chronic pain states that are poorly controlled by currently available therapies. Wieseler-Frank J, Maier SF, Watkins LR. Immune-to-brain communication dynamically modulates pain: physiological and pathological consequences. Brain Behav Immun. 2005 Mar;19(2):104–11.

Evolving evidence demonstrates that proinflammatory cytokines are a key mediator in the process of disc degeneration as well as in the pain experienced by those afflicted with lumbar herniated discs. Activated immune cells release proinflammatory cytokines, which signal the brain through humoral and neural routes. The brain responds by altering neural activity and promoting further production of proinflammatory cytokines within the brain and spinal cord. Increased local cytokine production by disc tissue irritates spinal nerve roots, resulting in pain and functional changes in neural activity. This review of the current literature explores the importance of cytokine production within the context of lumbar disc degeneration and lumbar spine pain. Furthermore, **the significance of the neural-immune interaction will be examined as it relates to pain management and to patient treatment**. Starkweather A, Witek-Janusek L, Mathews HL. Neural-immune interactions: implications for pain management in patients with low-back pain and sciatica. Biol Res Nurs. 2005 Jan;6(3):196–206.

The immune-to-brain communication pathway triggers the production of a constellation of CNS-mediated phenomena, collectively referred to as "sickness responses." These sickness responses are created by immune-to-brain signals activating CNS glia to release glial proinflammatory cytokines. The most recently recognized member of this constellation of changes is enhanced pain responsivity. The hypothesis is then developed that pathological, chronic pain may result from "tapping into" this ancient survival-oriented circuitry, including the activation of immune and glial cells and the release of immune/glial proinflammatory cytokines. This can occur at the level of peripheral nerves, dorsal root ganglia, spinal cord, and likely at higher brain areas. The implications of this model for human chronic pain syndromes and clinical resolution of these chronic pain states are then discussed. Watkins LR, Maier SF. Immune regulation of central nervous system functions: from sickness responses to pathological pain. J Intern Med. 2005 Feb;257(2):139–55.

Muscles and Chronic Pain

Fatty infiltrates in the cervical extensor musculature and widespread hyperalgesia were not features of the insidious-onset neck pain group in this study; whereas these features have been identified in patients with chronic WAD.

Elliott J, Sterling M, Noteboom JT, Darnell R, Galloway G, Jull G. Fatty infiltrate in the cervical extensor muscles is not a feature of chronic, insidious-onset neck pain. Clin Radiol. 2008 Jun;63(6):681–687.

There is significantly **greater fatty infiltration** in the neck extensor muscles, especially in the deeper muscles in the upper cervical spine, in subjects with persistent WAD when compared with healthy controls.

Elliott J, Jull G, Noteboom JT, Darnell R, Galloway G, Gibbon WW. Fatty infiltration in the cervical extensor muscles in persistent whiplash-associated disorders: a magnetic resonance imaging analysis. Spine. 2006 Oct 15;31(22):E847–55.

A quantitative measure of muscle/fat constituents has been developed, and results of this study indicate that relative fatty infiltration is **not a feature of age** in the upper cervical extensor muscles of women aged 18–45 years.

Elliott JM, Galloway GJ, Jull GA, Noteboom JT, Centeno CJ, Gibbon WW. Magnetic resonance imaging analysis of the upper cervical spine extensor musculature in an asymptomatic cohort: an index of fat within muscle. Clin Radiol. 2005 Mar;60(3):355–63.

Chronic tension-type headache (CTTH) patients demonstrate **muscle atrophy** of the rectus capitis posterior muscles.

Whether this selective muscle atrophy is a primary or secondary phenomenon remains unclear. In any case, muscle atrophy could possibly account for a reduction of proprioceptive output from these muscles, and thus contribute to the perpetuation of pain.

Fernández-de-Las-Peñas C, Bueno A, Ferrando J, Elliott JM, Cuadrado ML, Pareja JA. Magnetic resonance imaging study of the morphometry of cervical extensor muscles in chronic tension-type headache. Cephalalgia. 2007 Apr;27(4):355–62.

There is a relationship between chronic pain, somatic dysfunction, **muscle atrophy** and standing balance. We hypothesize a cycle initiated by chronic somatic dysfunction, which may result in muscle atrophy, which can be further expected to reduce proprioceptive output from atrophied muscles. The lack of proprioceptive inhibition of nociceptors at the dorsal horn of the spinal cord would result in chronic pain and a loss of standing balance.

McPartland JM, Brodeur RR, Hallgren RC. Chronic neck pain, standing balance, and suboccipital muscle atrophy—a pilot study. J Manipulative Physiol Ther. 1997 Jan;20(1):24–9.

The reduction in proprioceptive afferent activity in affected muscles may cause increased facilitation of neural activity that is perceived as pain. This preliminary work indicates **substantial infiltration of fatty tissue into suboccipital muscles** of some subjects being treated for chronic head and neck pain.

Hallgren RC, Greenman PE, Rechtien JJ. Atrophy of suboccipital muscles in patients with chronic pain: a pilot study. J Am Osteopath Assoc. 1994 Dec;94(12):1032–8.

The same pattern of muscular reaction was found in patients with rheumatoid arthritis as in patients with soft-tissue injuries of the neck (e.g., "whiplash injury"). In the ventral muscles and the obliquus capitis inferior, the occurrence of transformations correlated strongly with the duration of symptoms; in the ventral muscles the vast majority of transformations were encountered in patients with a shorter history of symptoms, whereas in the obliquus capitis inferior the reverse occurred. In the other dorsal muscles, no correlation with the duration of symptoms was found. Muscles in which transformations had ceased displayed, on average, a significantly higher percentage of fast type-IIB fibers than were found in muscles with ongoing transformations. ***This strongly indicates that the transformations proceeded in the direction from "slow oxidative" to "fast glycolytic."***

Uhlig Y, Weber BR, Grob D, Müntener M. Fiber composition

and fiber transformations in neck muscles of patients with dysfunction of the cervical spine. J Orthop Res. 1995 Mar;13(2):240–9.

§ 8:22 Posttraumatic stress disorder—Symptoms and the course of whiplash complaints

Individuals who had been involved in traffic accidents and had initiated compensation claim procedures with a Dutch insurance company were sent questionnaires (Q1) containing complaint-related questions and the Self-Rating Scale for PTSD. Of the 997 questionnaires that were dispatched, 617 (62%) were returned. Only car accident victims were included in this study (n=240). Complaints were monitored using additional questionnaires that were administered 6 months (Q2) and 12 months (Q3) after the accident.

PTSD was related to the presence and severity of concurrent post-whiplash syndrome. More specifically, the intensity of hyperarousal symptoms that were related to PTSD at Q1 was found to have predictive validity for the persistence and severity of post-whiplash syndrome at 6 and 12 months follow-up.

Results are consistent with the idea that PTSD hyperarousal symptoms have a detrimental influence on the recovery and severity of whiplash complaints following car accidents.

Buitenhuis J, de Jong PJ, Jaspers JP, Groothoff JW. Relationship between posttraumatic stress disorder symptoms and the course of whiplash complaints. J Psychosom Res. 2006 Nov;61(5):681–9.

To investigate differences in sensory and sympathetic nervous system (SNS) function between whiplash-injured persons with and without a posttraumatic stress reaction (PTSR) and explore associations between sensory, SNS function, and persistent PTSR at 6 months post-injury. Seventy-six acutely (<1 month) whiplash-injured persons (10 with PTSR persisting to 6 months post-injury, 14 with early PTSR that resolved, and 52 with no PTSR) were prospectively investigated. Those with persistent PTSR showed sensory hypersensitivity and impaired peripheral vasoconstriction, compared to those whose PTSR resolved and those without PTSR (P<.05). The early presence of sensory hypersensitivity was associated with PTSR at 6 months, but this relationship was mediated by pain and disability levels. Impaired vasoconstriction and higher pain and disability levels were associated with PTSR at 6 months. **Sensory disturbances following whiplash injury are associated with persistent**

PTSR but may be mediated by levels of pain and disability. Sterling M, Kenardy J. The relationship between sensory and sympathetic nervous system changes and posttraumatic stress reaction following whiplash injury-a prospective study. J Psychosom Res. 2006 Apr;60(4):387–93.

§ 8:23 Fibromyalgia

Fibromyalgia, in which there is no apperent peripheral pathology, may be a clinical manifestation of altered central nervous system processing. Woolf CJ. Somatic pain—pathogenesis and prevention. Br J Anaesth. 1995 Aug;75(2):169–76.

This central nervous system mechanism may explain fibromylagia and myofascial pain syndromes. Simms RW. Fibromyalgia is not a muscle disorder. Am J Med Sci. 1998 Jun;315(6):346–50.

The weight of evidence suggests that fibromyalgia is a chronic pain syndrome that has a central, rather than peripheral or muscular basis. Salerno A, Thomas E, Olive P, Blotman F, Picot MC, Georgesco M. Motor cortical dysfunction disclosed by single and double magnetic stimulation in patients with fibromyalgia. Clin Neurophysiol. 2000 Jun;111(6):994–1001.

An impairment in function descending pain-inhibiting pathways is likely to lead to: spontaneous deep pain (because of an increased background activity in nociceptive neurons supplying deep tissues), tenderness of deep tissues (because of a lowered mechanical threshold of the same neurons), and hyperalgesia of deep tissues (because of increased neuronal responses to noxious stimuli). Mense S. Neurobiological concepts of fibromyalgia—the possible role of descending spinal tracts. Scand J Rheumatol Suppl. 2000;113:24–9.

Adults with neck injuries had a tenfold increased risk of developing fibromyalgia within one year after their injury, compared with adults with lower extremity fractures. White KP, Carette S, Harth M, Teasell RW. Trauma and fibromyalgia: is there an association and what does it mean? Semin Arthritis Rheum. 2000 Feb;29(4):200–16.

Whiplash associated disorders carry a thirteen-fold risk for development of fibromyalgia. Buskila D, Neumann L, Vaisberg G, Alkalay D, Wolfe F. Increased rates of fibromyalgia following cervical spine injury. A controlled study of 161 cases of traumatic injury. Arthritis Rheum. 1997 Mar;40(3):446–52.

Trauma in the preceeding 6 months is significantly associated with the onset of fibromyalgia syndrome. Al-Allaf AW, Dunbar KL, Hallum NS, Nosratzadeh B, Templeton KD, Pullar T. A case-control study examining the role of physical trauma in the onset of fibromyalgia syndrome. Rheumatology (Oxford). 2002 Apr;41(4):450–3.

The findings indicate that CNS (central nervous system) dysfunction frequently occurs in patients with fibromyalgia, although proprioceptive disturbances might also explain some of the abnormalities observed. Rosenhall U, Johansson G, Orndahl G. Otoneurologic and audiologic findings in fibromyalgia. Scand J Rehabil Med. 1996 Dec;28(4):225–32.

Chronic pain in fibromyalgia and whiplash groups was associated with significantly higher muscle tension than in pain-free controls. Biomechanical output was significantly lower in patients with pain. Elert J, Kendall SA, Larsson B, Mansson B, Gerdle B. Chronic pain and difficulty in relaxing postural muscles in patients with fibromyalgia and chronic whiplash associated disorders. J Rheumatol. 2001. Jun;28(6):1361–8.

Compared with control subjects, the rCBF (regional cerebral blood flow) in FM patients was significantly reduced in the right thalamus (P = 0.006), but not in the left thalamus or head of either caudate nucleus. The thalamus is the switchboard of information into the cerebral cortex. **The finding of a reduction in thalamic rCBF is consistent with findings of functional brain imaging studies of other chronic clinical pain syndromes, while the finding of reduced pontine tegmental (part of the brain stem) rCBF is new.** See Kwiatek R, Barnden L, Tedman R, Jarrett R, Chew J, Rowe C, Pile K. Regional cerebral blood flow in fibromyalgia: single-photon-emission computed tomography evidence of reduction in the pontine tegmentum and thalami. Arthritis Rheum. 2000 Dec;43(12):2823–33.

Findings suggest that those with persistent moderate/severe symptoms at 6 months display, soon after injury, **generalized hypersensitivity** suggestive of changes in **central pain processing mechanisms**. This phenomenon did not occur in those who recover or those with persistent mild symptoms. This hyperalgesia persisted in those with moderate/severe symptoms at 6 months but resolved by 2 months in those who had recovered or reported persistent mild symptoms. Sterling M, Jull G, Vicenzino B, Kenardy J. Sensory hypersensitivity occurs soon after whiplash injury and is associated with poor recovery. Pain 2003;104:509–517.

Evidence is provided for **spinal cord hyperexcitability** in patients with chronic pain after whiplash injury and in fibromyalgia patients. This can cause exaggerated pain following low intensity nociceptive or innocuous peripheral stimulation. Spinal hypersensitivity may explain, at least in part, pain in the **absence of detectable tissue damage**. Banic B, Petersen-Felix S, Andersen OK, Radanov BP, Villiger PM, Arendt-Nielsen L, Curatolo M. Evidence for spinal cord hypersensitivity in chronic pain after whiplash injury and in fibromyalgia. Pain 2004;107: 7–15.

There is strong consistency in documentation that physical trauma such as a fall or motor vehicle accident, particularly a whiplash or spinal injury, can trigger Fibromyalgia in some patients. These studies, as well as the presentation of plausible etiological mechanisms, make a compelling argument that **trauma does, in fact, play an etiological role in the development of FMS** in some, but not all patients. Jain AK, Heffez DA, Carruthers BS, Leung FYK, van de Sande MI, Malone DG, Barron SR, Romano TJ, Donaldson CCS, Russell IJ, Dunne JV, Saul D, Gingrich E, Seibel DG. Fibromyalgia Syndrome: Canadian Clinical Working Case Definition, Diagnostic and Treatment Protocols—A Consensus Document. Journal of Musculoskeletal Pain 2003; Volume 11, Number 4, Pg. 44 – 45.

The evidence that motor vehicle collision trauma may trigger fibromyalgiaFM meets established criteria for determining causality, and has a number of important implications, both for patient care, and for research into the pathophysiology and treatment of these disorders. McLean SA, Williams DA, Clauw DJ. Fibromyalgia after motor vehicle collision: evidence and implications. Traffic Inj Prev. 2005 Jun;6(2) :97–104.

§ 8:24 Neuronal plasticity

Comment:

Neuronal plasticity—changes in the nervous system—can be good (improving your golf game by practicing) or bad (your body getting more efficient in transmitting pain signals). Joint mechanoreceptors and muscle spindles provide non-nociceptive information into the nervous system. Chronic muscle pain can be caused by dysfunction of the joints, as the joints normally provide non-nociceptive information into the nervous system. Joints that do not move are sensitized the same as in inflammation. Pain can be caused by a decrease in non-nociceptive input to the nervous system.

Central sensitization refers to enhanced excitability of dorsal horn neurons (sensory nerve cells in the posterior part of the spinal cord) and is characterized by increased spontaneous activity, enlarged receptive field (RF) areas, and an increase in responses evoked by large and small caliber, primary afferent fibers. **Sensitization of dorsal horn neurons often occurs following tissue injury and inflammation and is believed to contribute to hyperalgesia. Windup refers to the progressive increase in the magnitude of C-fiber evoked responses of dorsal horn neurons produced by repetitive activation of C-fibers.** Li J, Simone DA, Larson AA. Windup leads to characteristics of central sensitization. Pain. 1999 Jan;79(1):75–82.

Results suggest that after C-fiber injury, uninjured A-fiber central terminals can collaterally sprout into lamina II of the dorsal horn. This phenomenon may help to explain the pain associated with C-fiber neuropathy. Mannion RJ, Doubell TP, Coggeshall RE, Woolf CJ. Collateral sprouting of uninjured primary afferent A-fibers into the superficial dorsal horn of the adult rat spinal cord after topical capsaicin treatment to the sciatic nerve. J Neurosci. 1996 Aug 15;16(16):5189–95.

Patients with chronic cervicobrachialgia have pain thresholds and pain tolerances lower than normal. In a normal person, A-beta () afferent (large mylenated) fibers participate in transmitting low-threshold stimuli from mechanoreceptors and A-delta ()/C fibers participate in transmitting high threshold stimuli such as pain and thermal signals. Loss of input from A (afferent fibers may diminish the inhibition of the projecting neurons and give rise to "low-input" pain. With a phenotype change in the spinal cord, A afferent fibers that would normally evoke nonpainful sensations may elicit and maintain pain (allodynia). See Voerman VF, van Egmond J, Crul BJ. Elevated detection thresholds for mechanical stimuli in chronic pain patients: support for a central mechanism. Arch Phys Med Rehabil. 2000 Apr;81(4):430–5.

A-beta (β)-afferent input (large diameter nerve fibers that usually do not transmit pain) contributes to the allodynia experienced during inflammation. Ma QP, Woolf CJ. Basal and touch-evoked fos-like immunoreactivity during experimental inflammation in the rat. Pain. 1996 Oct;67(2–3):307–16.

If severe pain is allowed to persist for more than 24 hours, the neuroplastic changes associated with the development of incurable chronic pain syndrome begin to take place. Arnstein PM. The neuroplastic phenomenon: a physiologic link between chronic pain and learning. J Neurosci Nurs. 1997 Jun;29(3):179–86.

Summation of simultaneous nociceptive and non-nociceptive inputs plays an important role in the modulation of pain. See Melzack R, Wall PD. Pain mechanisms: a new theory. Science. 1965 Nov 19;150(699):971–9; Romaniello A, Svensson P, Cruccu G, Arendt-Nielsen L. Modulation of exteroceptive suppression periods in human jaw-closing muscles induced by summation of nociceptive and non-nociceptive inputs. Exp Brain Res. 2000 Jun;132(3):306–13.

In **chronic back pain**, the interrelationship between chemicals within and across brain regions was abnormal, and there was a specific relationship between regional chemicals and perceptual measures of pain and anxiety. These findings provide direct evidence of **abnormal brain chemistry in chronic back pain**. Grachev ID, Fredrickson BE, Apkarian AV. Abnormal brain chemistry in chronic back pain: an in vivo proton magnetic resonance spectroscopy study. Pain. 2000 Dec 15;89(1):7–18.

Deafferentation of inhibition (a decrease in pain inhibition) can cause neuropatic pain.

"Nerve injury might cause deafferentation and/or neuroma formation, or involve a constriction injury of the nerve. Neuroma formation or construction injury causes spontaneous activity in C fibresfibers and A-delta (d) fibresfibers, either at the site of injury or in dorsal root ganglion cells. This activity is transmitted to the nervous system where it excites and facilitates nociceptive neurons in lamina I and lamina V. That activity is perceived as pain, which by the mechanism involved is neurogenic pain. Facilitation of the central neurons becomes the basis for hyperalgesia, and also causes expansions of the receptive fields of adjacent neurons. The expanded fields capture evoked activity in A-beta (β) fibresfibers which is received by the facilitated neurons, and is perceived as allodynia . . . As well, or alternatively, inhibitory interneurones are stimulated by afferent activity and undergo excitotoxixity. **Loss of inhibitory interneurones results in**

disinhibitation of nociceptive neurons and expansion of receptive fields . . . On the other hand, additionally or alternatively, **deafferentation alone may result in disinhibition of interneurones, and thereby facilitation of nociceptive neurons and expansion of receptive fields**. Meanwhile, **deafferentatioin may result in spontaneous activity in nociceptive neurons, thereby causing central pain** . . . A CNS (central nervous system) lesion could evoke the same processes by causing disinhibition directly within the central nervous system. In order to accommodate visceral causes of SRPS, the model must assume that visceral disorders involve an injury to one or more of the nerves of the affected organ, or deafferentation of that organ . . . Central to the generation of 'sympathetic' features is disinhibition. This could be caused by central lesions of by deafferentation, and results in decreased vasoconstrictor drive, in the first instance. Subsequently, blood vessels develop denervation sensitivity. Meanwhile, in the case of peripheral lesions, spontaneous activity in nociceptive neurons may also cause antidromic vasodilation, which supplements or competes with sympathetically mediated vasodilatation or vasoconstriction . . . This model expects and requires no reinforcing effect of sympathetic activity on the processes that generate pain and other features. Such effects require more compelling data on the role of sympathetic nerves in CRPS (complex regional pain syndrome)." Bogduk N. Mechanisms of complex regional pain syndromes. International Spine Intervention Society 14th Scientific Meeting. Salt Lake City, 2006. pp 54–70.

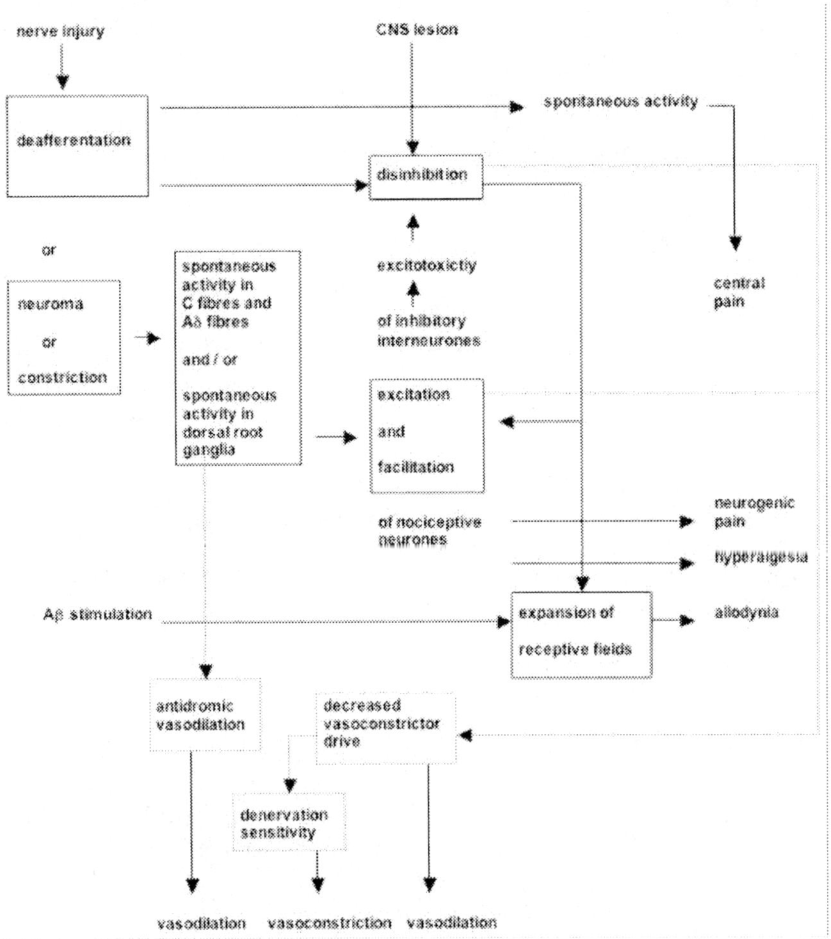

From Bogduk N. Mechanisms of complex regional pain syndromes. International Spine Intervention Society 14th Scientific Meeting. Salt Lake City, 2006; pp. 54–70.

§ 8:25 Receptive field enlargement

Peripheral inflammation results in an enlargement of the receptor fields of many neurons. Increases in neuronal activity in response to tissue injury lead to changes in gene expression and prolonged changes in the nervous system. **The functional result is hyperalgesia and spontaneous pain associated with tissue injury.** Dubner R, Ruda MA. Activity-dependent neuronal plasticity following tissue injury and inflammation. Trends Neurosci. 1992 Mar;15(3):96–103.

The sensory receptors of the joints are sensitized in a similar manner by immobilization and by inflammation, suggesting a relationship to pain. This is a peripheral sensitization mechanism. Okamoto T, Atsuta Y, Shimazaki S. Sensory afferent properties of immobilized or inflamed rat knees during continuous passive movement. J Bone Joint Surg Br. 1999 Jan;81(1):171–7.

§ 8:26 Factors that evoke pain

Davis et al. have identified the following factors that may evoke pain:

1) the loss of low-threshold mechanoreceptive neurons, such that nociceptive neuronal output is now prominent,

2) reduced tonic inhibition of thalamic or cortical neurons, and/or

3) unmasking or strengthening of nociceptive pathways.

Davis KD, Kiss ZH, Tasker RR, Dostrovsky JO. Thalamic stimulation-evoked sensations in chronic pain patients and in nonpain (movement disorder) patients. J Neurophysiol. 1996 Mar;75(3):1026–37.

§ 8:27 Factors that evoke pain—Genetic factors and pain

Genetics play a role in pain and pain inhibition. See Mogil JS, Sternberg WF, Marek P, Sadowski B, Belknap JK, Liebeskind JC. The genetics of pain and pain inhibition. Proc Natl Acad Sci U S A. 1996 Apr 2;93(7):3048–55; Mogil JS. The genetic mediation of individual differences in sensitivity to pain and its inhibition. Proc Natl Acad Sci U S A. 1999 Jul 6;96(14):7744–51.

Some patients may be predisposed genetically to a decreased amount of opioid receptors. Uhl GR, Sora I, Wang Z. The mu opiate receptor as a candidate gene for pain: polymorphisms, variations in expression, nociception, and opiate responses. Proc Natl Acad Sci U S A. 1999 Jul 6;96(14):7752–5.

Humans differ from one another in μOR densities. **Findings suggest 30–50% or larger ranges of individual human densities in μOR densities and ischemia can reduce the expression of mu-opioid receptors in the dorsal horn. The greater amount of opioid receptors one has, the most likely result will be in perceiving pain less.** See Yu W, Hao JX, Xu XJ, Hokfelt T, Elde R, Wiesenfeld-Hallin Z. Spinal cord ischemia reduces mu-opioid receptors in rats:

correlation with morphine insensitivity. Neuroreport. 1999 Jan 18;10(1):87–91.

Genetic factors of forebrain NMDA receptors (n-methyl-d-aspartate, receptors that glutamate attach to) can influence pain perception. Wei F, Wang GD, Kerchner GA, Kim SJ, Xu HM, Chen ZF, Zhuo M. Genetic enhancement of inflammatory pain by forebrain NR2B overexpression. Nat Neurosci. 2001 Feb;4(2):164–9.

The recently discovered peptide nociceptin/orphanin FQ (N/OFQ) and its receptor NOR share many structural similarities with the opioid peptides and their receptors. **The anatomical distributions of N/OFQ and NOR are similar to those of opioid peptides and receptors. The heptadecapeptide nociceptin/orphanin FQ is primarily pronociceptive in the female and primarily antinociceptive in the male.** See Flores CA, Wang XM, Zhang KM, Mokha SS. Orphanin FQ produces gender-specific modulation of trigeminal nociception: behavioral and electrophysiological observations. Neuroscience. 2001;105(2):489–98.

Findings suggest that N/OFQ has biphasic actions, depending on doses in the nociceptors and spinal synapses, and has postsynaptic antinociceptive actions in spinal cord by modulating SP signaling. Low doses of N/OFQ (i.t.) exerted nociceptive responses. Inoue M, Shimohira I, Yoshida A, Zimmer A, Takeshima H, Sakurada T, Ueda H. Dose-related opposite modulation by nociceptin/orphanin FQ of substance P nociception in the nociceptors and spinal cord. J Pharmacol Exp Ther. 1999 Oct;291(1):308–13.

§ 8:28 Factors that evoke pain—Weather and pain

The old-wives tale of aching bones forecasting the weather may be explained by science. **Decrease in temperature is associated with both increased pain and increased rigidity. Increase in relative humidity is associated with increased pain and rigidity in arthritis suffers.** See Aikman H. The association between arthritis and the weather. Int J Biometeorol. 1997 Jun;40(4):192–9.

Results demonstrated that weather consistently worsened pain for certain diagnoses. **Those patients most frequently reported weather-sensitive pain had a neural and or/bony component as the etiology of their pain conditions.** Hendler NH, Jamison RN, Morrison CH, Piper JK, Kahn Z. The relationship of diagnosis and weather sensitivity in chronic pain patients. J Neuromusculoskeletal Sys 1995; 3:10–5.

In patients with central pain, there is reorganization in the nervous system so that cold is relabeled to signal pain in the thalamus of patients. Lenz FA, Lee JI, Garonzik IM, Rowland LH, Dougherty PM, Hua SE. Plasticity of pain-related neuronal activity in the human thalamus. Prog Brain Res. 2000;129:259–73.

Painful osteoarthritis can cause muscle hyperalgesia and extended pain due to central sensitization. Bajaj P, Bajaj P, Graven-Nielsen T, Arendt-Nielsen L. Osteoarthritis and its association with muscle hyperalgesia: an experimental controlled study. Pain. 2001 Aug;93(2):107–14.

§ 8:29 Factors that evoke pain—Pain on movement

Comment:

The increase in sensory nerve endings suggests increase in blood flow, perhaps as an attempt to augment the nutrition of the degenerate disc.

The increase in the density of sensory nerves, and the presence of endplate cartilage defects, strongly suggests that the endplates and vertebral bodies are sources of pain; this may explain the severe pain on movement experienced by some patients with degenerative disc disease. Brown MF, Hukkanen MV, McCarthy ID, Redfern DR, Batten JJ, Crock HV, Hughes SP, Polak JM. Sensory and sympathetic innervation of the vertebral endplate in patients with degenerative disc disease. J Bone Joint Surg Br. 1997 Jan;79(1):147–53.

In a normal person, A afferent (large mylenated) fibers participate in transmitting low-threshold stimuli from mechanoreceptors, and A /C fibers participate in transmitting high threshold stimuli, such as pain and thermal signals. Loss of input from A afferent fibers may diminish the inhibition of the projecting neurons and give rise to "low-input" pain. **With a phenotype change in the spinal cord, A afferent fibers that would normally evoke nonpainful sensations may elicit and maintain pain (allodynia).** See Voerman VF, van Egmond J, Crul BJ. Elevated detection thresholds for mechanical stimuli in chronic pain patients: support for a central mechanism. Arch Phys Med Rehabil. 2000 Apr;81(4):430–5.

Nociceptive pain can be somatic or visceral in nature. Somatic pain tends to be well localized, constant pain that is described as sharp, aching, throbbing, or gnawing.

Nociceptive pain is caused by the stimulation of peripheral

of A-delta and C-polymodal pain receptors, by algogenic substances (eg. histamine bradykinin, substance P, etc.).

Neuropathic pain is described as "burning", "electric", "tingling", and "shooting."

Neuropathic pain is produced by damage to, or pathological changes in the peripheral or central nervous systems.

Allodynia is defined as pain resulting from a stimulus that ordinarily does not elicit a painful response.

Hyperalgesia is defined as an increased sensitivity to a normally painful stimuli.

Following a peripheral nerve injury (eg. **crush**, **stretch**, or axotomy) sensitization occurs which is characterized by spontaneous activity by the neuron, a lowered threshold for activation and increased response to a given stimulus. Should the injured nerve be a nociceptor then increased nervous discharge will equate to increased pain. Following nerve injury C-fiber nociceptors can develop new adrenergic receptors and sensitivity, which may help to explain the mechanism of sympathetically maintained pain. In addition to sensitization following damaged peripheral nerves, the formation of ectopic neuronal pacemakers can occur at various sites along the length of the nerve. Abnormal electrical connections can occur between adjacent demyelinated axons. These are referred to as ephapses. "Ephaptic cross talk" may result in the transfer of nerve impulses from one axon to another. Cross talk between A and C fibers develops in the dorsal root ganglion.

Following a peripheral nerve injury, anatomical and neurochemical changes can occur within the central nervous system that can persist long after the injury has healed.

Chronic Pain from a Whiplash Injury and Neuropathic pain

Whiplash injury has been shown to damage the facet joint by compression and/or stretching.

Injury to the vertebral joints, including the disc and facets, produces a nociceptive type of pain, and/or a neuropathic (nerve) type of pain.

The cervical facet capsular ligaments may be injured under combined shear, bending and compression load levels that occur in rear-end impacts (1). Facet joint components are at risk for injury during whiplash due to facet joint compression and excessive capsular ligament strain (2). The pinching of the lower cervical facet joints may lead to local tissue injury and nociceptive pain (3). Cervical facet capsular ligaments may be injured under loading conditions similar to those generated during whiplash (rear-end 8km/h [5mph] rear-end collision) (4). There does not need to be a complete failure of the tissues to cause injury or pain. Findings indicate that facet capsule strains comparable to those previously reported for whiplash kinematics and subcatastrophic failures of this ligament have the potential to produce pain symptoms and alter one element of nociception. Allodynia results showed immediate and sustained behavioral sensitivity following subcatastrophic vertebral distractions; pain symptoms were significantly greater than those for other injury groups. Further, spinal astrocytic activation was also greater for subcatastrophic injuries compared to lower distraction magnitudes (5).

When compared to the reported strains that facet joint capsules experienced in whiplash (35–60%) and the reported capsule subfailure strains (35–67%), high thresholds and after discharge strains are within that range. High threshold units likely signal nociception (pain sensation) while after discharge may signal capsule strain injury and contribute to persistent pain (6). Mechanical findings provide insight into the relationship between gross structural failure and painful loading for the facet capsular ligament. Gross failure occurred at 2.45+/-0.60 N and 0.92+/-0.17 mm. The yield point occurred at 1.68+/-0.56 N and 0.57+/-0.08 mm, which was significantly less than gross failure (p<0.001 for both measurements). The ligament yield point occurred at a distraction magnitude in which pain symptoms begin to appear (7).

Stretching the facet joint capsule beyond physiological range could result in **altered axonal morphology (the axon is part of the nerve)** that may be related to secondary or delayed axotomy changes similar to those seen in central nervous system injuries where axons are subjected to stretching and shearing. These may contribute to **neuropathic pain** and are potentially related to neck pain after whiplash events (8). Injured somatic tissues adjacent to nerve structures release inflammatory substances that can chemically irritate neural tissues (9–14). Inflammatory cytokines (IL-1beta, TNF-alpha, and IL-6) may the genesis of pain production in the facets (15,16) and [interleukin-6 (IL-6), interleukin-8 (IL-8) and prostaglandin E2 (PGE2), matrix metalloproteinases, nitric oxide] in disc herniations (17–19).

Central nervous system neurons become sensitized after peripheral nerve injury and expand their receptive fields (20, 21). Damage to the peripheral nervous system often leads to chronic neuropathic pain characterized by spontaneous pain and an exaggerated response to painful and/or innocuous stimuli. This pain condition is extremely debilitating and usually difficult to treat (22). Sensory hypoaesthesia and hypersensitivity co-exist in the chronic whiplash condition. Peripheral afferent nerve fiber involvement but could be a further manifestation of disordered central pain processing (23). A predominantly neuropathic pain component is related to a complex presentation of sensory hypersensitivity and higher pain/disability.(24) Whiplash is a heterogeneous condition with some individuals showing features suggestive of neuropathic pain, which is more difficult to treat.

(1) Siegmund GP, Myers BS, Davis MB, Bohnet HF, Winkelstein BA. Human Cervical Motion Segment Flexibility and Facet Capsular Ligament Strain under Combined Posterior Shear, Extension and Axial Compression. Stapp Car Crash J. 2000 Nov;44:159–70.

(2) Pearson AM, Ivancic PC, Ito S. Panjabi MM. Facet Joint Kinematics and Injury Mechanisms During Simulated Whiplash. Spine 2004,29.390–397.

(3) Cusick JF, Pintar FA, Yoganandan N. Whiplash syndrome: kinematic factors influencing pain patterns. Spine. 2001 Jun 1;26(11):1252–8.

(4) Siegmund GP, Myers BS, Davis MB, Bohnet HF, Winkelstein BA. Human cervical motion segmental flexibility and facet capsular ligament strain under combined posterior shear, extension and axial compression. Stapp Car Crash Journal 2000; 44:159–170.

(5) Lee KE, Davis MB, Mejilla RM, Winkelstein BA. In vivo cervical facet capsule distraction: mechanical implications for whiplash and neck pain. Stapp Car Crash J. 2004 Nov;48:373–95.

(6) Lu Y, Chen C, Kallakuri S, Patwardhan A, Cavanaugh JM. Neural response of cervical facet joint capsule to stretch: a study of whiplash pain mechanism. Stapp Car Crash J. 2005 Nov;49:49–65.

(7) Quinn KP, Winkelstein BA. Cervical facet capsular ligament yield defines the threshold for injury and persistent joint-mediated neck pain. J Biomech. 2007;40(10):2299–306.

(8) Kallakuri S, Singh A, Lu Y, Chen C, Patwardhan A, Cavanaugh JM. Tensile stretching of cervical facet joint capsule and related axonal changes. Eur Spine J. 2007 Dec 14;

(9) Cavanaugh J. Neural mechanisms of lumbar pain. Spine, 1995;20, 1804–1809.

(10) Garfin, S, Rydevik B, Brown R. Compressive neuropathy

of spinal nerve roots: A mechanical or biological problem? Spine. 1991; 16:162–166.

(11) Garfin S, Rydevik, B, Lind B, Massie, J. Spinal nerve root compression. Spine.1995; 20: 1810–1820.

(12) Murata Y, Rydevik B, Takahashi K, Larsson K, Olmarker K. Incision of the intervertebral disc induces disintegration and increases permeability of the dorsal root ganglion capsule. Spine. 2005; 30: 1712–1716.

(13) Takahashi N, Yabuki S, Aoki Y, Kikuchi S. Pathomechanisms of nerve root injury caused by disc herniation: An experimental study of mechanical compression and chemical irritation. Spine. 2003; 28: 435–441.

(14) Takebayashi T, Cavanaugh J, Ozaktay A, Kallakuri S, Chen C. Effect of nucleus pulposus on the neural activity of dorsal root ganglion. Spine. 2001; 26: 940–945.

(15) Igarashi A, Kikuchi S, Konno S, Olmarker K. Inflammatory cytokines released from the facet joint tissue in degenerative lumbar spinal disorders. Spine. 2004 Oct 1;29(19) :2091–5.

(16) Igarashi A, Kikuchi S, Konno S. Correlation between inflammatory cytokines released from the lumbar facet joint tissue and symptoms in degenerative lumbar spinal disorders. J Orthop Sci. 2007 Mar;12(2):154–60.

(17) Ahn SH, Cho YW, Ahn MW, Jang SH, Sohn YK, Kim HS. mRNA expression of cytokines and chemokines in herniated lumbar intervertebral discs. Spine. 2002 May 1;27(9) :911–7.

(18) Burke JG, Watson RW, McCormack D, Dowling FE, Walsh MG, Fitzpatrick JM. Intervertebral discs which cause low back pain secrete high levels of proinflammatory mediators. J Bone Joint Surg Br. 2002 Mar;84(2):196–201.

(19) Kang JD, Georgescu HI, McIntyre-Larkin L, Stefanovic-Racic M, Evans CH. Herniated cervical intervertebral discs spontaneously produce matrix metalloproteinases, nitric oxide, interleukin-6, and prostaglandin E2. Spine. 1995 Nov 15;20(22) :2373–8.

(20) Baron, R. (2000). Peripheral neuropathic pain: From mechanisms to symptoms. The Clinical Journal of Pain, 16(Suppl.), S12-S20.

(21) Devor M, Seltzer Z. Pathophysiology of damaged nerves in relation to chronic pain. In P. Wall & R. Melzack (Eds.), Textbook of pain (19994th ed., pp. 129–164). *Edinburgh: Churchill Livingstone.*

(22) Thacker MA, Clark AK, Marchand F, McMahon SB. Pathophysiology of peripheral neuropathic pain: immune cells and molecules. Anesth Analg. 2007 Sep;105(3):838–47.

(23) Chien A, Eliav E, Sterling M. Hypoaesthesia occurs with sensory hypersensitivity in chronic whiplash — Further evidence of a neuropathic condition. Man Ther. 2008 Feb 20;

(24) Sterling M, Pedler A. A neuropathic pain component is common in acute whiplash and associated with a more complex clinical presentation. Man Ther. 2008 Mar 19.

§ 8:30 Chiropractic adjustments and pain reduction

The current data support a neurophysiological mechanism underlying manipulation-induced analgesia. **Clinical and basic science literature suggests that the analgesic effects of manipulation are segmentally organized and probably result from large-diameter afferent stimulation. Further, this analgesic effect is nonopioid but involves spinal activation of serotoneric and noradrenergic-receptors**, implicating descending inhibitory pathways from the RVM and the noradrenergic cells in the brainstem. Sluka KA, Hoeger MK, Skyba DA. Basic Science Mechanisms of Nonpharmacological Treatments for Pain. Pain 2002-An Updated Review: ISAP Press 2002.

This study suggests that **cervical spine manipulation may alter cortical somatosensory processing and sensorimotor integration**. These findings may help to elucidate the mechanisms responsible for the effective relief of pain and restoration of functional ability documented following spinal manipulation treatment.

Haavik-Taylor H, Murphy B. Cervical spine manipulation alters sensorimotor integration: A somatosensory evoked potential study. Clin Neurophysiol. 2007 Feb;118(2):391–402.

§ 8:31 Chiropractic adjustments and pain reduction—Long term potentiation and long term depression

Long Term Potentiation is a form of nervous system hyperexcitability.

Long Term Depression can decrease the excitability.

Studies showing LTP in response to intense noxious stimulation and reports that A-delta-mechanosensitive afferent activation can reverse an existing LTP condition in dorsal horn neurons. The involvement of Long Term

Potentiation (LTP) in low back pain is discussed and a role for Long Term Depression (LTD) in spinal manipulative therapy is proposed. The need for future studies is identified in the areas of spatial and temporal changes in symptomatology post-SMT (spinal manipulative therapy) of the low back; combining, sequencing, and comparing several therapeutic approaches; and demonstrating LTD in spinal cord neurons post-SMT-like stimulation. **Activity-dependent neuronal plasticity such as LTP is known to be reversible, the idea is presented that SMT may act to reverse LTP within an already sensitized pain-signaling system.** ¶ Spinal manipulative therapy (SMT) may act to reverse LTP within an already sensitized pain-signaling system. Boal RW, Gillette RG. Central neuronal plasticity, low back pain and spinal manipulative therapy. J Manipulative Physiol Ther. 2004 Jun;27(5):314–26.

The suggestion from this review that Spinal Manipulative Therapy may influence dorsal horn neurons initiating LTD and dampening ongoing central sensitization is not intended to be an exclusive mechanism to explain all SMT therapeutic effects. Boal RW, Gillette RG. Central neuronal plasticity, low back pain and spinal manipulative therapy. J Manipulative Physiol Ther. 2004 Jun;27(5):314–26.

To summarize, sensory input — nociceptive and proprioceptive — produced as a result of peripheral tissue insult leads to physiological and anatomical changes at synapses in the central nervous system, a form of LTP.

As well as for pain, these synaptic events are a learned mechanism for the expression of (mal)adaptive changes in motor function — muscle tone, and postures and movements collectively known as 'behavior'. Unless and until movement can be carried out in the relative/total absence of pain, both the synaptic 'memory' and its behavioral consequences are likely to be self-reinforcing. Indeed, they have the potential to become chronic. This is generally averted by a combination of natural history and delivery of appropriate therapeutic interventions. An important neurological consequence of the latter is to drastically change — that is 'normalize' — the pattern of sensory input.

Zusman M. Mechanisms of musculoskeletal physiotherapy. Phys Ther Rev. 2004;9:39–49.

§ 8:32 Chiropractic adjustments and pain reduction—Dose-related response

In treating chronic neck and back pain patients, one or two

treatments may not be enough. Further, Chiropractic treatment may be based on the neuroplasticity of the nervous system. Several studies have shown that manual therapy is only slightly better than other therapies, or placebo, but the dosage of treatment with the manual therapy is minimal. The reported randomized control trails are usually done on an HMO patient database. Published studies with those HMO populations have shown that outcomes may be dose dependent. Instead of eight to 12 treatments per year, nine to 12 visits over three weeks may be needed to properly treat an episode of pain.

"This finding suggests that in the mature cortex, the apparently static structural attributes of the normal adult cortex depend on maintenance of patterns of afferent activity; with the corollary that changes in these patterns can induce structural plasticity." Tailby C, Wright LL, Metha AB, Calford MB. Activity-dependent maintenance and growth of dendrites in adult cortex. Proc Natl Acad Sci U S A. 2005 Mar 22;102(12):4631–6.

"In our experience, anything less than two weeks of daily manipulation is inadequate for chronic back pain patients." Kirkaldy-Willis WH, Cassidy JD. Spinal manipulation in the treatment of low-back pain. Can Fam Physician 1985;31:535–40.

"There was a positive, clinically important effect of the number of chiropractic treatments for chronic low back pain on pain intensity and disability at 4 weeks. Relief was substantial for patients receiving care **3 to 4 times per week for 3 weeks**." Haas M, Groupp E, Kraemer DF. Dose-response for chiropractic care of chronic low back pain. Spine J. 2004 Sep–Oct;4(5):574–83.

"Findings suggest the benefit of 9 to 12 visits over 3 weeks for the treatment of HA/neck pain and disability. **A larger number of visits than 12 in 3 weeks may be required for maximum relief and durability of outcomes**." Haas M, Groupp E, Aickin M, Fairweather A, Ganger B, Attwood M, Cummins C, Baffes L. Dose response for chiropractic care of chronic cervicogenic headache and associated neck pain: a randomized pilot study. J Manipulative Physiol Ther. 2004 Nov–Dec;27(9):547–53.

Chapter 9

Whiplash Diagnosis

§ 9:1 Physical evaluation—Manual palpation-facet joint pain

Comment:

Note that traditional orthopedic and neurological tests may pick up space occupying lesions, but may not detect the damage to the tissues caused in whiplash type injuries.

Palpation of cervical spine tenderness is a highly reliable examination tool. Hubka MJ, Phelan SP. Interexaminer reliability of palpation for cervical spine tenderness. J Manipulative Physiol Ther. 1994 Nov–Dec;17(9):591–5.

Manual palpation correctly identified all 15 patients with proven symptomatic zygapophysial joints, and specified correctly the segmental level of the symptomatic joint. None of the five patients with asymptomatic joints was misdiagnosed as having a symptomatic zygapophysial joint. Jull G, Bogduk N, Marsland A. The accuracy of manual diagnosis for cervical zygapophysial joint pain syndromes. Med J Aust. 1988 Mar 7;148(5):233–6.

Palpation over the facet joints was the most appropriate test. The tests for cervical spine rotation and cervical flexion/extension were not sufficiently sensitive. The test for formina intervebralia (neck rotated and laterally flexed) and upper limb tension test caused pain in musculoskletal structures, but they were intended to provoke pain from nervous system tissues. Sandmark H, Nisell R. Validity of five common manual neck pain provoking tests. Scand J Rehabil Med. 1995 Sep;27(3):131–6.

The neck compression, axial manual traction, and shoulder abduction test are valuable aids in the clinical examination of a patient with neck and arm pain. Viikari-Juntura E, Porras M, Laasonen EM. Validity of clinical tests in the diagnosis of root compression in cervical disc disease. Spine. 1989 Mar;14(3):253–7.

The Spurling test is not very sensitive, but it is specific for cervical radiculopathy. It is useful in confirming a cervical radiculopathy. (In undergoing the test, the patient laterally flexes and extends his neck, after which the examiner applies axial pressure on the spine). Tong HC, Haig AJ, Yamakawa K. The Spurling test and cervical radiculopathy. Spine. 2002 Jan 15;27(2):156–9.

Palpation is used to differentiate carpal tunnel syndrome from thoracic outlet syndrome. Palpatory examination assists initial treatment, including manipulation. Supplemental physical medicine modalities, such as ultrasound, may enhance the treatment response. Sucher BM. Palpatory diagnosis and manipulative management of carpal tunnel syndrome: Part 2. 'Double crush' and thoracic outlet syndrome. J Am Osteopath Assoc. 1995 Aug;95(8):471–9.

Objective, kinematic parameters can be generated, measured, and evaluated relative to palpatory findings of musculoskeletal impairment by identifying trends in ratios of cervical lateral flexion and axial rotation.

Bush TR, Vorro J. Kinematic measures to objectify head and neck motions in palpatory diagnosis: a pilot study. J Am Osteopath Assoc. 2008 Feb;108(2):55–62.

§ 9:2 Physical evaluation—Slump test

The results demonstrated that the addition of knee extension and left ankle dorsiflexion during the slump test produced a significant increase in the intensity of comparable cervical symptoms in the whiplash group. The whiplash group also showed a greater limitation in knee extension range of movement during the test than did the control group. Yeung E, Jones M, Hall B. The response to the slump test in a group of female whiplash patients. Aust J Physiother. 1997;43(4):245–252.

§ 9:3 Physical evaluation—Posture analysis

Normal postural alignment (without intervention) remains constant for at least two years. In a 2-year follow-up study, lateral resting posture is highly repeatable. Bullock-Saxton J. Postural alignment in standing: a repeatable study. Aust Physiother 1993; 39:25–29

Studies have demonstrated that repeat photographs of "natural head posture" are highly reproducible; cervical and cervico-thoracic posture reproducible the same day, one week, and one month later. See Lundstrom A, Forsberg CM, Westergren H, Lundstrom F. A comparison between estimated and registered natural head posture. Eur J Orthod. 1991 Feb; 13(1):59–64; Refshauge K, Goodsell LM.

Consistency of cervical and cervicothoracic posture in standing. Aust J Physiother 1994; 40:235–240;. Grimmer K. An investigation of poor cervical resting posture. Aust J Physiother. 1997; 43(1):7–16.

§ 9:4 Physical evaluation—Pain pressure thresholds (PPT) (Algometer)

The cervical region had the lowest pressure pain thresholds. The values increased in the thoracic and were highest in the lumbar region. **The average PPT at C6 was 255 kPa/cm2, T4 was 324 kPa/cm2, and 445 kPa/cm2 for L4. (1 pound per square inch = 6.89 kPa).** Keating L, Lubke C, Powell V, Young T, Souvlis T, Jull G. Mid-thoracic tenderness: a comparison of pressure pain threshold between spinal regions, in asymptomatic subjects. Man Ther. 2001 Feb;6(1):34–9.

The PPT (Algometer) is a reliable measure, and repeated algometry does not change pain threshold in healthy muscle over 3 consecutive days. The PPT can be used to evaluate the development and decline of experimentally induced muscle tenderness. Reliability is enhanced when all measurements are taken by one examiner. Nussbaum EL, Downes L. Reliability of clinical pressure-pain algometric measurements obtained on consecutive days. Phys Ther. 1998 Feb;78(2):160–9.

Pressure algometry and palpation are useful clinical tools in the evaluation of neck and jaw pain in acute whiplash injury. Kasch H, Stengaard-Pedersen K, Arendt-Nielsen L, Staehelin Jensen T. Pain thresholds and tenderness in neck and head following acute whiplash injury: a prospective study. Cephalalgia. 2001 Apr;21(3):189–97.

§ 9:5 Physical evaluation—Cervical range of motion (CROM) device

The cervical range of motion (CROM) device has moderate to high reliability among testers and between testers. **This method of evaluation can be used to obtain consistent, quantitative measurements in documenting changes in cervical range of motion.** See Tousignant M, de Bellefeuille L, O'Donoughue S, Grahovac S. Criterion validity of the cervical range of motion (CROM) goniometer for cervical flexion and extension. Spine. 2000 Feb 1;25(3):324–30; Dhimitri K, Brodeur S, Croteau M, Richard S, Seymour CJ. Reliability of the cervical range of motion device in measuring upper cervical motion. J Manual & Manipulative Therapy 1998; 6(1):31–6.

The greatest risk for long-term symptoms was seen among the group of patients with both point tenderness and limited range of motion. Hartling L, Brison RJ, Ardern C, Pickett W. Prognostic value of the Quebec Classification of Whiplash-Associated Disorders. Spine. 2001 Jan 1;26(1):36–41.

The extension test using a CROM was able to discriminate between whiplash and control patients. Verhagen AP, Lanser K, de Bie RA, de Vet HC. Whiplash: assessing the validity of diagnostic tests in a cervical sensory disturbance. J Manipulative Physiol Ther. 1996 Oct;19(8):508–12.

After 1 year, 11 (7.8%) persons with whiplash injury had not returned to usual level of activity or work. **The best single estimator of handicap was the cervical range-of-motion test, which had a sensitivity of 73% and a specificity of 91%.** Accuracy and specificity increased to 94% and 99% when combined with pain intensity and other complaints. Kasch H, Bach FW, Jensen TS. Handicap after acute whiplash injury: a 1-year prospective study of risk factors. Neurology. 2001 Jun 26;56(12):1637–43.

Although cervical spine motion ranges may remain within normal limits in patients, motion patterns were altered qualitatively and quantitatively. **Motion pattern analysis might prove a useful discrimination parameter in patients in whom anatomical lesions are not clearly identifiable.** Feipel V, Rondelet B, LePallec JP, DeWitte O, Rooze M. The use of disharmonic motion curves in problems of the cervical spine. Int Orthop. 1999;23(4):205–9.

In this study of X-ray analysis of normal vs feigned, restricted neck flexion and extension in healthy subjects, we have shown that the pattern of how each vertebral segment from C2–C3 to C6–C7 contributes to the total angular rotation from flexion to extension changes when subjects are asked to feign restricted neck range. When subjects feign restricted neck range, a change occurs from the normal pattern in that the upper cervical segments contribute more to the total angular rotation from flexion to extension and the C6–C7 segment contributes much less than it does in the normal state of flexion and extension.

Feigners of restricted neck range thus produce a pattern different from nonfeigning subjects.

Puglisi F, Strimpakos N, Papathanasiou M, Kapreli E, Bonelli A, Sgambetterra S, Ferrari R. Cervical spine segmental vertebral motion in healthy volunteers feigning restriction of neck flexion and extension. Int J Legal Med. 2007 Sep;121(5):337–40.

§ 9:6 Physical evaluation—Current perception threshold (CPT)

Quantititative sensory testing may be of help in patients with dysfunctional pain processing (decrease or increase sensitivities). Dotson RM. Clinical neurophysiology laboratory tests to assess the nociceptive system in humans. J Clin Neurophysiol. 1997 Jan;14(1):32–45; Dinh S, Marroquin E, Raj PP. Neuroselective quantification of allodynia by current perception threshold evaluation in RSD patients. Regional Anesthesia 1997; 22(2S):44.

Current perception threshold testing showed that the functions of A-beta, A-delta, and C fibers deteriorated in patients with lumbar radiculopathy. **This technique may be useful for quantifying sensory nerve dysfunction in patients with radiculopathy.** Yamashita T, Kanaya K, Sekine M, Takebayashi T, Kawaguchi S, Katahira G. A quantitative analysis of sensory function in lumbar radiculopathy using current perception threshold testing. Spine. 2002 Jul 15;27(14):1567–70.

A neurometer device is an electrical nerve stimulator used to determine the current perception threshold (CPT) evoked by stimulating A-beta fibers at 2,000 Hz, A-delta fibers at 250 Hz and C fibers at 5 Hz. CPT evaluation is used for analyzing peripheral nerve dysfunction. In this study, the sensory disturbance of the lower-extremity was quantitatively analyzed using CPT testing before and after lumbar discectomy. In 33 patients (L4/5: 16 and L5/S: 17), as subjective evaluations, tactile sensation and leg pain were assessed before and 2 weeks after surgery. In the subjectively improved group (n = 22), significant decreases in CPT at 2,000 and 250 Hz were noted postoperatively, whereas in the unchanged group (n = 11), no significant changes in CPT at any frequencies was noted. The leg pain improved in all patients. Likewise, CPT at 5 Hz, which stimulated C fiber, decreased significantly for both improved and unchanged groups. CPT measured by a **Neurometer is very useful in assessing lower-extremity sensory functions before and after surgery for lumbar disc herniation.** Imoto K, Takebayashi T, Kanaya K, Kawaguchi S, Katahira G, Yamashita T. Quantitative analysis of sensory functions after lumbar discectomy using current perception threshold testing. Eur Spine J. 2007 Jul;16(7):971–5.

CPT testing can distinguish demyelinating from axonal polyneuropathies. It may be particularly helpful in patients with predominantly sensory symptoms in

whom EMG/NCS data may be equivocal, or in patients who decline EMG/NCS studies. Menkes DL, Swenson MR, Sander HW. Current perception threshold: an adjunctive test for detection of acquired demyelinating polyneuropathies. Electromyogr Clin Neurophysiol. 2000 Jun;40(4):205–10.

According to the values obtained, R-CPT testing was reliable for the quantification of sensory function in healthy individuals. Lerner TH, Goldstein GR, Hittelman E. Quantitative sensory nerve conduction threshold (sNCT) evaluation of the trigeminal nerve at the mental foramen area. J Prosthet Dent. 2000 Jul;84(1):103–7.

§ 9:7 Physical evaluation—Proprioception

Subjects who have experienced a whiplash injury demonstrate a deficit in their ability to reproduce a target position of the neck. See Loudon JK, Ruhl M, Field E. Ability to reproduce head position after whiplash injury. Spine. 1997 Apr 15;22(8):865–8; Heikkila HV, Wenngren BI. Cervicocephalic kinesthetic sensibility, active range of cervical motion, and oculomotor function in patients with whiplash injury. Arch Phys Med Rehabil. 1998 Sep;79(9):1089–94.

Asymptomatic subjects are very good at reproducing the neutral position of the head. Christensen HW, Nilsson N. The ability to reproduce the neutral zero position of the head. J Manipulative Physiol Ther. 1999 Jan;22(1):26–8.

Changes in head and neck position have a greater effect on elbow joint position sense in people with whiplash-associated disorders. It has been shown that perception of elbow joint position is affected by changes in head and neck position. Further, people with whiplash-associated disorders (WAD) present with deficits in upper limb coordination and movement. This study is aimed to determine whether the effect of changes in head position on elbow joint position error (JPE) is more pronounced in people with WAD and to determine whether this is related to the participant's pain and anxiety levels. Nine people with chronic and disabling WAD and 11 healthy people participated in this experiment. The ability to reproduce a position at the elbow joint was assessed after changes in the position of the head and neck to 30 degrees and with the head in the midline. Pain was monitored in WAD participants. Absolute elbow JPE with the head in neutral was not different between WAD and control participants ($P=0.5$). Changes in the head and neck position increased absolute elbow JPE in the WAD group ($P<0.05$), but did not affect elbow

JPE in the control group (P=0.4). There was a connection between pain during testing and the effect of changes in head position on elbow JPE (P<0.05). **Elbow JPE is affected by movement of the head and neck,** with smaller angles of neck rotation in people with WAD than in healthy individuals. This observation may explain deficits in upper limb coordination in people with WAD, which may be due to the presence of pain or reduced range of motion in this population. Knox JJ, Beilstein DJ, Charles SD, Aarseth GA, Rayar S, Treleaven J, Hodges PW. Changes in head and neck position have a greater effect on elbow joint position sense in people with whiplash-associated disorders. Clin J Pain. 2006 Jul–Aug;22(6):512–8.

Changes in head and neck position affect elbow joint position sense. Changes in the position of the head and neck have been shown to introduce a systematic deviation in the end-point error of an upper limb pointing task. Although previous authors have attributed this to alteration of perceived target location, no studies have explored the effect of changes in head and neck position on the perception of limb position. This study investigated whether changes in head and neck position affect a specific component of movement performance, i.e., the accuracy of joint position sense (JPS) at the elbow. Elbow JPS was tested with the neck in four positions: neutral, flexion, rotation and combined flexion/rotation. A target angle was presented passively with the neck in neutral; after a rest period, this angle was reproduced actively with the head and neck in one of the test positions. The potential effects of distraction from head movement were controlled for by performing a movement control in which the head and neck were in neutral for the presentation and reproduction of the target angle but moved into flexion during the rest period. The absolute and variable joint position errors (JPE) were greater when the target angle was reproduced with the neck in the flexion, rotation, and combined flexion/rotation than when the head and neck were in neutral. **This study suggests that the reduced accuracy previously seen in pointing tasks with changes in head position may be partly because of errors in the interpretation of arm position.** Knox JJ, Hodges PW. Changes in head and neck position affect elbow joint position sense. Exp Brain Res. 2005 Aug;165(1):107–13.

§ 9:8 Physical evaluation—Cervical myleopathy

Modified JOA cervical spine myelopathy functional assessment scale*

Score	Definition
motor dysfunction upper extremities	
0	unable to move hands
2	unable to eat w/ a spoon but able to move hands
3	unable to button shirt but able to eat w/ a spoon
4	able to button shirt w/ great difficulty
5	able to button shirt w/ slight difficulty
6	no dysfunction
lower extremities	
0	complete loss of motor & sensory function
1	sensory preservation w/o ability to move legs
2	able to move legs but unable to walk
3	able to walk on flat floor w/ a walking aid (cane or crutch)
4	able to walk up- &/or downstairs w/ aid of a handrail
5	moderate-to-significant lack of stability but able to walk up- &/or downstairs w/o handrail
6	mild lack of stability but able to walk unaided w/smooth reciprocation
7	no dysfunction
sensory dysfunction, upper extremities	
0	complete loss of hand sensation
1	severe sensory loss or pain
2	mild sensory loss

Score	Definition
3	no sensory loss
sphincter dysfunction	
0	unable to micturate voluntarily
1	marked difficulty in micturition
2	mild-to-moderate difficulty in micturition
3	normal micturition

Sorar M, Seckin H, Hatipoglu C, Budakoglu II, Yigitkanli K, Bavbek M, Kars HZ. Cervical compression myelopathy: is fusion the main prognostic indicator? Neurosurg Spine. 2007 Jun;6(6):531–9.

Nurick **developed a system for grading the disability in** cervical **spondylotic** myelopathy **on the basis of gait abnormality**

Grade I No difficulty in walking

Grade II Mild gait involvement not interfering with employment

Grade III Gait abnormality preventing employment

Grade IV Able to walk only with assistance

Grade V Chairbound or bedridden

Nurick S. The pathogenesis of the spinal cord disorder associated with cervical spondylosis. Brain. 1972;95:87–100.

Cervical spondylotic myelopathy is the most common cause of spinal cord dysfunction in older persons. The aging process results in degenerative changes in the cervical spine that, in advanced stages, can cause compression of the spinal cord. Symptoms often develop insidiously and are characterized by neck stiffness, arm pain, numbness in the hands, and weakness of the hands and legs. The differential diagnosis includes any condition that can result in myelopathy, such as multiple sclerosis amyotrophic lateral sclerosis and masses (such as metastatic tumors) that press on the spinal cord. The diagnosis is confirmed by magnetic resonance imaging that shows narrowing of the spinal canal caused by osteophytes, herniated discs and ligamentum flavum hypertrophy. Choice of treatment remains controversial, surgical procedures designed to decompress the spinal cord and, in some cases, stabilize the spine are successful in many patients.

Clinical Presentation of Cervical Spondylotic Myelopathy

Common symptoms

Clumsy or weak hands

Leg weakness or stiffness

Neck stiffness

Pain in shoulders or arms

Unsteady gait

Common signs

Atrophy of the hand musculature

Hyperreflexia

Lhermitte's sign (electric shock-like sensation down the center of the back following flexion of the neck)

Sensory loss

Young WF. Cervical spondylotic myelopathy: a common cause of spinal cord dysfunction in older persons. Am Fam Physician. 2000 Sep 1;62(5):1064–70.

Differential Diagnoses of Cervical Spondylotic Myelopathy

Peripheral polyneuropathy

Motor neuron disease

Multiple sclerosis

Cerebrovascular disease

Syringomyelia

Rao R. Neck pain, cervical radiculopathy, and cervical myelopathy: pathophysiology, natural history, and clinical evaluation. J Bone Joint Surg Am. 2002 Oct;84-A(10):1872–81.

§ 9:9 X-rays—Multiple X-rays

Comment:

The treating doctor may take X-rays in his/her office as part of building a diagnosis. Note that the defense may say this duplication of the emergency room radiographs is a waste of money. The following study would appear to contradict this position.

Patients are evaluated with radiographs upon presenting for care for specific reasons: the patient had been involved in a trauma, and, according to the literature, significant injuries are often missed on initial examination and postural abnormalities observed on inspection. **It is not improper to take X-rays of the patient or to acquire another X-ray at a**

later date. Delayed instability may occur. Herkowitz HN, Rothman RH. Subacute instability of the cervical spine. Spine. 1984 May–Jun; 9(4):348–57; Delfini R, Dorizzi A, Facchinetti G, Faccioli F, Galzio R, Vangelista T. Delayed post-traumatic cervical instability. Surg Neurol. 1999 Jun; 51(6):588–94; discussion 594–5.

See also: Harger BL, Taylor JA, Haas M, Nyiendo J. Chiropractic radiologists: a survey of chiropractors' attitudes and patterns of use. J Manipulative Physiol Ther. 1997 Jun;20(5):311–4 ***(A survey of chiropractors' attitudes and patterns of use for X-rays indicates the majority use radiographs for pre and post analysis).***

§ 9:10 X-rays—Limitations of X-rays

A 50-year-old man visited the emergency department 12 hrs. after an alcohol-related motor vehicle accident, complaining of shoulder pain and neck stiffness. Cervical spine radiographs were obtained and interpreted as normal, and the patient was discharged. Subsequent review by a radiologist raised the question of a second cervical vertebra (C-2) abnormality, and the patient was recalled. Cervical computed tomography (CT) scan revealed an unstable oblique fracture of C-2 and a congenital nonfusion of the arch of C-1. The patient was placed in halo traction, and subsequent radiographs revealed a fracture of the transverse process of C-7. **The limitations of routine cervical radiographs are well-documented, but no feasible alternative exists as a screening procedure. Thus, a certain level of uncertainty must be accepted. Both physician and patient must recognize the limitations inherent in all medical practice, and that follow-up examination and treatment are essential.** Eckhardt WF, Doyle M, Woodward A, Freundlich I, Rockett FX. Cervical spine fracture following a motor vehicle accident. J Emerg Med. 1988 May–Jun;6(3):179–83.

In an analysis of emergency room cervical spine radiographs, 33.7% of the films were inadequate to exclude fracture or dislocation. Palmer SH, Maheson M. A radiological review of cervical spine injuries from an accident and emergency department: has the ATLS made a difference? J Accid Emerg Med. 1995 Sep;12(3):189–90.

Cross table lateral films missed 67% of the fractures and 45% of the subluxations. Woodring JH, Lee C. Limitations of cervical radiography in the evaluation of acute cervical trauma. J Trauma. 1993 Jan;34(1):32–9.

§ 9:11 X-rays—Sensitivity of X-rays to show lesions

Just because the X-rays show no structural damage does not mean that there are no lesions. **Mertz and Patrick inferred "minor ligamentous damage between the third and fourth cervical vertebrae" based on posttest X-rays in one of the two cadavers. As detailed cryosectioning was not performed, other soft tissue injuries went undetected.** See Yoganandan N, Pintar FA, Stemper BD, Schlick MB, Philippens M, Wismans J. Biomechanics of human occupants in simulated rear crashes: documentation of neck injuries and comparison of injury criteria. Stapp Car Crash Journal 2000;44:189–204.

". . . radiography identified the least number of lesions." Yoganandan N, Cusick JF, Pintar FA, Rao RD. Whiplash injury determination with conventional spine imaging and cryomicrotomy. Spine. 2001 Nov 15;26(22):2443–8.

Most injuries are not seen on plain film X-rays. Only 4 of 245 bone and discoligamentus lesions were detected by X-ray. Jonsson H Jr, Bring G, Rauschning W, Sahlstedt B. Hidden cervical spine injuries in traffic accident victims with skull fractures. J Spinal Disord. 1991 Sep;4(3):251–63.

§ 9:12 X-rays—Radiographic examination

Comment:

If X-rays don't show many lesions, why are they taken? X-rays may not show many injuries, but they may show mechanical alignment. **The findings on X-rays of the patient are one way to check for alignment**. Posture is the body at work against gravity. This is done by non-conscious mechanisms. **Average normal values and ideal normal values do exist in the literature for spinal alignment on radiographs**. In the cervical spine, averages range from 21–34 degrees with an ideal value of 43 degrees. In Gore's study, 9% of asymptomatic subjects had a kyphotic curve. This means in this study, 91% of asymptomatic normals had a lordotic curve. See Gore DR, Sepic SB, Gardner GM. Roentgenographic findings of the cervical spine in asymptomatic people. Spine. 1986 Jul–Aug;11(6):521–4; Owens EF, Hoiris KT. Cervical curve assessment using digitized radiographic analysis. Chiro Res J 1990; 4:47–62; Harrison DD, Janik TJ, Troyanovich SJ, Holland B. Comparisons of lordotic cervical spine curvatures to a theoretical ideal model of the static sagittal cervical spine. Spine. 1996 Mar 15;21(6):667–75.

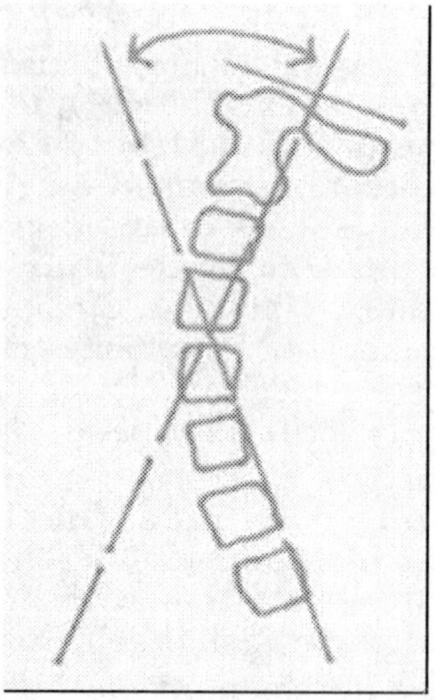

Above: The cervical spine absolute rotation angle (ARA) measures the posterior vertebral bodies of C2 and C7. The average measurements are a lordotic curve of 34 degrees and the ideal curve is 43 degrees. (Diagram adapted from Harrison DD et al. Comparisons of lordotic cervical spine curvatures to a theoretical ideal model of the sagittal cervical spine. Spine 1996;21:667–75)

§ 9:13 X-rays—Radiographic examination

Radiographic signs of instability: Lateral cervical X-ray

1) A decreased anterior disc height
2) An increased posterior disc height
3) Nonparallel facet planes
4) An increased interspinous space (fanning)
5) Anterior slippage of the upper vertebra
6) Kyphotic angulation
7) A disruption of the posterior cervical line of more than 1.5 mm

Foreman SM, Croft AC eds. Whiplash injuries: The Cervical Acceleration/Deceleration Syndrome. 3ed. Philadelphia: Lippincott Williams & Wilkins; 2002, p 52–53

We found a statistically significant association between **cervical pain and lordosis < 20 degrees** and a "clinically normal" range for cervical lordosis of 31 degrees to 40 degrees.

Maintenance of a lordosis in the range of 31 degrees to 40 degrees could be a clinical goal for treatment McAviney J, Schulz D, Bock R, Harrison DE, Holland B. Determining the relationship between cervical lordosis and neck complaints. J Manipulative Physiol Ther. 2005 Mar–Apr;28(3):187–93.

The loss of cervical lordosis increases the risk of injury to the cervical spine following axial loading. Oktenoglu T, Ozer AF, Ferrara LA, Andalkar N, Sarioglu AC, Benzel EC. Effects of cervical spine posture on axial load bearing ability: a biomechanical study. J Neurosurg. 2001 Jan;94(1 Suppl):108–14.

Degenerative changes are associated with a poor prognosis. The exact mode of injury is not associated with any specific radiographic appearance, except that "roll-overs" and side collisions are more likely to cause angulations in the cervical spine. Miles KA, Maimaris C, Finlay D, Barnes MR. The incidence and prognostic significance of radiological abnormalities in soft tissue injuries to the cervical spine. Skeletal Radiol. 1988;17(7):493–6.

§ 9:14 X-rays—Upper cervical region

Hyper-rotation of C0/C1 was shown in whiplash patients. Abnormal relative rotary values was recorded in 79%. This may show damage to the Alar and/or transverse ligament. Patijn J, Wilmink J, ter Linden FH, Kingma H. CT study of craniovertebral rotation in whiplash injury. Eur Spine J. 2001 Feb;10(1):38–43.

Functional loss of the alar ligaments indicates a potential for rotatory instability, which, however, must be determined in conjunction with other clinical findings, such as neurological dysfunction, pain, and deformity. Panjabi M, Dvorak J, Crisco JJ 3rd, Oda T, Wang P, Grob D. Effects of alar ligament transection on upper cervical spine rotation. J Orthop Res. 1991 Jul;9(4):584–93.

This study evaluated objective diagnostic methods for patients with possible upper cervical spine instability caused by trauma, and correlated them with subsequent neurosurgical findings and outcomes. **We conclude that functional MRI with lateral tilting and rotatory evaluation is a useful tool for investigating craniocervical instability. For patients who are recalcitrant to following a program of conservative therapy, surgical stabilization of the craniocervical junction appears to be justified.** See Volle E, Montazem A. MRI video diagnosis and surgical therapy of soft tissue trauma to the craniocervical junction. Ear Nose Throat J. 2001 Jan;80(1):41–4, 46–8.

Our diagnosis via functional magnetic resonance imaging (fMRI) with video did not focus on injuries to the ligamentous microstructure as visualized with high-resolution MRI. Our purpose was to demonstrate the cause of **instability** of the craniocervical junction by direct visualization during fMRI-video technique. Between December 1997 and March 1999, 200 patients were studied using fMRI on a 0.2-Tesla Magnetom Open. Routine evaluation of the extracranial vertebral circulation by MRI angiography as an additional preinvestigative requirement is recommended. The earliest examination time from injury to MRI evaluation was 3 months and the maximum, 5 years (average, 2.6 years). Among the 200 patients investigated, 30 showed instability of the ligamentous dens complex. Of the same 200, 8 (4%) had a complete rupture and 22 (11%) an incomplete rupture of the alar ligament, with instability signs. In another 45 patients (22.5%), fMRI-video showed evidence of instability, and all these patients had coexisting intraligamentous signal pattern variation, probably due to granulation tissue. Eighty patients of the 200 (40%) had signal indifference without demonstrable video instability signs, and 43 patients (21.5%) showed no evidence of instability and no signal variation in the alar ligaments. On the basis of recognition of instability and the malfunction of the ligaments, the fibrous capsula, and the tiny dens capsula, we now can distinguish between lesions caused by rotatory trauma to the craniocervical junction and those from classic whiplash injury.

Volle E. Functional magnetic resonance imaging—video diagnosis of soft-tissue trauma to the craniocervical joints and ligaments. Int Tinnitus J. 2000;6(2):134–9.

See also Levine AM, Edwards CC. Treatment of injuries in the C1–C2 complex. Orthop Clin North Am. 1986 Jan;17(1) :31–44, *which found the following:* ***Atlantoaxial offset = X + Y; Atlantoaxial offset < 5.7 mm => transverse ligament intact (stable); Atlantoaxial offset > 6.9 mm => transverse ligament ruptured (unstable).***

Whiplash trauma can damage soft tissue structures of the upper cervical spine, particularly the alar ligaments. Structural lesions in this area contribute to the understanding of the chronic whiplash syndrome.

Krakenes J, Kaale BR. Magnetic resonance imaging assessment of craniovertebral ligaments and membranes after whiplash trauma. Spine. 2006 Nov 15;31(24):2820–6.

This preliminary work indicates substantial **infiltration of fatty tissue into suboccipital muscles of some subjects being treated for chronic head and neck pain.** Hallgren RC, Greenman PE, Rechtien JJ. Atrophy of suboccipital muscles in patients with chronic pain: a pilot study. J Am Osteopath Assoc. 1994 Dec;94(12):1032–8.

§ 9:15 X-rays—Flexion/extension radiographs

Flexion/extension is the most sensitive load-direction for the tested discoligamentous instabilities. Richter M, Wilke HJ, Kluger P, Claes L, Puhl W. Load-displacement properties of the normal and injured lower cervical spine in vitro. Eur Spine J. 2000 Apr; 9(2):104–8.

The trauma group showed trends toward hypermobility in the upper and middle cervical levels. Dvorak J, Panjabi MM, Grob D, Novotny JE, Antinnes JA. Clinical validation of functional flexion/extension radiographs of the cervical spine. Spine. 1993 Jan;18(1):120–7.

Clinical instability in the neutral zone has been associated with clinical complaints, and flexion/extension radiographs may show some of this abnormal motion. Panjabi MM, Lydon C, Vasavada A, Grob D, Crisco JJ 3rd, Dvorak J. On the understanding of clinical instability. Spine. 1994 Dec 1;19(23):2642–50.

Increased flexibility implies yielding of the soft tissue structure and constitutes functional injury to the spine. Panjabi MM, Nibu K, Cholewicki J. Whiplash injuries and the potential for mechanical instability. Eur Spine J. 1998;7(6):484–92.

Flexion and extension views are essential to help define whiplash and other ligamentous injuries of the cervical spine. Griffiths HJ, Olson PN, Everson LI, Winemiller M. Hyperextension strain or "whiplash" injuries to the cervical spine. Skeletal Radiol. 1995 May;24(4):263–6.

The segmental extension-flexion motion of the cervical spine and the overall C1–C7 motion were measured on functional X-rays in 19 patients with post-traumatic headache and 19 age- and sex-matched controls. **The extension-flexion C1–C7 motion was reduced in patients with post-traumatic headache due to reduced motion in three segments: C2–C3, C5–C6 ($p < 0.05$), and C6–C7 ($p < 0.01$).** Jensen OK, Justesen T, Nielsen FF, Brixen K. Functional radiographic examination of the cervical spine in patients with post-traumatic headache. Cephalalgia. 1990 Dec;10(6):295–303.

§ 9:16 X-rays—More on X-ray examination

A normal sagittal spine configuration is desirable. A cervical lordosis, measured from C2 to C7, of 34 degrees is suggestive for clinical outcomes (range 16–66 degrees). See Harrison DD, Janik TJ, Troyanovich SJ, Holland B. Comparisons of lordotic cervical spine curvatures to a theoretical ideal model of the static sagittal cervical spine. Spine. 1996 Mar 15;21(6):667–75; Harrison DD, Troyanovich SJ, Harrison DE, Janik TJ, Murphy DJ. A normal sagittal spinal configuration: a desirable clinical outcome. J Manipulative Physiol Ther. 1996 Jul–Aug;19(6):398–405.

Lateral cervical X-ray analysis is reliable. Jackson BL, Harrison DD, Robertson GA, Barker WF. Chiropractic biophysics lateral cervical film analysis reliability. J Manipulative Physiol Ther. 1993 Jul–Aug;16(6):384–91.

There is very good reliability in cervical spine measurements (X-ray). Jackson BL, Barker W, Bentz J, Gambale AG. Inter- and intra-examiner reliability of the upper cervical X-ray marking system: a second look. J Manipulative Physiol Ther. 1987 Aug;10(4):157–63.

A kyphotic curve is a buckled configuration and withstands less loading. **This is a basis for the formation of osteophytes on the anterior margins of the vertebrae in kyphotic regions of the sagittal cervical spine.** See Harrison DE, Harrison DD, Janik TJ, William Jones E, Cailliet R, Normand M. Comparison of axial and flexural stresses in lordosis and three buckled configurations of the cervical spine. Clin Biomech (Bristol, Avon). 2001 May;16(4):276–84; Frost HM. From Wolff's law to the mechanostat: a new "face" of physiology. J Orthop Sci. 1998;3(5):282–6.

§ 9:17 MRI studies

IL-1beta and Tumor necrosis factor-alpha (TNF-a) are proinflammatory cytokines. Inflammation may be seen on MRI as **Modic Type 1** changes.

Trauma to the intervertebral disc could result in the production of inflammatory substances within the nucleus pulposus. Diffusion of such toxic chemicals through the vertebral endplate could then result in a local inflammatory reaction resulting in pain.

Braithwaite I, White J, Saifuddin A, Renton P, Taylor BA. Vertebral end-plate (Modic) changes on lumbar spine MRI: correlation with pain reproduction at lumbar discography. Eur Spine J. 1998;7(5):363–8

Type I changes consist of reduced signal intensity (SI) in the vertebral end-plates on T1- and increasedSI on T2-weighted sequences. Inflammation in the subchondral bone adjacent to the end-plate would result in reduced SI on T1-weighted MRI sequences and increased SI on T2-weighted MRI sequences, equivalent to a Type 1 Modic change. Modic changes type 1 are more strongly associated with pain compared to type 2. The reason for this may be that Modic changes type 1 reflects earlier and acute stages of inflammation, whereas Modic changes type 2 are thought to be a result of previous inflammation and more progressive degeneration.

Albert HB, Manniche C. Modic changes following lumbar disc herniation. Eur Spine J. 2007 Jul;16(7):977–82

Spinal structural abnormalities on radiographs and MRI are not always correlated with the perception of pain. See Boden SD, McCowin PR, Davis DO, Dina TS, Mark AS, Wiesel S. Abnormal magnetic-resonance scans of the cervical spine in asymptomatic subjects. A prospective investigation. J Bone Joint Surg Am. 1990 Sep;72(8):1178–84; Jensen MC, Brant-Zawadzki MN, Obuchowski N, Modic MT, Malkasian D, Ross JS. Magnetic resonance imaging of the lumbar spine in people without back pain. N Engl J Med. 1994 Jul 14;331(2):69–73; Lee CK, Vessa P, Lee JK. Chronic disabling low back pain syndrome caused by internal disc derangements. The results of disc excision and posterior lumbar interbody fusion. Spine. 1995 Feb 1;20(3):356–61; Schellhas KP, Smith MD, Gundry CR, Pollei SR. Cervical discogenic pain. Prospective correlation of magnetic resonance imaging and discography in asymptomatic subjects and pain sufferers. Spine. 1996 Feb 1;21(3):300–11; discussion 311–2; Savage RA, Whitehouse GH, Roberts N. The relationship between the magnetic resonance imaging appearance of the lumbar spine and low back pain, age and occupation in males. Eur Spine J. 1997;6(2):106–14; Wallis BJ, Lord SM, Bogduk N. Resolution of psychological distress of whiplash patients following treatment by radiofrequency neurotomy: a randomized, double-blind, placebo-controlled trial. Pain. 1997 Oct;73(1):15–22; Matsumoto M, Fujimura Y, Suzuki N, Nishi Y, Nakamura M, Yabe Y, Shiga H. MRI of cervical intervertebral discs in asymptomatic subjects. J Bone Joint Surg Br. 1998 Jan;80(1):19–24.

The relationship of lumbar MRI findings to symptoms is largely unknown. Beattie PF, Meyers SP, Stratford P, Millard RW, Hollenberg GM. Associations between patient report of symptoms and anatomic impairment visible on lumbar magnetic resonance imaging. Spine. 2000 Apr 1;25(7):819–28.

MRI studies may be performed in patients with suspected occult cervical injury with negative standard radiographs. MRI is more sensitive in detecting ligamentous injury not evident on plain radiographs. Geck MJ, Yoo S, Wang JC. Assessment of cervical ligamentous injury in trauma patients using MRI. J Spinal Disord. 2001 Oct;14(5):371–7.

Routine use of MRI is not justified but may be of use in those patients with persistent radiating pain. See Voyvodic F, Dolinis J, Moore VM, Ryan GA, Slavotinek JP, Whyte AM, Hoile RD, Taylor GW. MRI of car occupants with whiplash injury. Neuroradiology. 1997 Jan;39(1):35–40; Jonsson H Jr, Cesarini K, Sahlstedt B, Rauschning W. Findings and outcome in whiplash-type neck distortions. Spine. 1994 Dec 15;19(24):2733–43.

This study evaluated objective diagnostic methods for patients with possible upper cervical spine instability caused by trauma and correlated them with subsequent neurosurgical findings and outcomes. **We conclude that functional MRI with lateral tilting and rotatory evaluation is a useful tool for investigating craniocervical instability. For patients who are recalcitrant to following a program of conservative therapy, surgical stabilization of the craniocervical junction appears to be justified.** See Volle E, Montazem A. MRI video diagnosis and surgical therapy of soft tissue trauma to the craniocervical junction. Ear Nose Throat J. 2001 Jan;80(1):41–4, 46–8.

Alar ligament damage can take up to 2 years for complete healing. The increased [high] signal within the ligament noted on high resolution MRI is probably due to atrophy of fibres and fatty infiltration. Craniovertebral junction ligament injury may prove to be the structural substrate for the late whiplash syndrome. See Krakenes J, Kaale BR, Moen G, Nordli H, Gilhus NE, Rorvik J. MRI assessment of the alar ligaments in the late stage of whiplash injury — a study of structural abnormalities and observer agreement. Neuroradiology. 2002 Jul;44(7):617–24.

Combining MRI findings with a positive provocative vibratory test increased the sensitivity to 85.9% and accuracy 83.0%. Vanharanta H, Ohnmeiss DD, Aprill CN. Vibration pain provocation can improve the specificity of MRI in the diagnosis of symptomatic lumbar disc rupture. Clin J Pain. 1998 Sep;14(3):239–47.

Measuring differences in **neck extensor muscle** rCSA

(cross section area) with MRI in an asymptomatic population provides the basis for future study investigating relationships between muscular atrophy and symptoms in patients suffering from persistent neck pain. Elliott JM, Jull GA, Noteboom JT, Durbridge GL, Gibbon WW. Magnetic resonance imaging study of cross-sectional area of the cervical extensor musculature in an asymptomatic cohort. Clin Anat. 2007 Jan;20(1):35–40.

A quantitative measure of **muscle/fat constituents** has been developed, and results of this study indicate that relative fatty infiltration is not a feature of age in the upper cervical extensor muscles of women aged 18–45 years. Elliott JM, Galloway GJ, Jull GA, Noteboom JT, Centeno CJ, Gibbon WW. Magnetic resonance imaging analysis of the upper cervical spine extensor musculature in an asymptomatic cohort: an index of fat within muscle. Clin Radiol. 2005 Mar;60(3):355–63.

There is significantly greater **fatty infiltration** in the neck extensor muscles, especially in the deeper muscles in the upper cervical spine, in subjects with persistent WAD when compared with healthy controls. Future studies are required to investigate the relationships between muscular alterations and symptoms in patients suffering from persistent WAD. Elliott J, Jull G, Noteboom JT, Darnell R, Galloway G, Gibbon WW. Fatty infiltration in the cervical extensor muscles in persistent whiplash-associated disorders: a magnetic resonance imaging analysis. Spine. 2006 Oct 15;31(22):E847–55.

This study suggests that there is a relationship between **chronic pain, somatic dysfunction, muscle atrophy and standing balance**. We hypothesize a cycle initiated by chronic somatic dysfunction, which may result in muscle atrophy, which can be further expected to reduce proprioceptive output from atrophied muscles. The lack of proprioceptive inhibition of nociceptors at the dorsal horn of the spinal cord would result in chronic pain and a loss of standing balance. McPartland JM, Brodeur RR, Hallgren RC. Chronic neck pain, standing balance, and suboccipital muscle atrophy—a pilot study. J Manipulative Physiol Ther. 1997 Jan;20(1):24–9.

Chronic Tension Type Headache patients demonstrate muscle atrophy of the rectus capitis posterior muscles. Whether this selective muscle atrophy is a primary or secondary phenomenon remains unclear. In any case, muscle atrophy could possibly account for a reduction of proprioceptive output from these muscles, and thus contribute to the perpetuation of pain. Fernandez-de-Las-Penas C, Bueno A, Ferrando J, Elliott JM,

Cuadrado ML, Pareja JA.Magnetic resonance imaging study of the morphometry of cervical extensor muscles in chronic tension-type headache. Cephalalgia. 2007 Apr;27(4):355–62.

§ 9:18 MRI studies—MRI and cervical discogenic pain

MRI in its current state of technology does not reliably detect anular defects. Significant cervical anular tears often escape MRI detection, and MRI cannot reliably identify the source of cervical discogenic pain. **In more than half of the studies, three or more levels were identified as pain generators, suggesting that treatment decisions based on information from fewer discs injected during discography may be tenuous.** Schellhas KP, Smith MD, Gundry CR, Pollei SR. Cervical discogenic pain. Prospective correlation of magnetic resonance imaging and discography in asymptomatic subjects and pain sufferers. Spine. 1996 Feb 1; 21(3):300–11; discussion 311–2.

Production of proinflammatory mediators within the nucleus pulposus may be a major factor in the genesis of a painful lumbar disc. Burke JG, Watson RW, McCormack D, Dowling FE, Walsh MG, Fitzpatrick JM. Intervertebral discs which cause low back pain secrete high levels of proinflammatory mediators. J Bone Joint Surg Br. 2002 Mar;84(2):196–201.

Diagnostic blocks: a truth serum for malingering. Malingering is not a diagnosis; rather, it is a behavior for which there are no established diagnostic criteria. Guidelines have been published according to which malingering might be suspected, but those guidelines do not discriminate between patients who are malingering and patients with genuine sources of chronic pain. In such patients, while malingering cannot be proven, it can be refuted if a genuine source of pain can be established. In patients with no apparent cause of pain, the source of that pain can be established using controlled diagnostic blocks. A positive response to diagnostic blocks demonstrates that the complaint of pain is genuine and, by implication, refutes any contention that the patient is malingering. **When positive, diagnostic blocks provide objective data by which disputes based on opinion as to whether a patient is malingering can be resolved.** Negative responses do not exclude a genuine complaint of pain, for patients may have a source of pain that is not amenable to testing with diagnostic blocks. **Diagnostic blocks have proved particularly useful in the investigation of spinal pain for which the cause is not evident on conventional**

medical imaging. They can also confirm or refute purported mechanisms of certain clinical features in complex regional pain syndromes. Bogduk N. Diagnostic blocks: a truth serum for malingering. Clin J Pain. 2004 Nov–Dec;20(6):409–14.

§ 9:19 MRI studies—Functional imaging

fMRI, or functional MRI, has the highest spatial resolution of the imaging technologies that are used for functional mapping the brain. The signal generated from fMRI is due to the differences in magnetic properties of oxygenated versus deoxygenated hemoglobim (BOLD contrast). See Volkow ND, Rosen B, Farde L. Imaging the living human brain: magnetic resonance imaging and positron emission tomography. Proc Natl Acad Sci U S A. 1997 Apr 1;94(7):2787–8.

Kinematic Imaging

Biomechanical changes in the herniated disk were noted, with mildly increased spinal stenosis following flexion. The authors conclude that flexion and extension MR can be a valuable adjunct examination in the evaluation of patients in the clinical setting of subacute cervical spine trauma. As a result of their study, the authors believe that flexion-extension MRI can be very useful in cases of low-impact injuries in which there were clinical signs of cervical instability. Their procedure optimizes the detection of segment motions abnormalities and injuries of the disco-ligamentous complex. Biomechanical changes in herniated disc are also observed with their imaging protocol. This MR protocol is less reliable during the acute phase of injury (first 12 weeks) because of the presence of muscle spasm, which can exaggerate the biomechanical changes. They recommend the MR extension-flexion protocol during the sub acute phase (12–14 weeks after injury).

The presence of neurologic symptoms was exacerbated following flexion in 89% of subjects (89 of 100), compared to 24% of subjects during extension.

Disk herniations were observed in 28% of subjects, observed as extradural impression on the subarachnoid space, which was mildly accentuated following flexion in all of the injured subjects (28 of 28). Giuliano V, Giuliano C, Pinto F, Scaglione M. The use of flexion and extension MR in the evaluation of cervical spine trauma: initial experience in 100 trauma patients compared with 100 normal subjects. Emerg Radiol. 2002 Nov;9(5):249–53.

A 40-year-old man referred with complaints of neck pain, left arm pain, headaches, paresthesias in the index and middle fingers, with numbness in the C7 nerve root distribution. Conventional recumbent magnetic resonance imaging (MRI) was read by the radiologist as a small protrusion at C5-C6 that did not correlate with his symptoms. The patient had exhausted his treatment options. He underwent MRI in a weight-bearing, upright position with extension that revealed a positional cervical disc protrusion on the left at C6-C7. The protrusion was causing a proximal left C6-C7 neural foraminal stenosis and impingement that correlated with his symptoms. With this information, we were able to offer a targeted epidural block. **Imaging the spine in the weight-bearing position with extension or placing the spine in the position of pain may increase the diagnostic accuracy for the neuroradiologist and neuroimagist, who then can provide the spine surgeon or neurosurgeon potentially with additional information to further improve patient care.**

Gilbert JW, Wheeler GR, Lingreen RA, Johnson RR. Open stand-up MRI: a new instrument for positional neuroimaging. J Spinal Disord Tech. 2006 Apr;19(2):151–4.

Conventional magnetic resonance imaging (MRI) of complex cervical spine disorders may underestimate the magnitude of structural disease because imaging is performed in a nondynamic non-weight-bearing manner. Myelography provides additional information but requires an invasive procedure.

This was a prospective review of the first 20 upright weight-bearing cervical MRI procedures with patients in the flexed, neutral, and extended positions conducted in an open-configuration MRI unit.

This technique clearly illustrated the changes in spinal cord compression, angulation, and spinal column alignment that occur during physiologic movements with corresponding changes in midsagittal spinal canal diameter ($P < 0.05$). Image quality was excellent or good in 90% of the cases.

Dynamic weight-bearing MRI provides an innovative method for imaging complex cervical spine disorders. This technique is noninvasive and has adequate image quality that may make it a good alternative to cervical myelography.

Vitaz TW, Shields CB, Raque GH, Hushek SG, Moser R, Hoerter N, Moriarty TM. Dynamic weight-bearing cervical magnetic resonance imaging: technical review and preliminary results. South Med J. 2004 May;97(5):456–61.

The **potential relative beneficial aspects of upright, weight-bearing (pMRI), dynamic-kinetic (kMRI) spinal**

imaging on this system over that of recumbent MRI (rMRI) include: the revelation of occult disease dependent on true axial loading, the unmasking of kinetic-dependent disease, and the ability to scan the patient in the position of clinically relevant signs and symptoms. This imaging unit also demonstrated low claustrophobic potential and yielded relatively high-resolution images with little motion/chemical shift artifact.

Jinkins JR, Dworkin J. Proceedings of the State-of-the-Art Symposium on Diagnostic and Interventional Radiology of the Spine, Antwerp, September 7, 2002 (Part two). Upright, weight-bearing, dynamic-kinetic MRI of the spine: pMRI/kMRI. JBR-BTR. 2003 Sep-Oct;86(5):286–93.

The potential relative beneficial aspects of upright, weight-bearing (pMRI), dynamic-kinetic (kMRI) spinal imaging over that of recumbent MRI (rMRI) include the revelation of occult spinal disease dependent on true axial loading, the unmasking of kinetic-dependent spinal disease and the ability to scan the patient in the position of clinically relevant signs and symptoms. This imaging unit under study also demonstrated low claustrophobic potential and yielded comparatively high resolution images with little motion/magnetic susceptibility/chemical shift artifact. Overall, it was found that **rMRI underestimated the presence and maximum degree of gravity-dependent spinal pathology and missed altogether pathology of a dynamic nature**, factors that are optimally revealed with p/kMRI. Furthermore, p/kMRI enabled optimal linkage of the patient's clinical syndrome with the medical imaging abnormality responsible for the clinical presentation, thereby allowing for the first time an improvement at once in both imaging sensitivity and specificity.

Jinkins JR, Dworkin JS, Damadian RV. Upright, weight-bearing, dynamic-kinetic MRI of the spine: initial results. Eur Radiol. 2005 Sep;15(9):1815–25.

§ 9:20 Computer Tomography (CT)

The preferred screening modality in trauma patients at high and moderate risk for cervical spine fractures is computer tomography. Blackmore CC, Ramsey SD, Mann FA, Deyo RA. Cervical spine screening with CT in trauma patients: a cost-effectiveness analysis. Radiology. 1999 Jul;212(1):117–25.

§ 9:21 Computer Tomography (CT)—SPECT and PET scans

SPECT (single photon emission computed tomogra-

phy) may be seen in whiplash patients with the lesion most like damage to the vertebral endplates. Freeman MD, Sapir D, Boutselis A, Gorup J, Tuckmn G, Croft AC, Centeno C, Phillips A. Whiplash injury and occult vertebral fracture: a case of SPECT imaging of patients with persisting spine pain following a motor vehicle crash. Cervical Spine Research Society 29th Annual Meeting, Monterey, CA, Nov 29–Dec 1, 2001.

PET (positron emission tomography) or SPECT (single-photon emission computed tomography) are used for the measurements of molecular targets, such as receptors, transportors, and the enzymes that are involved in the synthesis and the metabolism of neurotransmitters. In PET and SPECT, radioisotopes bind selectively to molecules in the tissue. See Volkow ND, Rosen B, Farde L. Imaging the living human brain: magnetic resonance imaging and positron emission tomography. Proc Natl Acad Sci U S A. 1997 Apr 1;94(7):2787–8.

§ 9:22 Computer Tomography (CT)—Imaging for post-concussion syndrome

SPECT or PET (positron emission tomography) scans are performed in some patients to evaluate brain functioning. These scans evaluate brain functioning rather than the structure. These scans measure blood flow to brain regions or the use of nutrients by areas of the brain. Such scans help pinpoint areas of difficulty when an MRI or CT scan is normal.

As part of the family of nuclear imaging techniques, PET and SPECT scans use small amounts of radionuclides (radioactive isotopes) to measure cellular/tissue change. Radionuclides are absorbed by healthy tissue at a different rate than tissue undergoing a disease process. A deviation in normal rates of absorption may be an indication of abnormal metabolic activity, which could lead to structural change (e.g. vertebra). X-rays, CT Scans, and MRI can only image structure (e.g. anatomy), not function or metabolism.

A SPECT Scan is capable of providing information about blood flow to tissue. It is a sensitive diagnostic tool used to detect stress fracture, spondylosis, infection (e.g. discitis), and tumor (e.g. osteoid osteoma). Analyzing blood flow to an organ (e.g. bone) may help to determine how well it is functioning.

Following an inconclusive SPECT, a PET scan using the glucose analog 2-[fluorine-18]-fluoro-2-deoxy-D-glucose (FDG), a radionuclide injected intravenously, may be of use. Tissues absorb the radionuclide as it is circulated in the blood. As a camera rotates around the patient, it picks ups photons, the radionuclide particles. This information is transferred to a computer that converts the data onto film. The images are vertical and/or horizontal cross-sections of the body part and can be rendered into 3-D format.

Persistent Post-Concussion Syndrome (PPCS) is one of the most frustrating conditions to work with, simply because most imaging studies are not powerful enough to detect subtle brain tissue damage; MRI and CT scans usually show nothing in patients with long-term symptoms. SPECT scans show promise. **Of the 43 patients, SPECT found abnormalities in 53% of the subjects. MRI found abnormalities in just 9%, and CT only 4–6%. Thus, 23 patients had evidence of brain tissue damage on SPECT that was not detected by other imaging methods.**

Regarding the above discussion, see Kant R, Smith-Seemiller L, Isaac G, Duffy J. Tc-HMPAO SPECT in persistent post-concussion syndrome after mild head injury: comparison with MRI/CT. Brain Inj. 1997 Feb;11(2):115–24.

"None of the new brain imaging techniques nor quantitative EEG analyses have proved useful enough in the assessment of mild head injured, as well as whiplash, patients. The present study suggests an objective neurophysiological parameter, the P300 wave, as a possible diagnostic tool for the situation." Granovsky Y, Sprecher E, Hemli J, Yarnitsky D. P300 and stress in mild head injury patients. Electroencephalogr Clin Neurophysiol. 1998 Nov;108(6):554–9.

§ 9:23 Computer Tomography (CT)—Imaging for whiplash

The late whiplash syndrome shows slight abnormalities when examined with SPECT scans. The researchers concluded that the changes in brain structure were not due to direct head trauma, but "it may be that the perfusion deficits are caused by . . . a mechanism in the upper cervical spine." **The researchers speculate that these changes may be responsible for attentional dysfunction that is commonly found in whiplash patients.** Otte A, Mueller-Brand J, Fierz L. Brain SPECT findings in late whiplash syndrome. Lancet. 1995 Jun 10;345(8963):1513.

"Our hypothesis is that parieto-occipital hypometabolism may be caused by activation of nociceptive afferences from the upper cervical spine. By contrast, the areas of hypometabolism seen in areas other than parieto-occipital may mainly be explained by brain contusion and not by the effects of activated nociceptive afferences on brain metabolism. In addition, hypometabolism in parieto-occipital regions cannot be excluded in some cases as part or entirely a consequence of diffuse axonal lesions due to acceleration forces." **The authors also suggest that lowered glucose metabolism in these parts of the brain may also be responsible for some of the cognitive disturbances experienced by patients. SPECT and PET may provide important information for individual whiplash patients.** Otte A, Ettlin TM, Nitzsche EU, Wachter K, Hoegerle S, Simon GH, Fierz L, Moser E, Mueller-Brand J. PET and SPECT in whiplash syndrome: a new approach to a forgotten brain? J Neurol Neurosurg Psychiatry. 1997 Sep;63(3):368–72.

"We conclude that combined functional assessment using SPECT imaging and P300 recording in association with neuropsychological testing may be more appropriate than morphologic imaging alone for better evaluation of whiplash-associated complaints." Lorberboym M, Gilad R, Gorin V, Sadeh M, Lampl Y. Late whiplash syndrome: correlation of brain SPECT with neuropsychological tests and P300 event-related potential. J Trauma. 2002 Mar;52(3):521–6.

§ 9:24 Other imaging types—Surface electromyography

Surface electromyography may be a useful tool in objectively assessing musculoskeletal signs following whiplash. Nederhand MJ, IJzerman MJ, Hermens HJ, Baten CT, Zilvold G. Cervical muscle dysfunction in the chronic whiplash associated disorder grade II (WAD-II). Spine. 2000 Aug 1;25(15):1938–43.

Surface EMG findings could predict a worsening of complaints 1-year later. Lundblad I, Elert J, Gerdle B. Worsening of neck and shoulder complaints in humans are correlated with frequency parameters of electromyogram recorded 1-year earlier. Eur J Appl Physiol Occup Physiol. 1998 Dec; 79(1):7–16.

Surface EMG can interpret functional adaptation to muscle pain. Arendt-Nielsen L, Graven-Nielsen T, Svarrer H, Svensson P. The influence of low back pain on muscle activity and coordination during gait: a clinical and experimental study. Pain. 1996 Feb;64(2):231–40.

§ 9:25 Other imaging types—Bone scan

Bone scintigraphy (bone scan) may detect occult damage not visible on X-ray. Versijpt J, Dierckx RA, De Bondt P, Dierckx I, Lambrecht L, De Sadeleer C. The contribution of bone scintigraphy in occupational health or medical insurance claims: a retrospective study. Eur J Nucl Med. 1999 Aug;26(8):804–11.

§ 9:26 Other imaging types—Videofluoroscopy

Videofluroscopy allows the dynamic assessment to evaluate subtle variations of motion through the entire arc of motion. To show movements in the neutral zone, videofluoroscopy may show more then plain film radiographs. MRIs may show injury in certain conditions. **Videoflouroscopy can demonstrate different motion patterns between normal and pathologic spines.** See Hino H, Abumi K, Kanayama M, Kaneda K. Dynamic motion analysis of normal and unstable cervical spines using cineradiography. An in vivo study. Spine. 1999 Jan 15; 24(2):163–8.

Videoflouroscopy can demonstrate different motion patterns between normal and pathologic spines. Hino H, Abumi K, Kanayama M, Kaneda K. Dyamic motion analysis of normal and unstable cervical spines using cineradiography. An in vivo study. Spine. 1999 Jan 15;24(2):163–8.

In trauma patients with normal spine radiographs and an average Glascow Coma Scale of 9.2, nine patients on exam had evidence of cervical instability. Three patients would have been missed without videofluroscopy. **In these higher grade trauma patients, spinal lesions may be missed by conventional imaging.** Cox MW, McCarthy M, Lemmon G, Wenker J. Cervical spine instability: clearance using dynamic fluoroscopy. Curr Surg. 2001 Jan;58(1):96–100.

§ 9:27 Other imaging types—Provocative vibratory testing

Provocative vibratory testing was shown to agree with discographic pain provocation in 75% of the discs. Yrjama M, Tervonen O, Kurunlahti M, Vanharanta H. Bony vibration stimulation test combined with magnetic resonance imaging. Can discography be replaced? Spine. 1997 Apr 1;22(7):808–13.

Combining MRI findings with a positive provocative vibratory test increased the sensitivity to 85.9% and accuracy 83.0%. Vanharanta H, Ohnmeiss DD, Aprill CN. Vibration pain provocation can improve the specificity of MRI in the diagnosis of symptomatic lumbar disc rupture. Clin J Pain. 1998 Sep;14(3):239–47.

§ 9:28 Other imaging types—Criteria for serious injury

Bogduk and Yoganandan addressed the following in a 2001 paper (citation below):

"There is no universally accepted definition of what distinguishes major from minor injuries to the cervical spine." Fractures of the vertebral body, the pedicles, the odontoid process, the ring of the atlas, and dislocations are considered to be major injuries, as they threaten the stability of the cervical spine its neural contents. Fractures in an articular process or across the anterior edge of a vertebral body can be minor because they do not threaten spinal stability.

Minor injuries of the cervical spine are usually classified as "soft-tissue injuries," implying no bone injury, but rather injury to muscles or ligaments. X-rays cannot demonstrate these soft tissues. Computerized tomography (CT) and magnetic resonance imaging (MRI) also do not help in demonstrating these soft tissue injuries.

"CT may be used to better define fractures already evident on plain films, or to search for occult fractures, but it does not resolve soft-tissue injuries."

"MRI has the capacity to resolve certain soft-tissues, but no correlations have been established between neck pain and any feature evident on MRI."

Several factors render neck soft-tissue injuries controversial: They are not demonstrated on X-rays; soft-tissue injuries in the limbs, often (but not always), heal rapidly, in days or weeks; soft-tissue neck injuries are often associated with insurance claims. Compensation and monetary gain confounds the clinical picture; a proportion of these patients develop chronic symptoms that last well beyond the expected period in which soft-tissue injuries should have healed.

"However, the more that whiplash has been studied, the more has scientific inquiry dispelled incorrect notions that caused this controversy."

"The literature is replete with studies that have shown small injuries to intervertebral, discs, zygapophysial joints, and uncovertebral clefts, both in collagenous tissues and in cartilage and bones, that are plainly invisible on plain radiographs. Radiography simply lacks the sensitivity to detect these injuries, and therefore, cannot be used to exclude or refute them. Normal radiographs do not mean that there has been no injury."

"Extrapolation from the limbs about the nature of soft-tissue injuries and their period of healing is both inappropriate and false."

Muscle injury is not an acceptable model for the healing of ligaments, capsules, joints, and intervertebral discs. Although most sprained ankles recover within weeks, some do not, and many patients are left with chronic symptoms, even though compensation is not involved.

Knee meniscus injuries often do not resolve and cause chronic pain and disability.

Small articular fractures can cause chronic disability. "Intervertebral discs, like the menisci of the knee, are unlikely to heal spontaneously after injury, probably because of their relatively meager blood supply." "Clinical experience abounds with examples of soft tissue injuries to the limbs that do not summarily heal." "Correctly used, therefore, extrapolation would predict that at least some injuries of the cervical spine would not heal."

"Whereas muscle sprains should resolve rapidly, injuries to joints and discs may remain sources of chronic pain."

Formal studies refute that patients with neck pain exaggerate or perpetuate their symptoms for the purpose of financial gain, and their symptoms often persist after settlement of compensation claims.

Regarding the foregoing, see Bogduk N, Yoganandan N. Biomechanics of the cervical spine Part 3: minor injuries. Clin Biomech (Bristol, Avon). 2001 May;16(4):267–75.

Major injuries are defined as having either radiographic or CT evidence of instability, with or without associated localized or central neurological findings, or have the potential to produce neurological findings. *See* Daffner RH, Brown RR, Goldberg AL. A new classification for cervical vertebral injuries: influence of CT. Skeletal Radiol. 2000 Mar;29(3):125–32.

According to the Daffner study, **cervical injury should be classified as "major" if the following radiographic and/or computer tomography (CT) criteria are present:**

- displacement of more than 2 mm in any plane
- wide vertebral body in any plane
- wide interspinous/interlaminar space

- wide facet joints
- disrupted posterior vertebral body line
- wide disc space
- vertebral burst fracture
- locked or perched facets (unilateral or bilateral)
- "hanged man" fracture of C2
- dens fracture
- type III occipital condyle fracture

See Daffner RH, Brown RR, Goldberg AL. A new classification for cervical vertebral injuries: influence of CT. Skeletal Radiol. 2000 Mar;29(3):125–32.

Subluxation greater than 2 mm in men 18 to 40 years of age may be a useful variable for further study as an indicator of ligamentous injury. Interspinous distance and vertebral angulation appear less likely to have useful clinical application. Knopp R, Parker J, Tashjian J, Ganz W. Defining radiographic criteria for flexion-extension studies of the cervical spine. Ann Emerg Med. 2001 Jul;38(1):31–5.

Localized kinking (kyphosis) greater than 10 degrees and fanning between the spinous process greater than 12 mm are useful measurements to determine true whiplash injuries from minor ligamentous tears in about 80% of the cases. Griffiths HJ, Olson PN, Everson LI, Winemiller M. Hyperextension strain or "whiplash" injuries to the cervical spine. Skeletal Radiol. 1995 May;24(4):263–6.

A 3mm displacement on the lateral cervical radiograph, which is seen on occasion, was considered a "significant dislocation of a cervical vertebra." Bunketorp L, Nordholm L, Carlsson J. A descriptive analysis of disorders in patients 17 years following motor vehicle accidents. Eur Spine J. 2002 Jun;11(3):227–34.

According to Foreman et al., **the following are radiographic signs of instability:**

- A decreased anterior disc height
- An increased posterior disc height
- Nonparallel facet planes
- An increased interspinous space (fanning)
- Anterior slippage of the upper vertebra
- Kyphotic angulation
- A disruption of the posterior cervical line of more than 1.5 mm

See Foreman SM, Croft AC eds. Whiplash injuries: The Cervical Acceleration/Deceleration Syndrome. 3ed. Philadelphia: Lippincott Williams & Wilkins; 2002, p 52–53.

§ 9:29 Refuting common defense positions regarding X-rays—Cervical lordotic curve

Comment:

Note the variance in the findings of the following studies. It is important to note that the findings of Matsumumo were from X-rays taken of the subjects while sitting. Black states that different sitting positions can affect the cervical spine posture. The Harrison study had the subjects in a standing position.

As previously mentioned, the average cervical curve is 34 degrees (as measured from C2–C7) with a range of 16–66 degrees. *See* Harrison DD, Janik TJ, Troyanovich SJ, Holland B. Comparisons of lordotic cervical spine curvatures to a theoretical ideal model of the static sagittal cervical spine. Spine. 1996 Mar 15;21(6):667–75.

The defense may bring up a study (Matsumoto, et al.) that would suggest that non-lordotic cervical curvature and angular kyphosis in acute whiplash injury constitutes "normal" variants. In that study, the authors classified the groups as lordosis, straight, sigmoid, reversed sigmoid and kyphosis. The radiographs were taken in the sitting position. Flexion/extension views were not taken. Harrison's studies were taken in the standing position. See Matsumoto M, Fujimura Y, Suzuki N, Toyama Y, Shiga H. Cervical curvature in acute whiplash injuries: prospective comparative study with asymptomatic subjects. Injury. 1998 Dec;29(10):775–8.

Sitting can change the cervical spine posture. Head orientation appeared to be maintained by compensatory adjustments in both the upper and lower cervical spine, and changes in lumbar posture were associated with compensatory changes in overall cervical position. As the lumbar spine moved toward extension, the cervical spine flexed, and as the lumbar spine flexed, the cervical spine extended. However, there was variation among subjects as to whether cervical spine adjustments occurred primarily in the upper or lower cervical region. **Different sitting postures clearly resulted in changes in cervical spine position. Lumbar and pelvic position should be considered when control of cervical posture is desired.** See Black KM, McClure P, Polansky M. The influence of different sitting positions on cervical and lumbar posture. Spine. 1996 Jan 1;21(1):65–70.

Compare the following:

Studies have shown that positioning is repeatable

with a method error of only a few degrees. See Singer KP, Edmondston SJ, Day RE, Breidahl WH. Computer-assisted curvature assessment and Cobb angle determination of the thoracic kyphosis. An in vivo and in vitro comparison. Spine. 1994 Jun 15; 19(12):1381–4; Stagnara P, De Mauroy JC, Dran G, Gonon GP, Costanzo G, Dimnet J, Pasquet A. Reciprocal angulation of vertebral bodies in a sagittal plane: approach to references for the evaluation of kyphosis and lordosis. Spine. 1982 Jul–Aug; 7(4):335–42; Jackson BL, Barker W, Bentz J, Gambale AG. Inter- and intra-examiner reliability of the upper cervical X-ray marking system: a second look. J Manipulative Physiol Ther. 1987 Aug; 10(4):157–63; Plaugher G, Hendricks AH, Doble RW Jr, Bachman TR, Araghi HJ, Hoffart VM. The reliability of patient positioning for evaluating static radiologic parameters of the human pelvis. J Manipulative Physiol Ther. 1993 Oct; 16(8):517–22; Rochester RP, Owen EF. Patient placement error in rotation and its effect on the upper cervical measuring system. Chiropr Res J 1996; 3:40–54; Harrison DD, Jackson BL, Troyanovich S, Robertson G, de George D, Barker WF. The efficacy of cervical extension-compression traction combined with diversified manipulation and drop table adjustments in the rehabilitation of cervical lordosis: a pilot study. J Manipulative Physiol Ther. 1994 Sep; 17(7):454–64; Sandham A. Repeatability of head posture recordings from lateral cephalometric radiographs. Br J Orthod. 1988 Aug;15(3):157–62; Milne JS, Williamson J. A longitudinal study of kyphosis in older people. Age Ageing. 1983 Aug; 12(3):225–33.

§ 9:30 Refuting common defense positions regarding X-rays—"Slight head nodding"

A perpetuated fallacy is that "slight head nodding" can reverse the cervical curve. This comes from a 1963 study in which patients "with the chin slightly lowered" altered the cervical lordosis in 41% of the subjects, and in the other 59% did not alter the cervical configuration. The chin was lowered 1.5 to 2 vertebral bodies, calculating the head flexion to be 22 degrees. **The amount of flexion does not qualify as "slight head nodding."** Fineman S, Borrelli J, Rubinson BM, Epstein H, Jacobson HG. The cervical spine: transformation of the normal lordosis pattern into a linear pattern in the neutral posture. A roentgenographic demonstration. J Bone Joint Surg Am 1963; 45:1179–1183.

From page 88 in the AMA Guides to the Evaluation of Permanent Impairment, the total amount of head flexion is 60 degrees. This study used 33% of head flexion and should not be used to claim that "slight nodding" can cause large changes in lordosis. **Slight head nodding occurs in the upper cervical spine and does not affect curve measurements from C2 to C7.** See Wallace HL, Jahner S, Buckle K, Desai N. The relationship of changes in cervical curvature to visual analog scale, neck disability index scores, and pressure algometry in patients with neck pain. J Chiropr Res 1994; 9:19–23; Bland JH. Disorders of the cervical spine. Diagnosis and medical management. 2nd ed. Philadelphia: WB Saunders: 1994; Dvorak J, Panjabi MM, Novotny JE, Antinnes JA. In vivo flexion/extension of the normal cervical spine. J Orthop Res. 1991 Nov; 9(6):828–34; Torg JS, Sennett B, Vegso JJ. Spinal injury at the level of the third and fourth cervical vertebrae resulting from the axial loading mechanism: an analysis and classification. Clin Sports Med. 1987 Jan; 6(1):159–83.

A 1962 article claimed that **position changes of the head caused by muscle contraction could cause loss or reversal of cervical lordosis. The patients were instructed to posteriorly translate their heads with slight head chin flexion. This is not a typical cervical muscle contraction.** See Juhl JH, Miller SM, Roberts GW. Roentgenographic variations in the normal cervical spine. Radiology 1962; 78:591–597.

This study is not relevant to patient positioning. **It should not be claimed that slight head nodding, positioning errors, or muscle spasm drastically reduce the cervical lordosis.** See Harrison DE, Harrison DD, Janik TJ, Holland B, Siskin LA. Slight head extension: does it change the sagittal cervical curve? Eur Spine J. 2001 Apr;10(2):149–53

Chapter 10

Soft Tissue Treatment

Common treatments of whiplash injuries consist of benign neglect, activities as usual, neck collars, anti-inflammatory medication, muscles relaxant medication, pain medications, physical therapy modalities, and manual therapy.

A number of alternative and complementary medicine interventions have more evidence of efficacy than conventional medical care.

Contrary to popular beliefs, major complications of common treatments are exceedingly rare and probably equivalent on average across treatments.

Guzman J, Haldeman S, Carroll LJ, Carragee EJ, Hurwitz EL, Peloso P, Nordin M, Cassidy JD, Holm LW, Côté P, van der Velde G, Hogg-Johnson S; Bone and Joint Decade 2000–2010 Task Force on Neck Pain and Its Associated Disorders. Clinical practice implications of the Bone and Joint Decade 2000–2010 Task Force on Neck Pain and Its Associated Disorders: from concepts and findings to recommendations. Spine. 2008 Feb 15;33(4 Suppl):S199–213.

§ 10:1 Early mobilization

A study in 2000 showed that mobilization within 96 hours could reduce whiplash pain significantly more than mobilization initiated after 2 weeks. Rosenfeld M, Gunnarsson R, Borenstein P. Early intervention in whiplash-associated disorders: a comparison of two treatment protocols. Spine. 2000 Jul 15;25(14):1782–7.

Acute whiplash injuries are a common cause of soft tissue trauma, for which the standard treatment is rest and initial immobilization with a soft cervical collar. Because the efficacy of this treatment is unknown, a randomized study in 61 patients was carried out comparing the standard treatment with an alternative regimen of early active mobilization. **Results showed that eight weeks after the accident the degree of improvement seen in the actively treated group compared with the group given standard treatment was significantly greater for both cervical movement (p less than 0.05) and intensity of pain (p less than 0.0125).** *See* Mealy K, Brennan H, Fenelon GC. Early mobilization of acute whiplash injuries. Br Med J (Clin Res Ed). 1986 Mar 8; 292(6521):656–7.

Early mobilization may prevent scar transformation of hidden injuries. See Mealy K, Brennan H, Fenelon GC. Early mobilization of acute whiplash injuries. Br Med J (Clin Res Ed). 1986 Mar 8;292(6521):656–7; Pennie B, Agambar L. Patterns of injury and recovery in whiplash. Injury. 1991 Jan;22(1):57–9.

Early mobilization of the spine is better than restricted movement in the care of whiplash injuries. Reduced long-term pain and complaints were observed in the early mobilization group. Borchgrevink GE, Kaasa A, McDonagh D, Stiles TC, Haraldseth O, Lereim I. Acute treatment of whiplash neck sprain injuries. A randomized trial of treatment during the first 14 days after a car accident. Spine. 1998 Jan 1;23(1):25–31.

"Early mobilization after a whiplash injury may decrease neck-shoulder pain more than a standard program using a soft collar or initial rest." Kai Y, Oyama M, Kurose S, Inadome T, Oketani Y, Masuda Y. Neurogenic thoracic outlet syndrome in whiplash injury. J Spinal Disord. 2001 Dec; 14(6):487–93.

Note:

This does not mean at the start of treatment having a patient wear a soft cervical support a couple hours a day for a couple of days is inappropriate.

§ 10:2 Manual therapy

A recent study clearly shows that **a treatment strategy consisting mainly of spinal mobilization by a manual therapist is superior compared to analgesics, consulting and education provided by a general practitioner or combined exercise and massage by a physical therapist for patients with neck pain.** Patients with more severe complaints at baseline appear to benefit most from spinal mobilization. Manual therapy (spinal mobilization) is more effective and less costly than physical therapy and GP (general practitioner) care. See Hoving LJ. Neck pain in primary care: The effects of commonly applied interventions. PhD thesis. Institute for Research in Extramural Medicine, Vrije University, The Netherlands, 2001.

The purpose of this study was to assess the effects of early active mobilization versus standard treatment with a soft cervical collar. A prospective, randomized clinical trial with a total of 168 patients was performed. **Early mobilization is superior to the standard therapy regarding pain intensity and disability. They concluded that mobilization should be recommended as the new adequate standard-therapy in the acute management of whiplash injury.** Schnabel M, Vassiliou T, Schmidt T, Basler HD, Gotzen L, Junge A, Kaluza G. Results of early mobilization of acute whiplash injuries. Schmerz. 2002 Feb;16(1):15–21.

Manual therapy with specific adjuvant exercise appears to be beneficial in treating chronic low back pain. Despite changes in pain, perceived function did not improve. It is possible that impacting chronic low back pain alone does not address psychosocial or other factors that may contribute to disability. Further studies are needed to examine the long-term effects of these interventions and to address what adjuncts are beneficial in improving function in this population. Geisser ME, Wiggert EA, Haig AJ, Colwell MO. A randomized, controlled trial of manual therapy and specific adjuvant exercise for chronic low back pain. Clin J Pain. 2005 Nov–Dec;21(6):463–70.

Effectiveness of supervised physical training. Supervised training was significantly more favorable than home training, with a more rapid improvement in self-efficacy (P = 0.03), fear of movement/(re)injury (P = 0.03) and pain disability (P = 0.03) at three months. Further, supervised training significantly reduced the frequency of analgesic consumption (P = 0.03). The improvements were partly maintained at nine months, even though there was no amelioration in pain and physical disorders. Despite the favorable outcome, supervised intervention did not reduce sick leave. The findings indicate a treatment approach that is feasible in the rehabilitation of patients with subacute whiplash-associated disorders in the short term, but additional research is needed to extend these findings and elucidate treatment strategies that also are cost effective. Bunketorp L, Lindh M, Carlsson J, Stener-Victorin E. The effectiveness of a supervised physical training model tailored to the individual needs of patients with whiplash-associated disorders—a randomized controlled trial. Clin Rehabil. 2006 Mar;20(3):201–17.

To investigate whether vestibular rehabilitation for patients with whiplash-associated disorder and dizziness had any effect on balance measures and self-perceived handicap.

Randomized, controlled trial. Subjects: Twenty-nine patients, 20 women and 9 men, age range 22–76 years.

The patients were randomized to an intervention group or a control group. The intervention comprised vestibular rehabilitation. All patients were assessed at baseline, after 6 weeks and after 3 months with 4 different balance measures and the Dizziness Handicap Inventory.

After 6 weeks, the intervention group showed statistically significant improvements compared with the control group in the following measures: standing on one leg eyes open (p=0.02), blindfolded tandem stance (p=0.045), Dizziness Handicap Inventory total score (p=0.047), Dizziness Handicap Inventory functional score (p=0.005) and in Dizziness Handicap Inventory physical score (p=0.033). After 3 months, the intervention group showed statistically significant improvements compared with the control group in the following measures: standing on one leg eyes open (p=0.000), tandem stance (p=0.033) and Dizziness Handicap Inventory physical score (p=0.04).

Vestibular rehabilitation for patients with whiplash-associated disorder can decrease self-perceived handicap and increase postural control.

Ekvall Hansson E, Mansson NO, Ringsberg KA, Hakansson A. Dizziness among patients with whiplash-associated disorder: a randomized controlled trial. J Rehabil Med. 2006 Nov;38(6):387–90.

The Khan Kinetic Treatment (KKT) uses high-frequency small-amplitude sinusoidal waves to vibrate the vertebrae and repeatedly activate associated neuromuscular structures, which evoke multiple mechanisms of pain relief.

KKT treatment is best described by comparing known mechanisms of pain relief with a novel spinal injury model proposed by a group at the Yale University School of Medicine based on spine stability. Panjabi identified 3 subsystems contributing to spine stability: (1) the passive subsystem consisting of the vertebrae and facet joints, ligaments, and intervertebral disks; (2) the active subsystem consisting of the muscles and tendons surrounding the spinal column; (3) the neural and feedback subsystem consisting mainly of the control centers that excite and coordinate the active subsystem. A dysfunction in any one of these 3 subsystems can contribute to instability of the spine and, therefore, lead to subsequent injury and pain.

The KKT is a spinal and upper cervical treatment device consisting of a controller mounted on top of an impulse delivery mechanism, or device head, which is mounted on a movable armature to a fixed stand (similar to certain upper chiropractic procedures). The device head generates waveforms and the stylus located at the base of the device head mechanically transduces the waveforms through the skin and ultimately to the spine, causing minor vibration of the vertebrae and minor repetitive stretching/activation of the attached soft tissues.

Many manual therapy approaches recommend mobilization or manipulation interventions if patients lack spine mobility and present with no sign of contraindications. The treatment of choice for hypomobile joints of the spine causing pain is therapeutic manipulation, which causes spine segment mobility.

In contrast, hypermobile joints may be best dealt with using exercises specific to conditioning muscles that act to stabilize those same joints.

We theorize that the success of the KKT for both hyper and hypomobile joints works by replacing abnormal cervical instantaneous axes of rotation in hypermobile joints and help mobilize hypomobile joints to normal ranges.

When compared with a control group, **initial results show that KKT caused significant decreases in neck pain of neuromusculoskeletal origin and decreased** pain medication use but no changes in functional measures were found.

Desmoulin GT, Yasin NI, Chen DW. Spinal mechanisms of pain control. Clin J Pain. 2007 Sep;23(7):576–85.

Omega-3 fatty acids (fish oil) as an anti-inflammatory. Of the 250 patients, 125 returned a questionnaire at an average of 75 days on fish oil. Seventy-eight percent were taking 1200 mg, and 22% were taking 2400 mg of essential fatty acids (EFAs). Fifty-nine percent discontinued taking their prescription NSAID medications for pain. Sixty percent stated that their overall pain was improved, and 60% stated that their joint pain had improved. Eighty percent stated they were satisfied with their improvement, and 88% stated they would continue to take the fish oil. There were no significant side effects reported. Our results mirror other controlled studies that compared ibuprofen and omega-3 EFAs demonstrating equivalent effect in reducing arthritic pain. **Omega-3 EFA fish oil supplements appear to be a safer alternative to NSAIDs for treatment of nonsurgical neck or back pain in this selective group.** Maroon JC, Bost JW. Omega-3 fatty acids (fish oil) as an anti-inflammatory: an alternative to nonsteroidal anti-inflammatory drugs for discogenic pain. Surg Neurol. 2006 Apr;65(4):326–3.

§ 10:3 Chiropractic therapy

Spinal manipulation of dysfunctional cervical joints can lead to transient cortical plastic changes, as demonstrated by attenuation of cortical somatosensory evoked responses.

This study suggests that cervical spine manipulation may alter cortical somatosensory processing and sensorimotor integration. These findings may help to elucidate the mechanisms responsible for the effective relief of pain and restoration of functional ability documented following spinal manipulation treatment. Haavik-Taylor H, Murphy B. Cervical spine manipulation alters sensorimotor integration: A somatosensory evoked potential study. Clin Neurophysiol. 2007 Feb;118(2):391–402.

Chiropractic is a proven effective treatment in chronic whiplash cases. Patients were referred for chiropractic treatment on the average of 15.5 months (range 3–44) after their initial injury. **93% of patients improved following chiropractic treatment.** Woodward MN, Cook JC, Gargan MF, Bannister GC. Chiropractic treatment of chronic 'whiplash' injuries. Injury. 1996 Nov;27(9):643–5.

Another study of chiropractic treatment of whiplash injuries showed 74% of the patients improved following treatment. Khan S, Cook J, Gargan M, Bannister G. A symptomatic classification of whiplash injury and the implications for treatment. J Orthop Med 1999;21:22–5.

During the first week of treatment Grade III and IV mobilization along with TENS was the primary treatment. Following the first week the treatment was a form of high-velocity, low-amplitude manual therapy. Electrical muscle stimulation was also employed.

	Grade I	**Grade II**
Number	16	25
Mean visits	19.9	34.7
95% CI	16.4 – 23.4	29.8 – 39.7
Minimum	6	15
Maximum	30	66
SD	6.6	12
Mean Wks Treatment	10	18.2
95% CI	7.7 – 12.4	15.1 – 21.2
SD	4.5	7.3
X-ray curve	13.3	1.8
95% CI	9.7 – 16.8	3.9k – 7.5
SD	6.7	13.8
Initial Pain	7.1	7.7
95% CI	6.6 – 7.6	7.4 – 8.0

	Grade I	Grade II
SD	0.9	0.8
Final Pain	0.6	2.0
95% CI	0.1 – 1.0	1.4 – 2.5
SD	0.8	0.3

Mean, 95% confidence interval (CI) & standard deviations.

K — kyphosis (+Rx postural displacement found in neutral resting stance)

In this study Grade I patients almost completely recover with this type of treatment and Grade II patients improve substantially. Chiropractic therapy in acute whiplash patients Grade I & II appears to provide at least short-term benefits despite ongoing pending litigation.

Davis CG. Chiropractic Treatment in Acute Whiplash Injuries: Grades I & II. J. Vertebral Subluxation Res. May 19, 2008.

Chiropractic treatment of patients with low back pain derives more benefit and longer term satisfaction than treatment by hospitals. Meade TW, Dyer S, Browne W, Frank AO. Randomized comparison of chiropractic and hospital outpatient management for low back pain: results from extended follow up. BMJ. 1995 Aug 5;311(7001):349–51; Meade TW, Dyer S, Browne W, Townsend J, Frank AO. Low back pain of mechanical origin: randomized comparison of chiropractic and hospital outpatient treatment. BMJ. 1990 Jun 2;300(6737):1431–7.

At 8 weeks, the mean improvement in the Roland-Morris Disability Questionnaire RMDQ was 5.5 points greater for the chiropractic group (decrease in disability by 5.9) than for the pain-clinic group (0.36) (95% CI 2.0 points to 9.0 points; p = 0.004). Reduction in mean pain intensity at week 8 was 1.8 points greater for the chiropractic group than for the pain-clinic group (p = 0.023).

This study suggests that chiropractic management administered in an National Health Service setting may be effective for reducing levels of disability and perceived pain during the period of treatment for a subpopulation of patients with Chronic Low Back Pain.

Wilkey A, Gregory M, Byfield D, McCarthy PW. A comparison between chiropractic management and pain clinic management for chronic low-back pain in a national health service outpatient clinic. J Altern Complement Med. 2008 Jun;14(5):465–73.

Evidence that, in patients with chronic spinal pain syndromes, spinal manipulation, if not contraindicated, results in greater improvement than acupuncture and medicine. Giles LG, Muller R. Chronic spinal pain syndromes: a clinical pilot trial comparing acupuncture, a nonsteroidal anti-inflammatory drug, and spinal manipulation. Manipulative Physiol Ther. 1999 Jul–Aug;22(6):376–81.

Manipulative therapy for neurogenic cervicobrachial pain has been shown to help. Cowell IM, Phillips DR. Effectiveness of manipulative physiotherapy for the treatment of a neurogenic cervicobrachial pain syndrome: a single case study—experimental design. Man Ther. 2002 Feb;7(1):31–8.

The treatment of lumbar intervertebral disk herniation is both safe and effective. Cassidy JD, Thiel HW, Kirkaldy-Willis WH. Side posture manipulation for lumbar intervertebral disk herniation. J Manipulative Physiol Ther. 1993 Feb;16(2):96–103.

Manipulation produced a 12-month outcome that was equivalent to chemonucleolysis and can be considered as an option for treatment of lumbar disc herniation. Burton AK, Tillotson KM, Cleary J. Single-blind randomized controlled trial of chemonucleolysis and manipulation in the treatment of symptomatic lumbar disc herniation. Eur Spine J. 2000 Jun;9(3):202–7.

Intensive training, physiotherapy, or manipulation has demonstrated meaningful improvement in patients with chronic neck pain of greater than 3 months duration. Jordan A, Bendix T, Nielsen H, Hansen FR, Host D, Winkel A. Intensive training, physiotherapy, or manipulation for patients with chronic neck pain. A prospective, single-blinded, randomized clinical trial. Spine. 1998 Feb 1;23(3):311–8; discussion 319.

Saggital cervical tractions with a transverse load at midneck (2-way cervical traction), combined with cervical manipulation, can improve cervical lordosis. Harrison DE, Cailliet R, Harrison DD, Janik TJ, Holland B. A new 3-point bending traction method for restoring cervical lordosis and cervical manipulation: a nonrandomized clinical controlled trial. Arch Phys Med Rehabil. 2002 Apr;83(4):447–53.

Spinal manual therapy has been shown to be efficacious in the treatment of cervicogenic headache (CGH). Treatment aimed at relevant myofascial trigger points can also be useful. Specifically targeted diagnostic injection is required for definitive anatomical diagnosis. If such diagnostic procedures lead to a diagnosis of facet joint pain, treatment with radiofrequency neurotomy has proven efficacy. Jensen S. Neck related causes of headache. Aust Fam Physician. 2005 Aug;34(8):635–9.

§ 10:4 Chiropractic therapy—Manipulation therapy, generally

Spinal manipulation has been successful in treating cervical disc pain. See Brouillette DL, Gurske DT. Chiropractic treatment of cervical radiculopathy caused by a herniated cervical disc. J Manipulative Physiol Ther. 1994 Feb;17(2):119–23; Beneliyahu DJ. Chiropractic management and manipulative therapy for MRI documented cervical disk herniation. J Manipulative Physiol Ther. 1994 Mar–Apr;17(3):177–85; BenEliyahu DJ. Magnetic resonance imaging and clinical follow-up: study of 27 patients receiving chiropractic care for cervical and lumbar disc herniations. J Manipulative Physiol Ther. 1996 Nov–Dec;19(9):597–606; Davis CG. Chronic Cervical Spine Pain Treated with Manipulation Under Anesthesia. Journal of the Neuromusculoskeletal System. 1996; 4(3):102–115; Eriksen K. Management of cervical disc herniation with upper cervical chiropractic care. J Manipulative Physiol Ther. 1998 Jan;21(1):51–6; Herzog J. Use of cervical spine manipulation under anesthesia for management of cervical disk herniation, cervical radiculopathy, and associated cervicogenic headache syndrome. J Manipulative Physiol Ther. 1999 Mar–Apr;22(3):166–70; Polkinghorn BS. Treatment of cervical disc protrusions via instrumental chiropractic adjustment. J Manipulative Physiol Ther. 1998 Feb;21(2):114–21.

Cervical spine manipulation may help shoulder problems. See Smith TL. Cervical manipulation for shoulder injury. JNMS 2000; 24–6; Winters JC, Sobel JS, Groenier KH, Arendzen HJ, Meyboom-de Jong B. Comparison of physiotherapy, manipulation, and corticosteroid injection for treating shoulder complaints in general practice: randomized, single blind study. BMJ. 1997 May 3;314:1320–5.

Chiropractic manipulation can make a demonstrable difference in carpal tunnel syndrome. Valente R, Gibson H. Chiropractic manipulation in carpal tunnel syndrome. Manipulative Physiol Ther. 1994 May;17(4):246–9.

Cervical spine manipulation can improve pain and function of tennis elbow. Vicenzino B, Wright A. Effects of a novel manipulative physiotherapy technique on tennis elbow: a single case study. Man Ther. 2000 Nov;1(1):30–35.

Brachioradial puritus (BRP). Ten of 14 patients reported resolution of BRP following cervical spine manipulation. Tait CP, Grigg E, Quirk CJ. Brachioradial pruritus and cervical spine manipulation. Australas J Dermatol. 1998 Aug;39(3):168–70.

§ 10:5 Chiropractic therapy—Effects of manipulation

Spinal manipulation may impact most efficiently on the complex process of proprioception and dizziness of cervical origin. Heikkila H, Johansson M, Wenngren BI. Effects of acupuncture, cervical manipulation and NSAID therapy on dizziness and impaired head repositioning of suspected cervical origin: a pilot study. Man Ther. 2000 Aug;5(3):151–7.

Cervical spine manipulation improved muscle function, cervical range of motion and pain sensitivity, and might therefore be beneficial for treating patients with chronic neck pain. Suter E, McMorland G. Decrease in elbow flexor inhibition after cervical spine manipulation in patients with chronic neck pain. Clin Biomech (Bristol, Avon). 2002 Aug;17(7):541.

Passive muscle stretch, joint manipulation and muscle massage all result in a significant decrease in the excitability of neurons within the lower motorneuron pool and within the limits of pain. Vujnovich AL, Neural plasticity, muscle spasm and tissue manipulation: A review of the literature. J Man & Manipal Ther 1995:3(4):152–156).

Manipulation therapy improves pain tolerance. Spinal manipulative treatments show a consistent reflex response of multireceptor origin and may cause clinically observed benefits, including a reduction of pain and a decrease in hypertonicity of muscles. See Herzog W, Scheele D, Conway PJ. Electromyographic responses of back and limb muscles associated with spinal manipulative therapy. Spine. 1999 Jan 15;24(2):146–52; discussion 153; Gillette RG, Kramis RC, Roberts WJ. Suppression of activity in spinal nocireceptive 'low back' neurons by paravertebral somatic stimuli in the cat. Neurosci Lett. 1998 Jan 23;241(1):45–8; Terrett AC, Vernon H. Manipulation and pain tolerance. A controlled study of the effect of spinal manipulation on paraspinal cutaneous pain tolerance levels. Am J Phys Med. 1984 Oct;63(5):217–25.

Cervical spine manipulation produced significant improvement in pressure pain threshold, pain-free grip, neurodynamics and pain scores in patients with lateral

epicondylalgia. Vicenzino B, Collins D, Wright A. The initial effects of a cervical spine manipulative physiotherapy treatment on the pain and dysfunction of lateral epicondylalgia. Pain. 1996 Nov;68(1):69–74.

The PAG mediated descending pain inhibitory system is not the only mechanism associated with manipulative therapy-induced hypoalgesia. Vicenzino B, Cartwright T, Collins D, Wright A. An investigation of stress and pain perception during manual therapy in asymptomatic subjects. Eur J Pain. 1999 Mar;3(1):13–18.

The cerebral cortex is involved in pain activity. See Bushnell MC, Duncan GH, Hofbauer RK, Ha B, Chen JI, Carrier B. Pain perception: is there a role for primary somatosensory cortex? Proc Natl Acad Sci U S A. 1999 Jul 6;96(14):7705–9; Ploghaus A, Tracey I, Gati JS, Clare S, Menon RS, Matthews PM, Rawlins JN. Dissociating pain from its anticipation in the human brain. Science. 1999 Jun 18;284(5422):1979–81; Coghill RC, Sang CN, Maisog JM, Iadarola MJ. Pain intensity processing within the human brain: a bilateral, distributed mechanism. J Neurophysiol. 1999 Oct;82(4):1934–43.

Afferent input evokes changes in the central nervous system and causes changes in the brain depending on the side—ipsilateral or contralateral—being treated. Carrick FR. Changes in brain function after manipulation of the cervical spine. J Manipulative Physiol Ther. 1997 Oct;20(8):529–45.

Manipulation therapy produces changes in sudomotor, cutaneous vasomotor, respiratory, cardiac activity and antinociception, suggesting that activation is through a central control mechanism at a high level in the neuroaxis. Vicenzino B, Collins D, Benson H, Wright A. An investigation of the interrelationship between manipulative therapy-induced hypoalgesia and sympathoexcitation. J Manipulative Physiol Ther. 1998 Sep;21(7):448–53.

Neurons in lamina VI respond predominantly to nonnoxious manipulation of joints. Kandel & Swartz, Principals of Neural Science 2000.

Beta-endorphin levels have also been shown to increase. Vernon HT, Dhami MS, Howley TP, Annett R. Spinal manipulation and beta-endorphin: a controlled study of the effect of a spinal manipulation on plasma beta-endorphin levels in normal males. J Manipulative Physiol Ther. 1986 Jun;9(2):115–23.

§ 10:6 Chiropractic therapy—Safety of chiropractic treatment

Vertebrobasilar artery (VBA) stroke is a very rare event in the population. The increased risks of VBA stroke associated with chiropractic and primary care physician (PCP) visits is likely due to patients with headache and neck pain from VBA dissection seeking care before their stroke. We found no evidence of excess risk of VBA stroke associated chiropractic care compared to primary care.

Cassidy JD, Boyle E, Côté P, He Y, Hogg-Johnson S, Silver FL, Bondy SJ. Risk of vertebrobasilar stroke and chiropractic care: results of a population-based case-control and case-crossover study. Spine. 2008 Feb 15;33(4 Suppl):S176–83.

Chiropractic manipulative therapy of the cervical spine is several hundred times safer than taking non-steroidal anti-inflammatory drugs (NSAIDs). Dabbs V, Lauretti WJ. A risk assessment of cervical manipulation vs. NSAIDs for the treatment of neck pain. J Manipulative Physiol Ther. 1995 Oct;18(8):530–6.

Severe complication from cervical manipulations have been estimated at between 1 in 380,000 to over 1 in a million. See Eder M, Tilscher H. Diagnosis and Treatment. In: Chiropractic Therapy. Gengenbach MS ed. Aspen Pub. Gaithersburg, MD. 1990, pp. 60–61; Terrett AGJ, Kleynhans AM. Cerebralvascular complications of manipulation. In Haldeman S, ed. Modern Development in the Principles and Practice of Chiropractic. 2nd ed. New York: Appleton-Century-Crofts. 1992:579–98.

A recent study estimated that arterial dissection following spinal manipulation is approximately 1 in 8.06 million office visits, 1 in 5.85 million cervical manipulations, 1 in 1,430 chiropractic years and 1 in 48 chiropractic practice careers. Haldeman S, Carey P, Townsend M, Papadopoulos C. Arterial dissections following cervical manipulation: the chiropractic experience. CMAJ. 2001 Oct 2;165(7):905–6.

A positive pre-manipulative test is not an absolute contraindication to manipulation of the cervical spine. Licht PB, Christensen HW, Hoilund-Carlsen PF. Is there a role for premanipulative testing before cervical manipulation? J Manipulative Physiol Ther. 2000 Mar–Apr;23(3):175–9.

This study was unable to identify factors from the clinical history and physical examination of the patient that would assist a physician attempting to isolate the

patient at risk of cerebral ischemia after cervical manipulation. Haldeman S, Kohlbeck FJ, McGregor M. Unpredictability of cerebrovascular ischemia associated with cervical spine manipulation therapy: a review of sixty-four cases after cervical spine manipulation. Spine. 2002 Jan 1;27(1):49–55.

Note that this author has reviewed the 2003 article regarding risk of stroke and chiropractic treatment (Neurology 2003;60:1424–1428. *Spinal manipulative therapy is an independent risk factor for vertebral artery dissection*) and does not feel the findings are reliable. The real rate of strokes caused by chiropractic neck adjustments is the same as for spontaneous strokes. See Haldeman S, Carey P, Townsend M, Papadopoulos C. Arterial dissections following cervical manipulation: the chiropractic experience. CMAJ. 2001 Oct 2;165(7):905–6.

§ 10:7 Chiropractic therapy—Standard medical treatment compared

Standard medical treatment, rest and a collar resulted in 91% of the patients having more than low pain at 6 months. With active treatment patients, early home exercises and mobilization, 48% continued to have clinically important symptoms at 6 months. Rosenfeld M, Gunnarsson R, Borenstein P. Early intervention in whiplash-associated disorders: a comparison of two treatment protocols. Spine. 2000 Jul 15;25(14):1782–7.

§ 10:8 Chiropractic therapy—Treating spine for extremity problems

It is evident that arm and hand complaints have a cervical component. There is plenty of support in the medical literature. See e.g., Tinazzi M, Zanette G, Volpato D, Testoni R, Bonato C, Manganotti P, Miniussi C, Fiaschi A. Neurophysiological evidence of neuroplasticity at multiple levels of the somatosensory system in patients with carpal tunnel syndrome. Brain. 1998 Sep;121 (Pt 9):1785–94; Chang MH, Chiang HT, Ger LP, Yang DA, Lo YK. The cause of slowed forearm median conduction velocity in carpal tunnel syndrome. Clin Neurophysiol. 2000 Jun;111(6):1039–44; Upton AR, McComas AJ. The double crush in nerve entrapment syndromes. Lancet. 1973 Aug 18;2(7825):359–62; Wood VE, Biondi J. Double-crush nerve compression in thoracic-outlet syndrome. J Bone Joint Surg Am. 1990 Jan;72(1):85–7; Narakas AO. The role of thoracic outlet syndrome in the double crush syndrome.

Ann Chir Main Memb Super. 1990;9(5):331–40; Golovchinsky V. Relationship between damage of cervical nerve roots or brachial plexus and development of peripheral entrapment syndromes in the upper extremities (Double Crush Syndrome). J Neurol Orthop Med Surg 1995; 1:61–9; Dellon AL, Mackinnon SE. Chronic nerve compression model for the double crush hypothesis. Ann Plast Surg. 1991 Mar;26(3):259–64; Liu JE, Tahmoush AJ, Roos DB, Schwartzman RJ. Shoulder-arm pain from cervical bands and scalene muscle anomalies. J Neurol Sci. 1995 Feb;128(2):175–80; Rydevik BL. The effects of compression on the physiology of nerve roots. J Manipulative Physiol Ther. 1992 Jan;15(1):62–6; Rydevik B, Brown MD, Lundborg G. Pathoanatomy and pathophysiology of nerve root compression. Spine. 1984 Jan–Feb;9(1):7–15; Epstein NE, Epstein JA, Carras R. Coexisting cervical spondylotic myelopathy and bilateral carpal tunnel syndromes. J Spinal Disord. 1989 Mar;2(1):36–42; Hurst LC, Weissberg D, Carroll RE. The relationship of the double crush to carpal tunnel syndrome (an analysis of 1,000 cases of carpal tunnel syndrome). J Hand Surg [Br]. 1985 Jun;10(2):202–4; Raps SP, Rubin M. Proximal median neuropathy and cervical radiculopathy: double crush revisited. Electromyogr Clin Neurophysiol. 1994 Jun;34(4):195–6; Norlander S, Nordgren B. Clinical symptoms related to musculoskeletal neck-shoulder pain and mobility in the cervico-thoracic spine. Scand J Rehabil Med. 1998 Dec;30(4):243–51; Suter E, McMorland G. Decrease in elbow flexor inhibition after cervical spine manipulation in patients with chronic neck pain. Clin Biomechanics 2002;17:541–4.

Chronic cervical and lumbar pain has also been successfully treated with manipulation under anesthesia. *See* Davis CG. Chronic cervical spine pain treated with manipulation under anesthesia. JNMS: J Neuromusculoskeletal System 1996;4:102–15; Davis CG, Fernando CA, da Motta MA. Manipulation of the low back under general anesthesia: case studies and discussion. JNMS: J Neuromusculoskeletal System 1993; 1:126–34; West DT, Mathews RS, Miller MR, Kent GM. Effective management of spinal pain in one hundred seventy-seven patients evaluated for manipulation under anesthesia. J Manipulative Physiol Ther. 1999 Jun;22(5):299–308; Hughes BL. Management of cervical disk syndrome utilizing manipulation under anesthesia. J Manipulative Physiol Ther. 1993 Mar–Apr;16(3):174–81; Herzog J. Use of cervical spine manipulation under anesthesia for management of cervical disk herniation, cervical radiculopathy, and associated cervicogenic headache syndrome. J Manipulative Physiol Ther.

1999 Mar–Apr;22(3):166–70.; Gerber A, Miller LE. Management of chronic cervical sprain and strain due to whiplash mechanism. J Am Osteopath Assoc. 1960 Nov;60:212–6.

§ 10:9 Chiropractic therapy—Chiropractic adjustments and pain reduction

The current data support a neurophysiological mechanism underlying manipulation-induced analgesia. **Clinical and basic science literature suggests that the analgesic effects of manipulation are segmentally organized and probably result from large-diameter afferent stimulation. Further, this analgesic effect is nonopioid but involves spinal activation of serotoneric and noradrenergic-receptors**, implicating descending inhibitory pathways from the RVM and the noradrenergic cells in the brainstem. Sluka KA, Hoeger MK, Skyba DA. Basic Science Mechanisms of Nonpharmacological Treatments for Pain. Pain 2002-An Updated Review: ISAP Press 2002.

§ 10:10 Chiropractic therapy—Chiropractic adjustments and pain reduction—Long term potentiation and long term depression

Studies showing LTP in response to intense noxious stimulation and reports that A-delta-mechanosensitive afferent activation can reverse an existing LTP condition in dorsal horn neurons. The involvement of Long Term Potentiation (LTP) in low back pain is discussed and a role for Long Term Depression (LTD) in spinal manipulative therapy is proposed. The need for future studies is identified in the areas of spatial and temporal changes in symptomatology post-SMT (spinal manipulative therapy) of the low back; combining, sequencing, and comparing several therapeutic approaches; and demonstrating LTD in spinal cord neurons post-SMT-like stimulation. **Activity-dependent neuronal plasticity such as LTP is known to be reversible, the idea is presented that SMT may act to reverse LTP within an already sensitized pain-signaling system.** ¶ Spinal manipulative therapy (SMT) may act to reverse LTP within an already sensitized pain-signaling system. Boal RW, Gillette RG. Central neuronal plasticity, low back pain and spinal manipulative therapy. J Manipulative Physiol Ther. 2004 Jun;27(5):314–26.

The suggestion from this review that SMT may influence dorsal horn neurons initiating LTD and dampening ongoing central sensitization is not intended to be an exclusive mechanism to explain all SMT therapeutic effects. Boal RW, Gillette RG. Central neuronal plasticity, low back pain and spinal manipulative therapy. J Manipulative Physiol Ther. 2004 Jun;27(5):314–26.

§ 10:11 Chiropractic therapy—Chiropractic adjustments and pain reduction—Dose-related response

In treating chronic neck and back pain patients, one or two treatments may not be enough. Further, Chiropractic treatment may be based on the neuroplasticity of the nervous system. Several studies have shown that manual therapy is only slightly better than other therapies, or placebo, but the dosage of treatment with the manual therapy is minimal. The reported randomized control trails are usually done on an HMO patient database. Published studies with those HMO populations have shown that outcomes may be dose dependent. Instead of eight to 12 treatments per year, nine to 12 visits over three weeks may be needed to properly treat an episode of pain.

"This finding suggests that in the mature cortex, the apparently static structural attributes of the normal adult cortex depend on maintenance of patterns of afferent activity; with the corollary that changes in these patterns can induce structural plasticity." Tailby C, Wright LL, Metha AB, Calford MB. Activity-dependent maintenance and growth of dendrites in adult cortex. Proc Natl Acad Sci U S A. 2005 Mar 22;102(12):4631–6.

"In our experience, anything less than two weeks of daily manipulation is inadequate for chronic back pain patients." Kirkaldy-Willis WH, Cassidy JD. Spinal manipulation in the treatment of low-back pain. Can Fam Physician 1985;31:535–40.

"There was a positive, clinically important effect of the number of chiropractic treatments for chronic low back pain on pain intensity and disability at 4 weeks. Relief was substantial for patients receiving care **3 to 4 times per week for 3 weeks**." Haas M, Groupp E, Kraemer DF. Dose-response for chiropractic care of chronic low back pain. Spine J. 2004 Sep–Oct;4(5):574–83.

"Findings suggest the benefit of 9 to 12 visits over 3 weeks for the treatment of HA/neck pain and disability. **A larger number of visits than 12 in 3 weeks may be required for**

maximum relief and durability of outcomes." Haas M, Groupp E, Aickin M, Fairweather A, Ganger B, Attwood M, Cummins C, Baffes L. Dose response for chiropractic care of chronic cervicogenic headache and associated neck pain: a randomized pilot study. J Manipulative Physiol Ther. 2004 Nov–Dec;27(9):547–53.

§ 10:12 Medications—Generally

There is no beneficial effect from the medications, at least at the doses stated, in the management of delayed-onset muscle soreness. Aspirin (900 mg); codeine (60 mg); and paracetamol (1000 mg). Barlas P, Craig JA, Robinson J, Walsh DM, Baxter GD, Allen JM. Managing delayed-onset muscle soreness: lack of effect of selected oral systemic analgesics. Arch Phys Med Rehabil. 2000 Jul;81(7):966–72.

The results of 26 randomized trials suggest that NSAIDs might be effective for short-term symptomatic relief in patients with uncomplicated low back pain, but are less effective or ineffective in patients with low back pain with sciatica and patients with sciatica with nerve root symptoms. Koes BW, Scholten RJ, Mens JM, Bouter LM. Efficacy of non-steroidal anti-inflammatory drugs for low back pain: a systematic review of randomized clinical trials. Ann Rheum Dis. 1997 Apr;56(4):214–23.

There was a statistically significant but small effect in favor of nonsteroidal anti-inflammatory drugs as compared with a placebo. The evidence from the 51 trials included in this review suggests that nonsteroidal anti-inflammatory drugs (NSAIDs) are effective for short-term symptomatic relief in patients with acute low back pain. **Furthermore, there does not seem to be a specific type of nonsteroidal anti-inflammatory drug that is clearly more effective than others. Sufficient evidence of NSAIDs on chronic low back pain still is lacking.** van Tulder MW, Scholten RJ, Koes BW, Deyo RA. Nonsteroidal anti-inflammatory drugs for low back pain: a systematic review within the framework of the Cochrane Collaboration Back Review Group. Spine. 2000 Oct 1;25(19):2501–13.

§ 10:13 Medications—Problem with medications

People who often take acetaminophen (Tylenol) or non-steroidal anti-inflammatory drugs (NSAIDs) have an increased risk of end stage renal (kidney) disease. In one year: 105–365 pills a year, a 1.4 risk ratio; over 366 pills a year, a 2.1 risk ratio rate. Lifetime pills taken: 1000 to 4999 pills, a 2.0 risk (double the risk); over 5000 pills, a 2.4 times increase rate. Perneger TV, Whelton PK, Klag MJ. Risk of kidney failure associated with the use of acetaminophen, aspirin, and nonsteroidal anti-inflammatory drugs. N Engl J Med. 1994 Dec 22;331(25):1675–9.

It has been estimated that 1 in 1200 patients taking NSAIDs for at least 2 months will die from gastroduodenal complications who would not have died had they not taken NSAIDs. Tramer MR, Moore RA, Reynolds DJ, McQuay HJ. Quantitative estimation of rare adverse events which follow a biological progression: a new model applied to chronic NSAID use. Pain. 2000 Mar;85(1–2):169–82.

16,500 patients died a year from gastrointestional toxic effects of NSAIDs. Leukemia kills 20,197; AIDS kills 16,685; multiple myeloma 10,503; asthma 5,338; cervical cancer 4,441; and Hodgkin's disease 1,437 a year. Wolfe MM, Lichtenstein DR, Singh G. Gastrointestinal toxicity of nonsteroidal antiinflammatory drugs. N Engl J Med. 1999 Jun 17;340(24):1888–99.

Chiropractic manipulative therapy of the cervical spine is several hundred times safer than taking nonsteroidal anti-inflammatory drugs (NSAIDs). Dabbs V, Lauretti WJ. A risk assessment of cervical manipulation vs. NSAIDs for the treatment of neck pain. J Manipulative Physiol Ther. 1995 Oct;18(8):530–6.

§ 10:14 Other treatment types—Massage

Twenty-one female patients suffering from chronic tension headache received 10 sessions of upper body massage, consisting of deep tissue techniques in addition to softer techniques in the beginning. When found, trigger points were carefully and forcefully massaged. The range of cervical movements, surface EMG on mm. frontalis and trapezius, visual analogue scale (VAS) and Finnish Pain Questionnaire (FPQ), and the incidence of neck pain during a two week period before and after the treatment, and at 3 and 6 months during the follow-up period together with Beck depression inventory were taken for evaluation and follow-up. The range of movement in all directions increased, and FPQ, VAS and the number of days with neck pain decreased significantly. There was a significant change in EMG on the frontalis muscle, whereas changes in trapezius remained insignificant. Beck inventory showed an improvement after the treatment. **This study confirmed clinical**

and physiological effects of massage. Puustjarvi K, Airaksinen O, Pontinen PJ. The effects of massage in patients with chronic tension headache. Acupunct Electrother Res. 1990;15(2):159–62.

Massage therapy is effective in reducing pain, stress hormones and symptoms associated with chronic low back pain. Adults (M age=39.6 years) with low back pain, with a duration of at least 6 months, received two 30-min massage or relaxation therapy sessions per week for 5 weeks. **Participants receiving massage therapy reported experiencing less pain, depression, anxiety and their sleep had improved.** Hernandez-Reif M, Field T, Krasnegor J, Theakston H. Lower back pain is reduced and range of motion increased after massage therapy. Int J Neurosci. 2001;106(3–4):131–45.

§ 10:15 Other treatment types—Exercise

The evidence summarised in this systematic review indicates that specific exercises may be effective for the treatment of acute and chronic MND, with or without headache. To be of benefit, a stretching and strengthening exercise program should concentrate on the musculature of the cervical, shoulder-thoracic area, or both. A multimodal care approach of exercise, combined with mobilisation or manipulation for subacute and chronic MND with or without headache, reduced pain, improved function, and global perceived effect in the short and long term. The relative benefit of other treatments (such as physical modalities) compared with exercise or between different exercise programs needs to be explored. The quality of future trials should improve through more effective 'blinding' procedures and better control of compliance and co-intervention. Phase II trials would help identify the most effective treatment characteristics and dosages.

Kay TM, Gross A, Goldsmith C, Santaguida PL, Hoving J, Bronfort G; Cervical Overview Group. Exercises for mechanical neck disorders. Cochrane Database Syst Rev. 2005 Jul 20;(3):CD004250.

A total of 171 patients (80%) completed the study. There were no important statistical or clinical differences between the groups after 4 months of treatment. There was a small statistically significant effect at 12-month follow-up in both groups with home training regarding pain during rest ($p = 0.05$) and reported fatigue in the final week ($p = 0.02$).

No statistically significant differences were found between

the traditional physiotherapy group and the new sling exercise group, with or without home training. Since the groups were not compared with a control group without treatment, we cannot conclude that the studied treatments are effective for patients with whiplash-associated disorder, only that they did not differ in our study. Vikne J, Oedegaard A, Laerum E, Ihlebaek C, Kirkesola G. A Randomized Study of New Sling Exercise Treatment vs Traditional Physiotherapy for Patients with Chronic Whiplash-Associated Disorders with unsettled Compensation Claims. J Rehabil Med. 2007 Apr;39(3):252–259.

Exercises in an outpatient setting are widely used for the treatment of chronic low back pain. The efficacy of the active rehabilitation approach has been documented in randomized control studies, but these studies have seldom been focused on lumbar fatigability, which is now recognized as a frequent problem among patients with chronic low back pain. **The active, progressive treatment program was more successful in reducing pain and self-experienced disability, and also in improving lumbar endurance, than was the passive control treatment. However, the group difference in lumbar endurance tended to diminish at the 1-year follow-up.** Kankaanpaa M, Taimela S, Airaksinen O, Hanninen O. The efficacy of active rehabilitation in chronic low back pain. Effect on pain intensity, self-experienced disability, and lumbar fatigability. Spine. 1999 May 15;24(10):1034–42.

Exercise is effective for the management of chronic low back pain for up to 1 year after treatment and for fibromyalgia syndrome for up to 6 months (level 2). There is conflicting evidence (level 4b) about which exercise program is effective for chronic low back pain. For chronic neck pain, chronic soft tissue shoulder disorders, and chronic lateral epicondylitis, evidence of effectiveness of exercise is limited (level 3). Mior S. Exercise in the treatment of chronic pain. Clin J Pain. 2001 Dec;17(4 Suppl):S77–85.

Early active training program has a positive effect on the way patients cope with pain in their daily lives. Kjellby-Wendt G, Styf J, Carlsson SG. Early active rehabilitation after surgery for lumbar disc herniation: a prospective, randomized study of psychometric assessment in 50 patients. Acta Orthop Scand. 2001 Oct;72(5):518–24.

The introduction of low-impact aerobic exercise programs for patients with chronic low back pain may reduce the enormous costs associated with its treatment.

Mannion AF, Muntener M, Taimela S, Dvorak J. Comparison of three active therapies for chronic low back pain: results of a randomized clinical trial with one-year follow-up. Rheumatology (Oxford). 2001 Jul;40(7):772–8.

In older patients with CLBP (chronic low back pain), reduction of muscle strength was more marked in the spinal extensors than in the spinal flexors. **It was confirmed that trunk muscle strengthening exercises are useful for increasing muscle strength and improving symptoms in such patients.** Handa N, Yamamoto H, Tani T, Kawakami T, Takemasa R. The effect of trunk muscle exercises in patients over 40 years of age with chronic low back pain. J Orthop Sci. 2000;5(3):210–6.

Multifidus muscle recovery is not spontaneous on remission of painful symptoms. **Lack of localized, muscle support may be one reason for the high recurrence rate of low back pain following the initial episode.** Hides JA, Richardson CA, Jull GA. Multifidus muscle recovery is not automatic after resolution of acute, first-episode low back pain. Spine. 1996 Dec 1;21(23):2763–9.

§ 10:16 Other treatment types—Therapeutic ultrasound

This study was to investigate the effect of low-intensity pulsed ultrasound exposure on the healing of injured medial collateral ligaments. On the 12th day, the low-intensity pulsed, ultrasound-treated side exhibited significantly superior mechanical properties when compared with the control side in ultimate load, stiffness, and energy absorption ($P < .05$). However, the treatment did not afford any mechanical advantage when tested on the 21st day. The mean diameter of the fibril was significantly larger on the treatment side than on the control side ($P < .05$). **Conclusions: Low-intensity pulsed ultrasound exposure is effective for enhancing the early healing of medial collateral ligament injuries.** See Takakura Y, Matsui N, Yoshiya S, Fujioka H, Muratsu H, Tsunoda M, Kurosaka M. Low-intensity pulsed ultrasound enhances early healing of medial collateral ligament injuries in rats. J Ultrasound Med. 2002 Mar;21(3):283–8.

Seven days of continuous (non-pulsed) therapeutic ultrasound improved force production after contraction-induced muscle injury. See Karnes JL, Burton HW. Continuous therapeutic ultrasound accelerates repair of contraction-induced skeletal muscle damage in rats. Arch Phys Med Rehabil. 2002 Jan;83(1):1–4.

Therapeutic angiogenesis is the controlled induction or stimulation of new blood vessel formation to reduce unfavorable tissue effects caused by local hypoxia and to enhance tissue repair. The effects of ultrasound on wound healing, chronic ulcers, fracture healing and osteoradionecrosis may be explained by the enhancement of angiogenesis. The aim of this study was to identify which cytokines and angiogenesis factors are induced by ultrasound in vitro. **The results show that therapeutic ultrasound stimulates the production of angiogenic factors such as IL-8, bFGF and VEGF. This may be one of the mechanisms through which therapeutic ultrasound induces angiogenesis and healing.** See Reher P, Doan N, Bradnock B, Meghji S, Harris M. Effect of ultrasound on the production of IL-8, basic FGF and VEGF. Cytokine. 1999 Jun;11(6):416–23.

§ 10:17 Other treatment types—Acupuncture

Low frequency electroacupuncture stimulation significantly relieved the signs of mechanical allodynia. Hwang BG, Min BI, Kim JH, Na HS, Park DS. Effects of electroacupuncture on the mechanical allodynia in the rat model of neuropathic pain. Neurosci Lett. 2002 Mar 1;320(1–2):49–52.

Acupuncture is an effective short-term treatment for patients with chronic neck pain, but there is only limited evidence for long-term effects after five treatments. Irnich D, Behrens N, Molzen H, Konig A, Gleditsch J, Krauss M, Natalis M, Senn E, Beyer A, Schops P. Randomized trial of acupuncture compared with conventional massage and "sham" laser acupuncture for treatment of chronic neck pain. BMJ. 2001 Jun 30;322(7302):1574–8.

Manipulation was the only treatment to diminish the duration of dizziness/vertigo complaints during the past 7 days and increased the cervical range of motion. Both acupuncture and manipulation reduced dizziness/vertigo on the VAS scale and had positive effects on active head repositioning. Ketoprofen cutaneous application and acupuncture both alleviated pain. **Spinal manipulation may impact most efficiently on the complex process of proprioception and dizziness of cervical origin.** Heikkila H, Johansson M, Wenngren BI. Effects of acupuncture, cervical manipulation and NSAID therapy on dizziness and impaired head repositioning of suspected cervical origin: a pilot study. Man Ther. 2000 Aug;5(3):151–7.

Acupuncture and physiotherapy are effective forms of

treatment. See David J, Modi S, Aluko AA, Robertshaw C, Farebrother J. Chronic neck pain: a comparison of acupuncture treatment and physiotherapy. Br J Rheumatol. 1998 Oct;37(10):1118–22.

§ 10:18 Other treatment types—Botox

Comment:

Botox is a diluted version of the *botulinum* toxin. It paralyzes muscles.

Botulinum toxin was not proven effective in treatment of neck pain in chronic whiplash syndrome. Increased muscle tenderness alone might not be the major cause of neck pain in whiplash syndrome. Padberg M, de Bruijn SF, Tavy DL. Neck pain in chronic whiplash syndrome treated with botulinum toxin. A double-blind, placebo-controlled clinical trial. J Neurol. 2007 Mar;254(3):290–5.

BTX-A treatment of subjects with chronic WAD II neck pain resulted in a significant ($p < 0.01$) improvement in ROM and subjective pain, compared to a placebo group, but only a trend to improvement in subjective functioning. Freund BJ, Schwartz M. Treatment of whiplash associated neck pain [corrected] with botulinum toxin-A: a pilot study. J Rheumatol. 2000 Feb;27(2):481–4.

The most frequent adverse event was dysphagia, which occurred on average 9.7 days after injection and lasted, on average, for 3.5 weeks. While secondary nonresponse was seen in approx. 5% of patients, antibody tests revealed neutralizing serum antibodies in only 2%. **On the basis of the present data, therapy of cervical dystonia with BoNT/A seems to be safe and yields good stable results, even after 5 years of treatment.** Kessler KR, Skutta M, Benecke R. Long-term treatment of cervical dystonia with botulinum toxin A: efficacy, safety, and antibody frequency. German Dystonia Study Group. J Neurol. 1999 Apr;246(4):265–74.

The electrophysiological studies confirmed biological sensitivity to the toxin in all patients, showing a significant change beginning at two weeks and returning to baseline at 12 weeks. Houser MK, Sheean GL, Lees AJ. Further studies using higher doses of botulinum toxin type F for torticollis resistant to botulinum toxin type A. J Neurol Neurosurg Psychiatry. 1998 May;64(5):577–80.

In 18 BTXA-resistant patients, most patients continued to respond to BTXF for 1 year or longer, but four patients became resistant to BTXF. BTXF-resistant patients received a higher dose per treatment and a higher cumulative dose than BTXF-responsive patients. **BTXF can be used for long-term treatment of dystonia. It seems prudent to limit BTX doses of all serotypes to the lowest necessary for clinical efficacy.** Chen R, Karp BI, Hallett M. Botulinum toxin type F for treatment of dystonia: long-term experience. Neurology. 1998 Nov;51(5):1494–6.

The greatest concern with the use of BOTOX is probably the formation of blocking antibodies leading to nonresponse of subsequent treatment. Prevalence of resistance is less than 5%. Klein AW. Complications and adverse reactions with the use of botulinum toxin. emin Cutan Med Surg. 2001 Jun;20(2):109–20.

This study found that botulinum toxin A (BTA), which binds to GD1a, stains both motor and sensory nerve nodes of Ranvier. De Angelis MV, Di Muzio A, Lupo S, Gambi D, Uncini A, Lugaresi A. Anti-GD1a antibodies from an acute motor axonal neuropathy patient selectively bind to motor nerve fiber nodes of Ranvier. J Neuroimmunol. 2001 Dec 3;121(1–2):79–82.

The results show that a single dose treatment without physical therapy is not effective for chronic neck pain. Wheeler AH, Goolkasian P, Gretz SS. Botulinum toxin A for the treatment of chronic neck pain. Pain. 2001 Dec;94(3):255–60.

§ 10:19 Other treatment types—Traction

Manual cervical traction can help decrease muscle tightness. Manual cervical traction reduced the excitability of the alpha-motorneuro pool (which is in the spinal cord). This effect is mediated by the central nervous system. Bradnam L, Rochester L, Vujnovich A. Manual cervical traction reduces alpha-motoneuron excitability in normal subjects. Electromyogr Clin Neurophysiol. 2000 Jul–Aug;40(5):259–66.

A study comparing three types of traction (static, intermittent, and manual) in patients with cervical spine disorders were compared to a non-traction group. **Those receiving the intermittent traction showed significant improvement compared to the control group in terms of pain and increased range of motion.** Zylbergold RS, Piper MC. Cervical spine disorders. A comparison of three types of traction. Spine. 1985 Dec;10(10):867–71.

Static traction should be applied for 15–20 minutes at a time twice a day, depending on tolerance. Jackson R. The cervical syndrome. 4th ed. Springfield, Ill: Charles C. Thomas, 1978.

Cervical traction may help the symptoms in whiplash patients. Olson VL. Whiplash-associated chronic headache treated with home cervical traction. Phys Ther. 1997 Apr;77(4):417–24; Olson VL. Chronic whiplash associated disorder treated with home cervical traction. J Back Musculockletal Rehab 1997;9:181–90.

Traction therapy might improve conduction disturbance primarily by increasing the amount of blood flow from the nerve roots to the spinal parenchyma. Hattori M, Shirai Y, Aoki T. Research on the effectiveness of intermittent cervical traction therapy, using short-latency somatosensory evoked potentials. J Orthop Sci. 2002;7(2):208–16.

§ 10:20 Other treatment types—Electrical stimulation/ TENS

Pain control in patients with deafferenting (decrease in sending non-painful impulses into the nervous system) injuries is frequently refractory to treatment with standard analgesics. **Electrical stimulation excites mylenated (large diameter) afferents, which inhibit the transmission of nociceptive (painful) information in the central nervous system.** Davar G, Maciewicz RJ. Deafferentation pain syndromes. Neurol Clin. 1989 May;7(2):289–304.

Central neuron sensitization is reduced by electrical stimulation. TENS (transcutaneous electrical nerve stimulation) (4 hz or 100 hz, 20 min.) reduces central neuron sensitization. Ma YT, Sluka KA. Reduction in inflammation-induced sensitization of dorsal horn neurons by transcutaneous electrical nerve stimulation in anesthetized rats. Exp Brain Res. 2001 Mar;137(1):94–102.

Low frequency, high intensity electrical stimulation (2 hz, 20 min.) activates the endogenous opioid systems, producing antinociceptive effects. Nam TS, Choi Y, Yeon DS, Leem JW, Paik KS. Differential antinociceptive effect of transcutaneous electrical stimulation on pain behavior sensitive or insensitive to phentolamine in neuropathic rats. Neurosci Lett. 2001 Mar 23;301(1):17–20.

TENS protocol has different degrees of antinociceptive influence on chronic and acute pain. (80 hz, 60 min).

Cheing GL, Hui-Chan CW. Transcutaneous electrical nerve stimulation: nonparallel antinociceptive effects on chronic clinical pain and acute experimental pain. Arch Phys Med Rehabil. 1999 Mar;80(3):305–12.

TENS suppresses the central amplification of somatosensory input. Urasaki E, Wada S, Yasukouchi H, Yokota A. Effect of transcutaneous electrical nerve stimulation (TENS) on central nervous system amplification of somatosensory input. J Neurol. 1998 Mar;245(3):143–8.

TENS-mediated hypoalgesia is a consequence of mostly peripheral effects at 110 hz. Walsh DM, Lowe AS, McCormack K, Willer JC, Baxter GD, Allen JM. Transcutaneous electrical nerve stimulation: effect on peripheral nerve conduction, mechanical pain threshold, and tactile threshold in humans. Arch Phys Med Rehabil. 1998 Sep;79(9):1051–8.

Electrical stimulation of peripheral nerves leads to inhibitory input to the pain pathways at the spinal cord level. Hanai F. Effect of electrical stimulation of peripheral nerves on neuropathic pain. Spine. 2000 Aug 1;25(15):1886–92.

The overall results showed a significant decrease in pain with ENS therapy using a random-effects model ($p<0.0005$). These results indicate that ENS **is an effective treatment modality for chronic musculoskeletal pain** and that previous, equivocal results may have been due to underpowered studies.

Johnson M, Martinson M. Efficacy of electrical nerve stimulation for chronic musculoskeletal pain: a meta-analysis of randomized controlled trials. Pain. 2007 Jul;130(1–2):157–65.

§ 10:21 Other treatment types—Laser therapy

Pain, paravertebral muscle spasm, lordosis angle, and range of motion and function were observed to improve significantly in the low-power-laser group (LPL). **LPL seems to be successful in relieving pain and improving function in osteoarthritic diseases.** Ozdemir F, Birtane M, Kokino S. The clinical efficacy of low-power laser therapy on pain and function in cervical osteoarthritis. Clin Rheumatol. 2001;20(3):181–4.

The Ga-Al-As diode lasers (780nm, 2500 mW) resulted in a better quantitative healing in traumatized muscles. (This study was done on rabbits). G. Morrone, G.A. Guzzardella, L. Orienti, G. Giavaresi, M. Fini, M. Rocca, P. Torricelli, L. Martini, R. Giardino. Muscular Trauma Treated with a Ga-Al-As Diode Laser: In Vivo Experimental Study. Lasers Med Sci 13 (1998) 4, 293–298.

Laser therapy is effective on pain, muscle spasm, morning stiffness, and total tender point number in fibromyalgia. A. Gür, M. Karakoç, K. Nas, R. Çevik, J. Saraç, E. Demir.: Efficacy of Low Power Laser Therapy in Fibromyalgia: A Single-blind, Placebo-controlled Trial. Lasers Med Sci 17 (2002) 1, 57–61.

§ 10:22 Other treatment types—A note on surgery

Surgery for patients with cervical radiculopathy without myleopathy indicated a significant improvement in pain, neurological symptoms, functional status, and ability to perform activities of daily living. A significant number of patients who underwent surgery reported persistent, excruciating, or horrible pain on follow-up (25%). Sampath P, Bendebba M, Davis JD, Ducker T. Outcome in patients with cervical radiculopathy. Prospective, multicenter study with independent clinical review. Spine. 1999 Mar 15;24(6):591–7.

In managing lumbar radicular pain with interlaminar lumbar epidural steroid injections, the evidence is strong for short-term relief and limited for long-term relief. In managing cervical radiculopathy with cervical interlaminar epidural steroid injections, the evidence is moderate. The evidence for lumbar transforaminal epidural steroid injections in managing lumbar radicular pain is strong for short-term and moderate for long-term relief. The evidence for cervical transforaminal epidural steroid injections in managing cervical nerve root pain is moderate. The evidence is moderate in managing lumbar radicular pain in post lumbar laminectomy syndrome. The evidence for caudal epidural steroid injections is strong for short-term relief and moderate for long-term relief, in managing chronic pain of lumbar radiculopathy and postlumbar laminectomy syndrome.

There is moderate evidence for interlaminar epidurals in the cervical spine and limited evidence in the lumbar spine for long-term relief. The evidence for cervical and lumbar transforaminal epidural steroid injections is moderate for long-term improvement in managing nerve root pain. The evidence for caudal epidural steroid injections is moderate for long-term relief in managing nerve root pain and chronic low back pain.

Abdi S, Datta S, Trescot AM, Schultz DM, Adlaka R, Atluri SL, Smith HS, Manchikanti L. Epidural steroids in the management of chronic spinal pain: a systematic review. Pain Physician. 2007 Jan;10(1):185–212.

§ 10:23 Other treatment types—Radiofrequency neurotomy—Lumbar spine

Repeated radiofrequency neurotomies are an effective long-term palliative management of lumbar facet pain. Each radiofrequency neurotomy had a **mean duration of relief of 10.5 months** and was successful more than **85%** of the time.

Schofferman J, Kine G. Effectiveness of repeated radiofrequency neurotomy for lumbar facet pain. Spine. 2004 Nov 1;29(21):2471–3.

Of the 209 patients, 174 completed the study, and 35 were lost to follow-up or did not provide complete data for assessment. Of the 174 patients with complete data, 55 (**31.6%**) experienced **no benefit** from the procedure. One hundred and nineteen patients (**68.4%**) **had good** (> 50.) **to excellent** (> 80%) pain relief lasting from 6 to 24 months.

Proper patient selection and anatomically correct radiofrequency denervation of the lumbar zygapophysial joints provide long-term pain relief in a routine clinical setting.

Gofeld M, Jitendra J, Faclier G. Radiofrequency denervation of the lumbar zygapophysial joints: 10-year prospective clinical audit. Pain Physician. 2007 Mar;10(2):291–300.

§ 10:24 Other treatment types—Radiofrequency neurotomy—Cervical spine

Among patients with dominant headache, comparative blocks revealed that the prevalence of C2-C3 zygapophysial joint pain was 50%. Among those without C2-C3 zygapophysial joint pain, placebo-controlled blocks revealed the prevalence of lower cervical zygapophysial joint pain to be 49%. Overall, the **prevalence of cervical zygapophysial joint pain** (C2-C3 or below) **was 60%** (95% confidence interval, 46%, 73%).

Cervical zygapophysial joint pain is common among patients with chronic neck pain after whiplash. This nosologic entity has survived challenge with placebo-controlled, diagnostic investigations and has proven to be of major clinical importance.

Lord SM, Barnsley L, Wallis BJ, Bogduk N. Chronic cervical zygapophysial joint pain after whiplash. A placebo-controlled prevalence study. Spine. 1996 Aug 1;21(15):1737–44; discussion 1744–5.

With intraarticular facet joint injections, the evidence for short- and long-term pain relief is limited for cervical pain and moderate for lumbar pain. For medial branch blocks, the evidence is moderate for short- and long-term pain relief. For medial branch neurotomy, the **evidence is moderate for short- and long-term pain relief.**

Boswell MV, Colson JD, Sehgal N, Dunbar EE, Epter R. A systematic review of therapeutic facet joint interventions in chronic spinal pain. Pain Physician. 2007 Jan;10(1):229–53.

The median time that elapsed before the pain returned to at least 50 percent of the preoperative level was **263 days** in the active-treatment group and 8 days in the control group (P=0.04). At 27 weeks, seven patients in the active-treatment group and one patient in the control group were free of pain. Five patients in the active-treatment group had numbness in the territory of the treated nerves, but none considered it troubling.

In patients with chronic cervical zygapophyseal-joint pain confirmed with double-blind, placebo-controlled local anesthesia, percutaneous radio-frequency neurotomy with multiple lesions of target nerves can provide lasting relief. Lord SM, Barnsley L, Wallis BJ, McDonald GJ, Bogduk N. Percutaneous radio-frequency neurotomy for chronic cervical zygapophyseal-joint pain. N Engl J Med. 1996 Dec 5;335(23):1721–6.

Complete relief of pain was obtained in 71% of patients after an initial procedure. No patient who failed to respond to a first procedure responded to a repeat procedure, but if pain returned after a successful initial procedure, relief could be reinstated by a repeat procedure. **The median duration of relief after a first procedure was 219 days when failures are included but 422 days when only successful cases are considered. The median duration of relief after repeat procedures was at least 219 days**; several patients had ongoing relief at the time of follow-up. Outcome did not differ according to the operator, the type of electrode used, litigation status, or the type of diagnostic block used.

Radiofrequency neurotomy provides clinically significant and satisfying periods of freedom from pain, and its effects can be reinstated if pain recurs.

McDonald GJ, Lord SM, Bogduk N. Long-term follow-up of patients treated with cervical radiofrequency neurotomy for chronic neck pain.Neurosurgery. 1999 Jul;45(1):61–7; *discussion 67–8*.

Of 114 patients, who had positive response to diagnostic block, 46 patients did not respond favorably to pulsed RF application (pain reduction less than 50%). In 68 patients, the procedure was successful and lasted on average 3.93+/-1.86

months. Eighteen patients had the procedure repeated with the same duration of pain relief that was achieved initially. Previous surgery, duration of pain, sex, levels (cervical vs. lumbar) and stimulation levels did not influence outcomes.

The results of our study showed that the application of pulsed RF to medial branches of the dorsal rami in patients with chronic facet joint arthropathy **provided temporary pain relief in 68 of 118 patients.**

Mikeladze G, Espinal R, Finnegan R, Routon J, Martin D. Pulsed radiofrequency application in treatment of chronic zygapophyseal joint pain. Spine J. 2003 Sep-Oct;3(5):360–2.

Forty-six patients completed the study. The overall reduction in cervical whiplash symptoms and visual analogue pain scores were significant immediately after treatment (nonlitigants vs. litigants: 2.0 vs. 2.5, P = 0.36) and at 1 year (nonlitigants vs. litigants: 2.9 vs. 4.0, P = 0.05). One-year follow-up scores were higher than immediate post-treatment scores (nonlitigants vs. litigants: 2.5 vs. 3.6). The difference between litigants and nonlitigants in the degree of symptomatology or response to treatment did not reach significance.

These results demonstrate that the potential for secondary gain in patients who have cervical facet arthropathy as a result of a whiplash injury does not influence response to treatment. These data contradict the common notion that litigation promotes malingering. This study also confirms the efficacy of radiofrequency medial branch neurotomy in the treatment of traumatic cervical facet arthropathy.

Sapir DA, Gorup JM. Radiofrequency medial branch neurotomy in litigant and nonlitigant patients with cervical whiplash: a prospective study. Spine. 2001 Jun 15;26(12):E268–73.

Less than half the patients reported relief of pain for more than one week, and less than one in five patients reported relief for more than one month, irrespective of the treatment received. The median time to a return of 50 percent of the preinjection level of pain was 3 days in the 21 patients in the corticosteroid group and 3.5 days in the 20 patients in the local-anesthetic group (P = 0.42).

Intraarticular injection of betamethasone is not effective therapy for pain in the cervical zygapophyseal joints after a whiplash injury. Barnsley L, Lord SM, Wallis BJ, Bogduk N. Lack of effect of intraarticular corticosteroids for chronic pain in the cervical zygapophyseal joints. N Engl J Med. 1994 Apr 14;330(15):1047–50.

§ 10:25 Other treatment types—Treating Benign Paroxysmal Positional Vertigo (BPPV)

The liberatory manoeuvre should be tried in patients with horizontal canal vertigo. It should not be performed in patients with severe cervical arthrosis, vertebrobasilar insufficiency, or when the patient has neck pain during the manoeuvre. De la Meilleure G, Dehaene I, Depondt M, Damman W, Crevits L, Vanhooren G. Benign paroxysmal positional vertigo of the horizontal canal. J Neurol Neurosurg Psychiatry. 1996 Jan;60(1):68–71.

There is some evidence that the Epley manoeuvre is a safe effective treatment for posterior canal BPPV; however, this is based on the results of only two small, randomized, controlled trials with relatively short follow-up. Hilton M, Pinder D. The Epley (canalith repositioning) manoeuvre for benign paroxysmal positional vertigo. Cochrane Database Syst Rev. 2002;(1):CD003162. *Review.*

§ 10:26 Other treatment types—Complementary treatments for back or neck pain

Those reporting back or neck pain in the last 12 months, 37% had seen a conventional provider and 54% had used complementary therapies to treat their condition. Chiropractic, massage, and relaxation techniques were the most commonly used complementary treatments for back or neck pain (20%, 14%, and 12%, respectively, of those with back or neck pain). Chiropractic, massage, and relaxation techniques were rated as "very helpful" for back or neck pain among users (61%, 65%, and 43%, respectively), whereas conventional providers were rated as "very helpful" by 27% of users. We estimate that nearly one-third of all complementary provider visits in 1997 (203 million of 629 million) were made specifically for the treatment of back or neck pain. The conclusions reached were that; Chiropractic, massage, relaxation techniques, and other complementary methods all play an important role in the care of patients with back or neck pain Wolsko PM, Eisenberg DM, Davis RB, Kessler R, Phillips RS. Patterns and perceptions of care for treatment of back and neck pain: results of a national survey. Spine. 2003 Feb 1;28(3):292–7.

§ 10:27 Other treatment types—Heat for back pain

The evidence base to support the common practice of

superficial heat and cold for low back pain is limited and there is a need for future higher-quality randomised controlled trials. There is moderate evidence in a small number of trials that heat wrap therapy provides a small short-term reduction in pain and disability in a population with a mix of acute and sub-acute low-back pain, and that the addition of exercise further reduces pain and improves function.

French SD, Cameron M, Walker BF, Reggars JW, Esterman AJ. Superficial heat or cold for low back pain. Cochrane Database Syst Rev. 2006 Jan 25;(1):CD004750.

In this small study, continuous low-level heat wrap therapy was of **significant benefit** in the prevention and early phase treatment of low back Delayed Onset Muscle Soreness. Mayer JM, Mooney V, Matheson LN, Erasala GN, Verna JL, Udermann BE, Leggett S. Continuous low-level heat wrap therapy for the prevention and early phase treatment of delayed-onset muscle soreness of the low back: a randomized controlled trial. Arch Phys Med Rehabil. 2006 Oct;87(10):1310–7.

Combining continuous low-level heat wrap therapy with directional preference-based exercise during the treatment of acute low back pain **significantly improves functional outcomes** compared with either intervention alone or control. Either intervention alone tends to be more effective than control.

Mayer JM, Ralph L, Look M, Erasala GN, Verna JL, Matheson LN, Mooney V. Treating acute low back pain with continuous low-level heat wrap therapy and/or exercise: a randomized controlled trial. Spine J. 2005 Jul-Aug;5(4):395–403.

Overnight use of heatwrap therapy **provided effective pain relief** throughout the next day, reduced muscle stiffness and disability, and improved trunk flexibility. Positive effects were sustained more than 48 hours after treatments were completed.

Nadler SF, Steiner DJ, Petty SR, Erasala GN, Hengehold DA, Weingand KW. Overnight use of continuous low-level heatwrap therapy for relief of low back pain. Arch Phys Med Rehabil. 2003 Mar;84(3):335–42.

Continuous low-level heatwrap therapy was **shown to be effective** for the treatment of acute, nonspecific LBP.

Nadler SF, Steiner DJ, Erasala GN, Hengehold DA, Abeln SB, Weingand KW. Continuous low-level heatwrap therapy for treating acute nonspecific low back pain. Arch Phys Med Rehabil. 2003 Mar;84(3):329–34.

Chapter 11

Outcome Assessments

§ 11:1 Overview

In personal injury cases, outcome assessments can help tell part of the story. In presenting a case there is a need to describe what the injury is, how the injury happened, how the injury affected the patient's life, and whether the treatment was necessary for the person's complaints.

Outcome assessments include pain drawings, manual palpation, algometer readings (pressure pain thresholds), visual analog pain scales (VAS), neck & low back disability indices, cervical range of motion (CROM), sensory threshold perception (CPT), electromyography (EMG), nerve conduction velocities (NCV), imaging studies and other tests.

§ 11:2 Pain drawings

The pain drawing is a stable instrument for use in chronic back pain patients. Ohnmeiss DD. Repeatability of pain drawings in a low back pain population. Spine. 2000 Apr 15;25(8):980–8.

§ 11:3 Palpation

Palpation of cervical spine tenderness is a highly reliable examination tool. Hubka MJ, Phelan SP. Interexaminer reliability of palpation for cervical spine tenderness. J Manipulative Physiol Ther. 1994 Nov–Dec;17(9):591–5.

Manipulative physiotherapists can reliably palpate lumbar spinal levels. Downey BJ, Taylor NF, Niere KR. Manipulative physiotherapists can reliably palpate nominated lumbar spinal levels. Man Ther. 1999 Aug;4(3):151–6.

Palpation over the facet joins in the cervical spine was found to be the most appropriate screening test to corroborate self-reported dysfunctions of the neck. Sandmark H, Nisell R. Validity of five common manual neck pain provoking tests. Scand J Rehabil Med. 1995 Sep;27(3):131–6.

Manual diagnosis can be as accurate as radiologically controlled diagnostic blocks for the level of facet pain. Jull G, Bogduk N, Marsland A. The accuracy of manual diagnosis for cervical zygapophysial joint pain syndromes. Med J Aust. 1988 Mar 7;148(5):233–6.

In this study we examined whether results from a clinical test of passive mobility of soft tissue structures in **the upper cervical spine**, corresponded with signs of physical injuries, as judged by magnetic resonance imaging (MRI).

Each ligament and membrane was classified in one out of four possible predefined categories, referred to as MR grade 0–3. The following classification system was applied: Grade 0 reflected a normal structure. The alar and transverse ligaments were classified as grade 1 when less than one third of the cross section area showed increased signal intensity, as grade 2 when more than one third, but less than two thirds, showed increased signal intensity, and as grade 3 when more than two thirds of the cross section area showed increased signal intensity.

The posterior atlanto-occipital membrane was evaluated indirectly by changes in the adjacent dura mater. An irregularity or thinning of the dura was classified as grade 1, discontinuity as grade 2, and discontinuity with a dural flap as grade 3. Grade 1–3 classification of the tectorial membrane was diagnosed when less than one third, between one third and two thirds, and more than two thirds of the membrane was absent, and only the dura mater was remaining.

Results were based on examinations of 122 study participants, 92 with and 30 without a diagnosis of whiplash-associated disorder, type 2.

Tests of passive intervertebral movements (PIMs) of the cervical spine are frequently used for patients with neck pain.

The test for each single structure considered in the present study has specific test movements, and aims at clarifying the ability to withstand passive stretching. A specialist in manual therapy (BRK) performed the clinical examination while the patient was sitting in a chair. Passive stretching of the ligament and membrane was performed through the passive range of motion, or until a muscular contraction occurred due to pain in the area. The predefined clinical categories (category 0–3) were as follow: Category 0 indicated a normal ligament or membrane function. In category 1, a minor increase in motion between test points was found, in category 2 a moderately abnormal motion was found, and in category 3 an extensive increase in motion between test points was found.

The results for the membranes appeared somewhat better than for the ligaments. When there was disagreement, the classifications obtained by the clinical test were significantly lower than the MRI grading, but mainly within one grade difference. When combining grade 0–1 (normal) and 2–3 (abnormal), the agreement improved considerably (range 0.70–0.90).

Although results from the clinical test seem to be slightly more conservative than the MRI assessment, we believe that a clinical test can serve as valuable clinical tool in the assessment of WAD patients.

Results from the present study indicate that it is possible to detect joint dysfunction in the upper cervical spine by a clinical examination.

Kaale BR, Krakenes J, Albrektsen G, Wester K. Clinical assessment techniques for detecting ligament and membrane injuries in the upper cervical spine region-A comparison with MRI results. Man Ther. 2007 Oct 10.

§ 11:4 Soft tissue tenderness grading

Palpation:		
Grade	0	No tenderness
Grade	I	Tenderness with no physical response
Grade	II	Tenderness with grimace and/or flinch
Grade	III	Tenderness with withdrawal (positive jump sign)
Grade	IV	Withdrawal to non-noxious stimuli (superficial palpation, gentle percussion)

See Wolfe F, Smythe HA, Yunus MB, Bennett RM, Bombardier C, Goldenberg DL, Tugwell P, Campbell SM, Abeles M, Clark P, et al. The American College of Rheumatology 1990 Criteria for the Classification of Fibromyalgia. Report of the Multicenter Criteria Committee. Arthritis Rheum. 1990 Feb;33(2):160–72; Hubbard DR, Berkoff GM. Myofascial trigger points show spontaneous needle EMG activity. Spine. 1993 Oct 1;18(13):1803–7.

§ 11:5 Motor and sensory impairment

Cervical flexor endurance (CFE) in whiplash patients. CFE was measured using a stopwatch while the subject, in crook lying, held their head against gravity to fatigue. **CFE discriminated whiplash patients who were within six months of injury.** Kumbhare DA, Balsor B, Parkinson WL, Harding Bsckin P, Bedard M, Papaioannou A, Adachi JD. Measurement of cervical flexor endurance following whiplash. Disabil Rehabil. 2005 Jul 22;27(14):801–7.

Isometric **cervical strength** was measured in the directions of flexion, extension, right and left lateral flexion in 97 patients

(51 women and 46 men) using a wall-mounted dynamometer. Compared to published values of normal subjects, **whiplash patients suffered sharp reductions of about 90%** in both genders and in all directions. Prushansky T, Gepstein R, Gordon C, Dvir Z. Cervical muscles weakness in chronic whiplash patients. Clin Biomech (Bristol, Avon). 2005 Oct;20(8):794–8.

This study demonstrates a pathophysiological link between neck muscle fatigue and impaired postural control and also that physiotherapy can relieve symptoms and signs of impaired neck muscle function by reducing muscle fatigability. Stapley PJ, Beretta MV, Dalla Toffola E, Schieppati M. Neck muscle fatigue and postural control in patients with whiplash injury. Clin Neurophysiol. 2006 Mar;117(3):610–22.

Quantitative motor unit action potentials (QMUAP) in whiplash patients with neck and upper-limb pain. QEMG changes suggest neural injury in symptomatic side C6 and C7 innervated muscles, even in the absence of spontaneous activity. In acute and chronic pain patients, a higher percentage of polyphasic MUAPs is noted in the symptomatic side C6 muscle. **In chronic pain patients higher MUAP frequencies are noted in the symptomatic side C6 muscle.** Chu J, Eun SS, Schwartz I. Quantitative motor unit action potentials (QMUAP) in whiplash patients with neck and upper-limb pain. Electromyogr Clin Neurophysiol. 2005 Sep–Oct;45(6):323–8.

§ 11:6 Motor and sensory impairment—Muscle strength (AMA guides)

Percentage of Motor Deficits:	
(5) (Normal) Active movement against gravity with full resistance	0
(4) Active movement against gravity with some resistance	1–25
(3) Active movement against gravity only, without resistance	26–50
(2) Active movement with gravity eliminated	52–75
(1) Slight contraction and no movement	76–99

Percentage of Motor Deficits:	
(0) No contraction	100

See AMA Guides 5th ed. Pg 424

§ 11:7 Motor and sensory impairment—Muscle testing by Kendall & Kendall 1963

Functioning:	
(5)	The ability to hold the test position against gravity and maximum pressure. (100%)
(5, 4+)	Moderate pressure. (95–90%)
(4, 4-)	Minimum pressure. (80–70%)
(3)	The ability to hold the test position against gravity. (50%)
(3-)	The gradual release from the test position against gravity, or the ability to complete the arc of motion with gravity lessened. (40%)
(2+, 2)	The ability to move through a partial arc of motion with gravity lessened: moderate arc, 30% or poor +; small arch 20%, or poor. (30–20%)
(2-)	Muscle can be seen or palpated, a feeble contraction. (10%)
(1)	No visible movement of the part. (5%)
(0)	No contraction felt in the muscle. (0%)

See Muscles: Testing and Function. Kendall FP, McCreary EK, eds. Williams & Wilkins, Baltimore, 1983, pg. 12.

§ 11:8 Motor and sensory impairment—Sensory loss impairment

(5)	No loss of sensibility, abnormal sensation or pain	0
(4)	Distorted superficial tactile sensibility (diminished light touch)	1–25
(3)	Diminished light touch and 2-point discrimination	26–60
(2)	Decreased protective sensibility, abnormal sensations, moderate pain	61–80
(1)	Absent protective sensibility, severe pain, prevents most activity	81–99
(0)	Absent sensibility, abnormal sensations, severe pain prevents activity	100

See AMA Guides 5th ed.

§ 11:9 Deep tendon reflexes

(4+)	Very brisk, hyperactive
(3+)	Brisker than average
(2+)	Average, normal
(1+)	Diminished, low normal
(0)	No response

See AMA Guides 5th ed.

§ 11:10 Nerve root levels

Biceps	C5, 6
Brachioradialis	C5, 6
Triceps	C6, 7, 8
Patellar	L2, 3, 4
Achilles	L5, S1

See AMA Guides 5th ed.

§ 11:11 Posture

Normal postural alignment (without intervention) remains constant for at least two years. Bullock-Saxton J. Postural alignment in standing: a repeatability study. Australian J Physiotherapy 1993; 39:25–9.

§ 11:12 Algometer

Pressure threshold measurements (Algometer) are useful for documentation and identification of tender spots, as well as quantification of the degree of pain. See Fischer AA. Pressure algometry over normal muscles. Standard values, validity and reproducibility of pressure threshold. Pain. 1987 Jul;30(1):115–26; Fischer AA. Clin J Pain 1987; 2:207–14.

§ 11:13 Quantitative sensory tests

Quantitative sensory tests can be used for initial assessment, monitoring the clinical course, and determining the response to interventions. Dotson RM. Clinical neurophysiology laboratory tests to assess the nociceptive system in humans. J Clin Neurophysiol. 1997 Jan;14(1):32–45.

Electrocutaneous detection and pain thresholds A non-noxious method of electrocutaneous stimulation was used in a method of limits procedure using the Neurometer device (Neurotron, Baltimore, USA). Sites tested were those innervated by C5/6 (anterior shoulder, inferior to shoulder joint line), C7 (distal phalanx of index finger); C8 (distal phalanx of 5th digit) and tibialis anterior as a remote site. Three different sinusoidal frequencies (2000 Hz, 250 Hz and 5 Hz) were applied to each site in order to evoke a response from a different subpopulation of sensory fiber. The subjects reported when they first perceived the sensation (perception threshold) and again at the intensity at which they can no longer feel the sensation (disappearance threshold).

Hypersensitivity to a variety of stimuli has been shown in whiplash associated disorders and may be indicative of peripheral nerve involvement. This cross-sectional study utilized Quantitative sensory testing (QST) including vibration, thermal, electrical detection thresholds as an indirect measure of primary afferents that mediate innocuous and painful sensation.

The whiplash group demonstrated elevated vibration, heat and electrical detection thresholds at most hand sites compared to controls ($p<0.05$). Electrical detection thresholds in the lower limb were no different from controls ($p=0.83$). Mechanical and cold pain thresholds were lower in the whiplash group ($p<0.05$) with no group difference in heat pain thresholds ($p>0.1$).

A combination of pain threshold and detection measures best predicted the whiplash group. Sensory hypoaesthesia and hypersensitivity co-exist in the chronic whiplash condition. These findings may indicate peripheral afferent nerve fiber involvement but could be a further manifestation of disordered central pain processing.

Chien A, Eliav E, Sterling M. Hypoaesthesia occurs with sensory hypersensitivity in chronic whiplash — Further evidence of a neuropathic condition. Man Ther. 2008 Feb 20.

§ 11:14 Range of motion

Asymmetrical loss of range of motion is a Category II (5–8%) total body impairment rating. (DRE) Diagnosis Related Estimates Method of Assigning Impairment Rating Based on the AMA Guide to Permanent Impairment, 2001 pp. 373–431.

Total Cervical Range of Motion (CROM) was significantly lower and the MCV was significantly higher in patients compared with healthy subjects. Age and gender affected TCROM significantly in both groups while MCV remained unaffected, respectively. Atypical patients were identified by having a TCROM < 58 degrees and or MCV > 22%, both scores corresponding to 2 SDs below and above group means, respectively. These benchmarks resulted in classifying as atypical 6% of the CW group who also scored drastically higher in the NDI and SCL-R-90 questioners. Prushansky T, Pevzner E, Gordon C, Dvir Z. Performance of cervical motion in chronic whiplash patients and healthy subjects: the case of atypical patients. Spine. 2006 Jan 1;31(1):37–43.

The WAD group displayed a reduced flexion-extension range ($P = 1.9 \times 10(-4)$), and larger head repositioning error (HRE) during flexion-extension and repositioning tasks (P =

0.009) than controls. Neither group nor task affected maximal motion velocity. Neutral HRE of the flexion-extension component was larger in blindfolded condition (P =0.03). Ipsilateral bending and axial rotation HRE components were smaller than the flexion-extension component (P = 7.1 × 10(-23)). For pure rotation repositioning, axial rotation HRE was significantly larger than flexion-extension and ipsilateral bending repositioning error (P = 3.0 × 10(-23)). Ipsilateral bending component of HRE was significantly larger combined tasks than for pure rotation tasks (P = 0.004). In patients with WAD, range of motion and head repositioning accuracy were reduced. However, the differences were small. Vision suppression and task type influenced HRE. Feipel V, Salvia P, Klein H, Rooze M. Head repositioning accuracy in patients with whiplash-associated disorders. Spine. 2006 Jan 15;31(2):E51–8.

There was no evidence of position sense impairment in the mildly disabled whiplash subjects. The performance of the cranio-cervical flexion action had no effect on position sense. Thus, clinical improvements observed from using this action may be more associated with mechanical stabilization. Armstrong BS, McNair PJ, Williams M. Head and neck position sense in whiplash patients and healthy individuals and the effect of the cranio-cervical flexion action. Clin Biomech (Bristol, Avon). 2005 Aug;20(7):675–84.

The extension test cervical range of motion was able to discriminate between whiplash and control patients. Verhagen AP, Lanser K, de Bie RA, de Vet HC. Whiplash: assessing the validity of diagnostic tests in a cervical sensory disturbance. J Manipulative Physiol Ther. 1996 Oct;19(8):508–12.

After 1 year, 11 (7.8%) persons with whiplash injury had not returned to usual level of activity or work. The best single estimator of handicap was the cervical range-of-motion test, which had a sensitivity of 73% and a specificity of 91%. Accuracy and specificity increased to 94% and 99% when combined with pain intensity and other complaints. Initiation of lawsuit within first month after injury did not influence recovery. Kasch H, Bach FW, Jensen TS. Handicap after acute whiplash injury: a 1-year prospective study of risk factors. Neurology. 2001 Jun 26;56(12):1637–43.

§ 11:15 Proprioception

Subjects who have experienced a whiplash injury demonstrate a deficit in their ability to reproduce a target

position of the neck. See Loudon JK, Ruhl M, Field E. Ability to reproduce head position after whiplash injury. Spine. 1997 Apr 15;22(8):865–8; Heikkila H, Astrom PG. Cervicocephalic kinesthetic sensibility in patients with whiplash injury. Scand J Rehabil Med. 1996 Sep;28(3):133–8.

Traumatic chronic cervical pain patients have shown impaired cervicocephalic kinesthetic sensibility. Non-traumatic neck pain patients show little evidence of impaired cervicocephalic kinesthetic sensibility. Rix GD, Bagust J. Cervicocephalic kinesthetic sensibility in patients with chronic, nontraumatic cervical spine pain. Arch Phys Med Rehabil. 2001 Jul;82(7):911–9.

Elbow JPE is affected by movement of the head and neck, with smaller angles of neck rotation in people with WAD than in healthy individuals. This observation may explain deficits in upper limb coordination in people with WAD, which may be due to the presence of pain or reduced range of motion in this population.

Knox JJ, Beilstein DJ, Charles SD, Aarseth GA, Rayar S, Treleaven J, Hodges PW. Changes in head and neck position have a greater effect on elbow joint position sense in people with whiplash-associated disorders. Clin J Pain. 2006 Jul-Aug;22(6):512–8.

The absolute and variable joint position errors (JPE) were greater when the target angle was reproduced with the neck in the flexion, rotation, and combined flexion/rotation than when the head and neck were in neutral. This study suggests that the reduced accuracy previously seen in pointing tasks with changes in head position may be partly because of errors in the interpretation of arm position.

Knox JJ, Hodges PW. Changes in head and neck position affect elbow joint position sense. Exp Brain Res. 2005 Aug;165(1):107–13.

§ 11:16 Pain and disability scales

How are these scales used? Explain briefly how they are obtained from patient.

Visual analog pain scale. 0–10 pain scale, 0 meaning no pain, 10 the worst imaginable pain. Huskisson EC. Measurement of pain. Lancet. 1974 Nov 9;2(7889):1127–31.

§ 11:17 Pain and disability scales—The Oswestry low back pain disability index

0–20%	Minimal Disability
20–40%	Moderate Disability
40–60%	Severe Disability
60–80%	Crippled
80–100%	Bed Bound or Exaggerating

Fairbank JC, Couper J, Davies JB, O'Brien JP. The Oswestry low back pain disability questionnaire. Physiotherapy. 1980 Aug;66(8):271–3.

§ 11:18 Pain and disability scales—Neck disability index (NDI)

Note:

The NDI is reliable. It is based on the Oswestry Disability Index. Interpretation of scoring NDI raw scores:

0 – 4 = no disability

5 – 14 = mild disability

15 – 24 = moderate disability

25 – 34 = severe disability

above 34 = complete disability

Vernon H, Mior S. The Neck Disability Index: a study of reliability and validity J Manipulative Physiol Ther. 1991 Sep;14(7):409–15.

§ 11:19 Pain and disability scales—Patient specific functional scale

Pain bothersomeness was more responsive than pain intensity, which was more responsive than the SF-36 pain measure. The Patient Specific Functional Scale was the most responsive disability measure, followed by the spine-specific measures, with the SF-36 physical summary measure the least responsive.

Pain bothersomeness and the **Patient Specific Functional Scale** provide the most responsive measures of pain and disability, respectively, in patients with chronic whiplash.

Stewart M, Maher CG, Refshauge KM, Bogduk N, Nicholas M. Responsiveness of pain and disability measures for chronic whiplash. Spine. 2007 Mar 1;32(5):580–5.

§ 11:20 X-rays

A normal sagittal spine configuration is desirable. A cervical lordosis, measured from C2 to C7, of 34 degrees is suggestive for clinical outcomes (range 16–66 degrees). See Harrison DD, Janik TJ, Troyanovich SJ, Holland B. Comparisons of lordotic cervical spine curvatures to a theoretical ideal model of the static sagittal cervical spine. Spine. 1996 Mar 15;21(6):667–75; Harrison DD, Troyanovich SJ, Harrison DE, Janik TJ, Murphy DJ. A normal sagittal spinal configuration: a desirable clinical outcome. J Manipulative Physiol Ther. 1996 Jul–Aug;19(6):398–405.

Lateral cervical X-ray analysis is reliable. Jackson BL, Harrison DD, Robertson GA, Barker WF. Chiropractic biophysics lateral cervical film analysis reliability. J Manipulative Physiol Ther. 1993 Jul–Aug;16(6):384–91.

There is very good reliability in cervical spine measurements (X-ray). Jackson BL, Barker W, Bentz J, Gambale AG. Inter- and intra-examiner reliability of the upper cervical X-ray marking system: a second look. J Manipulative Physiol Ther. 1987 Aug;10(4):157–63.

§ 11:21 Gargan & Bannister's rating system

The following is based on the Gargan & Bannister study, to grade severity of symptoms at follow-up:

Grade	Description
A	Symptom free
B	Minor, nuisance, no disruption of work or recreation
C	Moderate, Intrusive; Intermittent loss of work and recreation
D	Severe, Disruptive; loss of job and recreation

Gargan MF, Bannister GC. Long-term prognosis of soft-tissue injuries of the neck. J Bone Joint Surg Br. 1990 Sep;72(5):901–3.

§ 11:22 Questionnaires for neuropathic pain

A score of 12 or greater on the LANSS is an indication of neuropathic pain.

Questionnaires have been developed to differentiate neuropathic pain from non-neuropathic pain, e.g., the LANSS Pain Scale (Bennett 2001) and the Neuropathic Pain Questionnaire (Krause and Backonja 2003) or to measure various characteristics, e.g., the Neuropathic Pain Scale (Galer and Jensen 1997) and the Neuropathic Pain Inventory (Bouhassira et al. 2004).

Bennett M. The LANSS Pain Scale: the Leeds assessment of neuropathic symptoms and signs. Pain. 2001 May;92(1–2):147–57.

Backonja MM, Krause SJ. Neuropathic pain questionnaire—short form. Clin J Pain. 2003 Sep-Oct;19(5):315–6

Bouhassira D, Attal N, Fermanian J, Alchaar H, Gautron M, Masquelier E, Rostaing S, Lanteri-Minet M, Collin E, Grisart J, Boureau F. Development and validation of the Neuropathic Pain Symptom Inventory. Pain. 2004 Apr;108(3):248–57.

Bennett reported a sensitivity and specificity of 83% and 87% respectively for the LANSS scale.

Neuropathic pain has been defined by the International Association for the Study of Pain (IASP) as pain that is initiated or caused by a primary lesion or dysfunction in the nervous system.

Over 90% of the patients with a LANSS score = 12 reported that the pain impaired sleep.

Pain symptoms known to be associated with neuropathic pain such as allodynia, hyperalgesia, shooting pain, electric shock sensations, and burning and throbbing pain were significantly more prevalent in patients with a LANSS pain score =12.

Hans G, Masquelier E, De Cock P. The diagnosis and management of neuropathic pain in daily practice in Belgium: an observational study. BMC Public Health. 2007 Jul 24;7(147):170.

Chapter 12

Prognosis

§ 12:1 Factors of prognosis

Pain has a central role to play as a prognostic factor for the development of chronic whiplash symptoms. High initial neck pain intensity, neck pain related disability, and cold hyperalgesia all had moderate evidence for an association with the development of chronic whiplash symptoms.

Williams M, Williamson E, Gates S, Lamb S, Cooke M. A systematic literature review of physical prognostic factors for the development of Late Whiplash Syndrome. Spine. 2007 Dec 1;32(25):E764–80.

According to the logistic regression in patients referred from primary care the following initial variables are in significant relationship with poor outcome at 1 year: **impaired neck movement**, **history of pretraumatic headache**, **history of head trauma**, **higher age**, **initial neck pain intensity**, **initial headache intensity**, **nervousness score**, neuroticism score and test score on focused attention. Employing these variables, correct prediction of outcome at 1 year was found in 88% of patients recruited from the insurance company.

Radanov BP, Sturzenegger M. Predicting recovery from common whiplash. Eur Neurol. 1996; 36(1):48–51.

At 2 years, with regard to baseline findings the following significant differences were found:

Symptomatic patients were **older**, had higher incidence of **rotated or inclined head position** at the time of impact, had **higher prevalence of pretraumatic headache**, showed **higher intensity of initial neck pain** and **headache**, **complained of a greater number of symptoms**, **had a higher incidence of symptoms of radicular deficit** and **higher average scores on a multiple symptom analysis**, and **displayed more degenerative signs (osteoarthrosis) on X ray**. In addition, symptomatic patients scored higher with regard to impaired well-being and performed worse on tasks of attentional functioning and showed more concern with regard to long-term suffering and disability.

Radanov BP, Sturzenegger M, Di Stefano G. Long-term outcome after whiplash injury. A 2-year follow-up considering features of injury mechanism and somatic, radiologic, and psychosocial findings. Medicine (Baltimore). 1995; 74(5):281–297.

Three features of accident mechanisms were associated with more severe symptoms: an **unprepared occupant**; **rear-end collision**, with or without subsequent frontal impact; and **rotated or inclined head position** at the moment of impact.

Sturzenegger M, DiStefano G, Radanov BP, Schnidrig A. Presenting symptoms and signs after whiplash injury: the influence of accident mechanisms. Neurology. 1994 Apr;44(4):688–93.

Persons whose **heads are turned at the time of a rear impact collision** risk a much more serious whiplash injury with potentially chronic symptoms. First, there is an initial stretch in the neck ligaments, which is not present when the head is facing forward. During the rear impact, the ligaments are stretched further. This over-stretching of the ligaments can cause ligament tears and spinal instability, leading to neck pain. Second, rear impact with rotated head posture causes three-dimensional head and neck motions, as compared to only two dimensional motions in the head forward posture. These three-dimensional motions cause more complex types of neck injuries.

Panjabi MM, Ivancic PC, Maak TG, Tominaga Y, Rubin W. Multiplanar cervical spine injury due to head-turned rear impact. Spine. 2006 Feb 15;31(4):420–9.

A **head turned posture increases facet capsular ligament neck strain** compared to a neutral head posture — a finding consistent with the greater symptom severity and duration observed in whiplash neck injury patients who have their head turned at impact.

Siegmund GP, Davis MB, Quinn KP, Hines E, Myers BS, Ejima S, Ono K, Kamiji K, Yasuki T, Winkelstein BA. Head-turned postures increase the risk of cervical facet capsule injury during whiplash. Spine. 2008 Jul 1;33(15):1643–9.

A **rotated head** at impact is clearly unfavourable, as has been shown in the present study similar to other studies, both with respect to initial injury rate as well as long-term problems (Sturzenegger et al. 1994 and 1995, Jakobsson 2004).

Bunketorp O, Jakobsson L, Norin H. Comparison of frontal and rear-end impacts for car occupants with whiplash associated disorders: symptoms and clinical findings. IRCOBI Conference — Graz (Austria) September 2004:245–256.

Muscle weakness and paresthesias, documented in whiplash patients, have been associated with **neural compression within the cervical intervertebral foramen**.

Extrapolation of the present results indicated that the highest potential for ganglia compression injury was at the lower cervical spine, C5-C6 and C6-C7. Acute ganglia compression may produce a sensitized neural response to repeat compression, leading to chronic radiculopathy following rear impact.

Panjabi MM, Maak TG, Ivancic PC, Ito S. Dynamic intervertebral foramen narrowing during simulated rear impact. Spine. 2006 Mar 1;31(5):E128–34.

A **rotated head posture** at the time of vehicular rear impact has been correlated with a **higher incidence and greater severity of chronic radicular symptoms** than accidents occurring with the occupant facing forward. Analysis of the results indicated that the greatest potential for **cervical ganglion compression injury** existed at C5-6 and C6-7. Greater potential for ganglion compression injury existed at C3-4 and C4-5 during head-turned rear impact than during head-forward rear impact. Results of present results indicated potential ganglion compression in patients with a non-stenotic foramen at C5-6 and C6-7; in patients with a stenotic foramen the injury risk greatly increases and spreads to include the C3-4 through C6-7 as well as C4-5 through C6-7 nerve roots.

Tominaga Y, Maak TG, Ivancic PC, Panjabi MM, Cunningham BW. Head-turned rear impact causing dynamic cervical intervertebral foramen narrowing: implications for ganglion and nerve root injury. J Neurosurg Spine. 2006 May;4(5):380–7.

Whiplash patients who had been sitting with their **head/neck turned** to one side at the moment of collision **more often had high-grade lesions of the alar and transverse ligaments** ($p < 0.001$, $p = 0.040$, respectively). Severe injuries to the transverse ligament and the posterior atlanto-occipital membrane were more common in front than in rear end collisions ($p < 0.001$, $p = 0.001$, respectively). In conclusion, the difference in MRI-verified lesions between WAD patients and control persons, and in particular the association with head position and impact direction at time of accident, indicate that these lesions are caused by the whiplash trauma.

Kaale BR, Krakenes J, Albrektsen G, Wester K. Head position and impact direction in whiplash injuries: associations with MRI-verified lesions of ligaments and membranes in the upper cervical spine. J Neurotrauma. 2005 Nov;22(11):1294–302.

A history of neck injury is a risk factor in chronic neck pain. Croft PR, Lewis M, Papageorgiou AC, Thomas E, Jayson MI, Macfarlane GJ, Silman AJ. Risk factors for neck pain: a longitudinal study in the general population. Pain. 2001 Sep;93(3):317–25.

Onset of neck pain after a motor vehicle accident: a case-control study. In total, 26% of drivers reported post-accident neck pain. Women, younger individuals, and those with a history of neck pain were more likely to report neck pain following their accident (OR 1.50, 95% CI 0.98, 2.28; OR 1.62, 95% CI 0.96, 2.74; OR 1.75, 95% CI 1.09, 2.81, respectively). In addition, a number of accident-related and psychosocial factors were independently associated with **reporting post-accident neck pain**: **collision from behind** (OR 2.55, 95% CI 1.41, 4.62); **vehicle stationary at impact** (OR 1.93, 95% CI 1.12, 3.33); **collision severity** (upper vs. lowest quartile tertile: OR 16.1, 95% CI 8.64, 30.1); **not being at fault** (OR 2.61, 95% CI 1.49, 4.59); and **monotonous work** (OR 2.19, 95% CI 1.19, 4.04). Based on these eight factors, the likelihood of having neck pain increased from 7% with < or = 2 risk factors to 62% with > or = 5. Development of neck pain after a motor vehicle accident is a complex phenomenon resulting from the combined effects of constitutional, mechanical, and psychosocial factors. **Using eight such variables, it is possible to identify those at high risk of developing neck pain.** Wiles NJ, Jones GT, Silman AJ, Macfarlane GJ. Onset of neck pain after a motor vehicle accident: a case-control study. J Rheumatol. 2005 Aug;32(8):1576–83.

A consecutive series of 96 patients who were seen in the emergency room in the acute phase after the injury were followed prospectively for one year. Age, gender, and whether or not pain in the neck preceded the accident was recorded. Cases involving fractures or dislocations of the cervical spine, head trauma, or pre-existing neurological disorders were not included. The mean interval between the accident and the initial examination was 3+/-2(S.D.) days. Coping was measured using the Coping Strategies Questionnaire (CSQ). The outcome parameter was self-reported neck pain at one year after the motor vehicle accident. At one year, 34% of the patients had neck pain. Women developed chronic neck pain more often than men (71% versus 29%); they also had significantly higher coping activity, such as diverting attention, praying or hoping (p<0.05), catastrophising and increasing behavioral activities (p<0.0001). **Women** reported pain in the neck or shoulder more often before the accident and this was the only statistically significant predictor of chronic symptoms when analyzed by logistic regression (odds ratio 4.5). To conclude, we found **no evidence that the different coping patterns during the early phase after a whiplash injury influenced the prognosis**. Lu Y, Chen C, Kallakuri S, Patwardhan A, Cavanaugh JM. Neurophysiological and biomechanical characterization of goat cervical facet joint capsules. J Orthop Res. 2005 Jul;23(4):779–87.

Although a higher score on the Tampa Scale of Kinesiophobia (TSK-DV) was found to be associated with a longer duration of neck symptoms, **information on early kinesiophobia was**

not found to improve the ability to predict the duration of neck symptoms after motor vehicle collisions. Buitenhuis J, Jaspers JP, Fidler V. Can Kinesiophobia Predict the Duration of Neck Symptoms in Acute Whiplash? Clin J Pain. 2006 Mar;22(3):272–277.

The correlations between the sensory and affective dimensions of pain were non-significant, which indicates that they are **two independent constructs that describe various dimensions of whiplash-related pain**. **High pain intensity** and pain affect, **more widespread pain**, and high fear of movement/(re)injury corresponded to low self-efficacy. Multiple regression analyses showed that **self-efficacy was the most important predictor of persistent disability** contributing to 42% of the variation in the PDI score. The treatment approach for patients with subacute WAD should incorporate the multidimensional nature of pain and to prevent disability **special effort should be made to enhance the patient's self-efficacy beliefs**. Bunketorp L, Lindh M, Carlsson J, Stener-Victorin E. The perception of pain and pain-related cognitions in subacute whiplash-associated disorders: Its influence on prolonged disability. Disabil Rehabil. 2006 Mar;28(5):271–9.

The number of cases is small, but the similarity of the symptoms — and signs — following whiplash injury may suggest an **element of organic origin in the whiplash syndrome**. Sjaastad O, Fredriksen TA, Batnes J, Petersen HC, Bakketeig LS. Whiplash in individuals with known pre-accident, clinical neck status. J Headache Pain. 2006 Feb;7(1):9–20.

Fair or poor health before the collision was associated with severe neck pain in females (odds ratio 4.0, 95% confidence interval 1.8–8.9). Other associated factors in females included low education and prior neck pain. Low family income was associated with severe neck pain in males (odds ratio 2.3, 95% confidence interval 1.5–3.4), as was **prior headache and being unaware of the head position at the time of collision**. The results suggest that **neck pain intensity** in WAD seems to be influenced by several factors other than characteristics related to the injury event itself. Holm LW, Carroll LJ, Cassidy JD, Ahlbom A. Factors influencing neck pain intensity in whiplash-associated disorders. Spine. 2006 Feb 15;31(4):E98–104.

A total of 200 patients were recruited to the study, of which 30 were lost to follow up. Four variables, midline tenderness (p = 0.008; 95% CI 0.9 to 6.1), x-ray request (p = 0.004; 0.9 to 6.1), wearing a seat belt (p = 0.038; 0.2 to 6.2), and having seen their GP post injury (p = 0.001; CI -10.5 to 6.6), were found to be associated with a higher neck disability index (NDI) score at follow up. Significant correlation was identified with a high pain score and an increasing age of patient and high NDI scores. **No correlation was found between the impact speed, speed of vehicle struck, or time since incident with the NDI. Two thirds of patients had some disability at 4–6 weeks after injury**; 91 patients (54.5%) saw their GP in the intervening period between attending the department and telephone follow up, and 87/170 patients had no idea about their prognosis. **This study identifies that there is significant disability associated with whiplash-associated disorder.** Clear prognostic information would be a useful development. Crouch R, Whitewick R, Clancy M, Wright P, Thomas P. Whiplash associated disorder: incidence and natural history over the first month for patients presenting to a UK emergency department. Emerg Med J. 2006 Feb;23(2):114–8.

Injury- and patient-related factors with possible influence to the timing of recovery were analysed with univariate and multivariate statistical methods. Logistic regression showed significant association between high physical demand patient occupation and recovery within 6 months from injury (P = 0.036, coefficient 1.5, odds ratio 4.47) while initiation of physiotherapy treatment was associated with prolongation of symptoms for more than 6 months following injury (P < 0.001, coefficient -2.6, odds ratio 0.08).

An association between development of **arm pain** (P = 0.01), **upper limb numbness or paraesthesia** (P = 0.03) and **bilateral trapezius pain** (P = 0.04) and persistence of whiplash-related symptoms was also observed. These findings must be taken into account in evaluation and treatment of patients with acute whiplash injuries pursuing litigation.

Karnezis IA, Drosos GI, Kazakos KI. Factors affecting the timing of recovery from whiplash neck injuries: study of a cohort of 134 patients pursuing litigation. Arch Orthop Trauma Surg. 2007 Oct;127(8):633–6.

Widespread pain was associated with negative consequences with respect to pain intensity, prevalence of other symptoms including depressive symptoms, some aspects of coping, life satisfaction and general health. Peolsson M, Borsbo B, Gerdle B. Generalized pain is associated with more negative consequences than local or regional pain: A study of chronic whiplash-associated disorders. J Rehabil Med. 2007 Apr;39(3):260–9.

§ 12:2 Factors of prognosis—Body mass index and recovery from whiplash injuries

The results do not support the hypothesis that individuals who are overweight or obese have a worse prognosis for whiplash.

Yang X, Cote P, Cassidy JD, Carroll L. Association between Body Mass Index and Recovery from Whiplash Injuries: A Cohort Study. Am J Epidemiol. 2007 May 1;165(9):1063–9.

§ 12:3 Factors of prognosis—Neck ligament strength is decreased following whiplash trauma

For all whiplash-exposed ligaments, the average failure elongation exceeded the average physiological elongation. The highest average failure force of 204.6 N was observed in the ligamentum flavum, significantly greater than in middle-third disc and interspinous and supraspinous ligaments. The highest average failure elongation of 4.9 mm was observed in the interspinous and supraspinous ligaments, significantly greater than in the anterior longitudinal ligament, middle-third disc, and ligamentum flavum. The average energy absorbed ranged from 0.04 J by the middle-third disc to 0.44 J by the capsular ligament. The ligamentum flavum was the stiffest ligament, while the interspinous and supraspinous ligaments were most flexible. The whiplash-exposed ligaments had significantly lower ($P = 0.036$) failure force, 149.4 vs. 186.0 N, and a trend ($P = 0.078$) towards less energy absorption capacity, 308.6 vs. 397.0 J, as compared to the control data.

The present decreases in neck ligament strength due to whiplash provide support for the ligament-injury hypothesis of whiplash syndrome.

Tominaga Y, Ndu AB, Coe MP, Valenson AJ, Ivancic PC, Ito S, Rubin W, Panjabi MM. Neck ligament strength is decreased following whiplash trauma. BMC Musculoskelet Disord. 2006 Dec 21;7:103.

Average elongation of the whiplash-exposed facet capsular ligaments was significantly greater than that of the control ligaments at tensile forces of 0 and 5 N. No significant differences between spinal levels were observed.

Facet capsular ligament injuries, in the form of increased laxity, may be one component perpetuating chronic pain and clinical instability in whiplash patients.

Ivancic PC, Ito S, Tominaga Y, Rubin W, Coe MP, Ndu AB, Carlson EJ, Panjabi MM. Whiplash causes increased laxity of cervical capsular ligament. Clin Biomech (Bristol, Avon). 2008 Feb;23(2):159–65.

§ 12:4 Damage to disc, facet, alar ligament

A complete review of whiplash-type injuries indicates most minor injuries will heal in 2–3 months, and 25% will become chronic. Injuries involving the disc, zygapophysial (facet) joints or alar ligaments will not resolve spontaneously, and will become chronic. These patients may improve over a period of two years and are unlikely to improve after 2 years. Barnsley L, Lord S, Bogduk N. Whiplash injury. Pain. 1994 Sep;58(3):283–307.

The greatest risk for long-term symptoms was seen among the group of patients with both point tenderness and limited range of motion. Hartling L, Brison RJ, Ardern C, Pickett W. Prognostic value of the Quebec Classification of Whiplash-Associated Disorders. Spine. 2001 Jan 1;26(1):36–41.

§ 12:5 Long-term consequence of whiplash

In drivers with reported whiplash injury, the risk of neck or shoulder pain 7 years after the collision was **increased nearly three-fold** compared to unexposed subjects. Berglund A, Alfredsson L, Cassidy JD, Jensen I, Nygren A. The association between exposure to a rear-end collision and future neck or shoulder pain: a cohort study. J Clin Epidemiol. 2000 Nov;53(11):1089–94.

When exposed subjects with whiplash injury were compared to unexposed subjects, increased risks in the range of 1.6–3.7 were seen for headache, thoracic and low back pain, as well as for fatigue, sleep disturbances and ill health. Berglund A, Alfredsson L, Jensen I, Cassidy JD, Nygren A. The association between exposure to a rear-end collision and future health complaints. J Clin Epidemiol. 2001 Aug;54(8):851–6.

§ 12:6 Whiplash acceleration degeneration of the joints, disc

The long-term effects of trauma (whiplash in this case) on the cervical spine demonstrated that patients injured in such accidents develop spondylosis approximately six times more frequently than age and gender-matched controls, and in cases where a loss of consciousness was reported, these patients were 10 times more likely to

develop such degenerative changes. Hohl M. Soft-tissue injuries of the neck in automobile accidents. Factors influencing prognosis. J Bone Joint Surg Am. 1974 Dec;56(8):1675–82.

A trauma to the spine may accelerate normal age-related deterioration of the discs. A 2-year follow-up period is too brief. Previous studies indicating posttraumatic degenerative changes based on plain radiographs had a 10-year follow-up. Pettersson K, Hildingsson C, Toolanen G, Fagerlund M, Bjornebrink J. Disc pathology after whiplash injury. A prospective magnetic resonance imaging and clinical investigation. Spine. 1997 Feb 1;22(3):283–7; discussion 288.

Radiographic degenerative changes in the cervical spine appeared 10 years earlier in the whiplash group. Gargan MF. Bannister GC. The comparative effects of whiplash injuries. J Orthopedic Medicine 1997; 19:15–17.

The loss of cervical lordosis increases the risk of injury to the cervical spine following axial loading. Oktenoglu T, Ozer AF, Ferrara LA, Andalkar N, Sarioglu AC, Benzel EC. Effects of cervical spine posture on axial load bearing ability: a biomechanical study. J Neurosurg. 2001 Jan;94(1 Suppl):108–14.

The connection between subjects in whiplash trauma and the progression of disc disease requiring the surgical procedure of anterior discectomy is twice the rate seen in the general population. **They found that the mean age of the whiplashed surgical group was 45 +/- 12 years, whereas the mean age of the non-whiplashed surgical group was 55 +/-14 years (p<0.001).** Hamer AJ, Gargan MF, Bannister GC, Nelson RJ. Whiplash injury and surgically treated cervical disc disease. Injury. 1993 Sep;24(8):549–50.

The results of this study suggest that the altered composition of collagens observed in the degenerate porcine nucleus pulposus results from changes in cell phenotype: Notochondral cells were replaced by fibroblast-like cells. **It is likely that trauma to the anulus fibrosus can initiate a progressive degenerative process in the disc tissue.** Kaapa E, Han X, Holm S, Peltonen J, Takala T, Vanharanta H. Collagen synthesis and types I, III, IV, and VI collagens in an animal model of disc degeneration. Spine. 1995 Jan 1;20(1):59–66; discussion 66–7.

Genetic risk factors likely play a significant role in lumbar disc disease. Paassilta P, Lohiniva J, Goring HH, Perala M, Raina SS, Karppinen J, Hakala M, Palm T, Kroger H, Kaitila I, Vanharanta H, Ott J, Ala-Kokko L. Identification of a novel common genetic risk factor for lumbar disc disease. JAMA. 2001 Apr 11;285(14):1843–9.

Minor damage to a vertebral endplate leads to progressive structural changes in the adjacent intervertebral discs. Adams MA, Freeman BJ, Morrison HP, Nelson IW, Dolan P. Mechanical initiation of intervertebral disc degeneration. Spine. 2000 Jul 1;25(13):1625–36.

This is the first study documenting synergism of a signaling response to biomechanical and biochemical stimuli in human disc cells. IL-1beta appeared to "sensitize" annulus cells to mechanical load. **This increased responsiveness to mechanical load in the face of inflammatory cytokines may imply the sensitivity of annulus cells to shear increases during inflammation and may affect initiation and progression of disc degeneration.** Elfervig MK, Minchew JT, Francke E, Tsuzaki M, Banes AJ. IL-1beta sensitizes intervertebral disc annulus cells to fluid-induced shear stress. J Cell Biochem. 2001;82(2):290–8.

§ 12:7 Pre-existing degenerative changes

Patients with pre-existing spondylosis generally fared worse in whiplash injuries. See Watkinson A, Gargan MF, Bannister GC. Prognostic factors in soft tissue injuries of the cervical spine. Injury. 1991 Jul;22(4):307–9; Parmar HV, Raymakers R. Neck injuries from rear impact road traffic accidents: prognosis in persons seeking compensation. Injury. 1993 Feb;24(2):75–8.

§ 12:8 Risk factors in whiplash

The following is a list of possible factors that may have an effect on the patient. Some of the factors may be more important in acute injury and some for chronic problems:

§ 12:9 Risk factors in whiplash—Rear impacts

Rear impacts are more likely to cause injury.

Balla JI. The late whiplash syndrome. Aust N Z J Surg. 1980 Dec; 50(6):610–4; Croft AC. The case against litigation neurosis in mild brain injuries and cervical acceleration/deceleration trauma. J Neuromusculoskeletal Syst 1(4):149–155, 1993; Otte D. Rether JR: Risks and mechanisms of injuries to the cervical spine in traffic accidents. International IRCOBI/AAAM Conference on the Biomechanics of Impacts, Goetborg, Sweden 1985; Dvorak J, Panjabi MM. Functional anatomy of the alar ligaments. Spine. 1987 Mar; 12(2):183–9; Deans GT, Magalliard JN, Kerr M, Rutherford WH. Neck sprain—a major cause of disability following car accidents. Injury. 1987 Jan; 18(1):10–2; Nygren A, Gustafsson H, Tingvall C. Effects of different types of head restraints in rear-end collisions. 10th International Technical Conference on Experimental Safety Vehicles, Oxford, England 85–90, 1985; Deans GT, McGalliard JN, Rutherford WH. Incidence and duration of neck pain among patients injured in car accidents. Br Med J (Clin Res Ed). 1986 Jan 11;292(6513):94–5; Olsnes BT. Neurobehavioral findings in whiplash patients with long-lasting symptoms. Acta Neurol Scand. 1989 Dec; 80(6):584–8; Yoganandan N, Haffner M, Maiman DJ, et al. Epidemiology and injury biomechanics of motor vehicle related trauma to the human spine. SAE 892438, in Proceedings of the 33rd Stapp Car Crash Conference, Detroit, MI, Society of Automotive Engineers, 223–242, 1989; Data Link. Car crash outcomes in rear impacts. Appendix A to Current Issues of Occupant Protection in Car Rear Impacts. Washington, D.C., Data Link, inc., 1989; Balla JI. Report to the Motor Accidents Board of Victoria on whiplash injuries. In (Chapter 10) Headache and cervical disorders. In Hopkins A, ed., Headache: Problems in Diagnosis and Management. London, Saunders, 1988, pp 256–269; Juhl M, Seerup KK. Cervical spine injuries: epidemiological investigation. Medical and social consequences. International IRCOBI Conference on the Biomechanics of Impacts, Salon-de-Provence, France, 49–57, 1981; Bourbeau R, Desjardins D, Maag U, Laberge-Nadeau C. Neck injuries among belted and unbelted occupants of the front seat of cars. J Trauma. 1993 Nov; 35(5):794–9; Jakobsson L, Norin H, Jernstrom C, et al. Analysis of different head and neck responses in rear-end car collisions using a new humanlike mathematical model. International IRCOBI Conference on the Biomechanics of Impacts. Lyon, France, Sept. 21–23, 1994.

§ 12:10 Risk factors in whiplash—Limited ROM; neurological symptoms

Regarding limited range of motion and/or neurological symptoms, see:

Gay JR, Abbott KG. Common whiplash injuries of the neck. JAMA 152:1698, 1953; Norris SH, Watt I. The prognosis of neck injuries resulting from rear-end vehicle collisions. J Bone Joint Surg 1983; 65B:1675–82; Kasch H, Bach FW, Jensen TS. Handicap after acute whiplash injury: a 1-year prospective study of risk factors. Neurology. 2001 Jun 26; 56(12):1637–43;

Hartling L, Brison RJ, Ardern C, Pickett W. Prognostic value of the Quebec Classification of Whiplash-Associated Disorders. Spine. 2001 Jan 1; 26(1):36–41.

§ 12:11 Risk factors in whiplash—Loss of cervical curve

Regarding loss of cervical curve, see:

Ettlin TM, Kischka U, Reichmann S, Radii EW, Heim S, Wengen D, Benson DF. Cerebral symptoms after whiplash injury of the neck: a prospective clinical and neuropsychological study of whiplash injury. J Neurol Neurosurg Psychiatry. 1992 Oct; 55(10):943–8; Pennie B, Agambar L. Patterns of injury and recovery in whiplash. Injury. 1991 Jan; 22(1):57–9; Gay JR, Abbott KG. Common whiplash injuries of the neck. JAMA 152:1698, 1953.

§ 12:12 Risk factors in whiplash—Previous whiplash injury

Regarding previous whiplash injury, see:

Khan S, Bannister G, Gargan M, Asopa V, Edwards A. Prognosis following a second whiplash injury. Injury. 2000 May; 31(4):249–51.

§ 12:13 Risk factors in whiplash—Previous spondylosis (degeneration on radiographs)

Regarding prior spondylosis, see:

Norris SH, Watt I. The prognosis of neck injuries resulting from rear-end vehicle collisions. J Bone Joint Surg Br. 1983 Nov; 65(5):608–11; Macnab I. Acceleration injuries of the cervical spine. J Bone Joint Surg 46A (8):1797–1799, 1964; Bohrer SP, Chen YM, Sayers DG. Cervical spine flexion patterns. Skeletal Radiol. 1990;19(7):521–5; Pennie B, Agambar L. Patterns of injury and recovery in whiplash. Injury. 1991 Jan; 22(1):57–9; Nygren A, Gustafsson H, Tingvall C. Effects of different types of head restraints in rear-end collisions. 10th International Technical Conference on Experimental Safety Vehicles, Oxford, England 85–90, 1985; Deans GT, McGalliard JN, Rutherford WH. Incidence and duration of neck pain among patients injured in car accidents. Br Med J (Clin Res Ed). 1986 Jan 11; 292(6513):94–5; Watkinson A, Gargan MF, Bannister GC. Prognostic factors in soft tissue injuries of the cervical spine. Injury. 1991 Jul; 22(4):307–9; Parmar HV, Raymakers R. Neck injuries from rear impact road traffic accidents: prognosis in persons seeking compensation. Injury. 1993 Feb; 24(2):75–8.

§ 12:14 Risk factors in whiplash—Initial back pain

Regarding initial back pain, see:

Radanov BP, Di Stefano G, Schnidrig A, Sturzenegger M. Psychosocial stress, cognitive performance and disability after common whiplash. J Psychosom Res. 1993 Jan; 37(1):1–10.

§ 12:15 Risk factors in whiplash—Decreased spinal canal width

A decreased spinal canal width is a poor prognostic factor, see:

Pettersson K, Karrholm J, Toolanen G, Hildingsson C. Decreased width of the spinal canal in patients with chronic symptoms after whiplash injury. Spine. 1995 Aug 1;20(15):1664–7.

§ 12:16 Risk factors in whiplash—Head rotation or head turned at time of impact

A turned or rotated head is a poor prognostic factor.

Regarding head rotation issues, see:

Pennie B, Agambar L. Patterns of injury and recovery in whiplash. Injury. 1991 Jan;22(1):57–9; Parmar HV, Raymakers R. Neck injuries from rear impact road traffic accidents: prognosis in persons seeking compensation. Injury. 1993 Feb; 24(2):75–8; Saldinger P, Dvorak J, Rahn BA, Perren SM. Histology of the alar and transverse ligaments. Spine. 1990 Apr; 15(4):257–61; Sturzenegger M, DiStefano G, Radanov BP, Schnidrig A. Presenting symptoms and signs after whiplash injury: the influence of accident mechanisms. Neurology. 1994 Apr; 44(4):688–93.

§ 12:17 Risk factors in whiplash—Preparedness for collision

Unprepared occupants fare worse in whiplash injuries.

Regarding victim's preparedness for collision, see:

Ono K, Kanno M.: Influences of the physical parameters on the risk to neck injuries in low impact speed rear-end collisions. International IRCOBI Conference on the Biomechanics of Impacts, Eindhoven, Netherlands, 201–212, 1993; Thomson RW, Romilly DP, Navin FPD, Macnabb MJ. Energy attenuation within the vehicle during low speed collisions. Report to Transport Canada, University of British Columbia, Aug, 1989; Galasko CS, Murray PM, Pitcher M, Chambers H, Mansfield S, Madden M, Jordon C, Kinsella A, Hodson M. Neck sprains after road traffic accidents: a modern epidemic. Injury. 1993 Mar; 24(3):155–7; Kumar S, Narayan Y, Amell T. Role of awareness in head-neck acceleration in low velocity rear-end impacts. Accid Anal Prev. 2000 Mar;32(2):233–41; Ryan GA, Taylor GW, Moore VM, Dolinis J. Neck strain in car occupants. The influence of crash-related factors on initial severity. Med J Aust. 1993 Nov 15; 159(10):651–6; Stemper BD, Yoganandan N, Cusick JF, Pintar FA. Stabilizing effect of precontracted neck musculature in whiplash. Spine. 2006 Sep 15;31(20) :E733–8.

§ 12:18 Risk factors in whiplash—Front seat position

Regarding front seat position, see:

Parmar HV, Raymakers R. Neck injuries from rear impact road traffic accidents: prognosis in persons seeking compensation. Injury. 1993 Feb;24(2):75–8; Dvorak J, Panjabi MM. Functional anatomy of the alar ligaments. Spine. 1987 Mar; 12(2):183–9.

§ 12:19 Risk factors in whiplash—Nonfailure of seat back

Regarding non-failure of back seats, see:

Foret-Bruno JY, Dauvilliers F, Tarriere C. Influence of the seat and head rest stiffness on the risk of cervical injuries. 13th International Technical Conference on Experimental Safety Vehicles. S-8-W-19, 968–974, 1991; States JD, Balcerak JD, Williams JS, et al. Injury frequency and head restraint effectiveness in rear end impact accidents. In Proceedings of the 16th Stapp Car Crash Conference, Detroit, MI, 228–257, 1972.

§ 12:20 Risk factors in whiplash—Shoulder harness/ seatbelt use

Regarding shoulder harness and/or seatbelt use, see:

Olsnes BT. Neurobehavioral findings in whiplash patients with long-lasting symptoms. Acta Neurol Scand. 1989 Dec; 80(6):584–8; Data Link: Car crash outcomes in rear impacts. Appendix A to Current Issues of Occupant Protection in Car Rear Impacts. Washington, D.C., Data Link, inc., 1989; *Mertz*

HJ Jr., Patrick LM. *Investigation of the kinematics and kinetics of whiplash. In Proceedings, 11th Stapp Car Crash Conference, SAE 670919, Detroit MI, Society of Automotive Engineers, 1967.*

§ 12:21 Risk factors in whiplash—Head restraint geometry

Regarding head restraint geometry, see:

Magnusson T. Extracervical symptoms after whiplash trauma. Cephalalgia. 1994 Jun;14(3):223–7; discussion 181–2; Neck strain in car occupants. The influence of crash-related factors on initial severity. Med J Aust. 1993 Nov 15;159(10):651–6; Croft AC. The cervical acceleration/deceleration syndrome. In Steigerwald DP, Croft AC (eds): Whiplash and Temporomandibular Joint Dysfunction: an Interdisciplinary Approach to Case Management. Encinitas, Keiser Publishing Co., 1992.

§ 12:22 Risk factors in whiplash—Short and long-term consequences of injury

Regarding short and long term consequences of injury, see:

Kraft M. A comparison of short- and long-term consequences of AIS 1 neck injuries, in rear impacts. International IRCOBI Conference on the Biomechanics of Impact. September 16–18, 1998, Goteborg, Sweden, 235–48; Kraft M. When do AIS 1 neck injuries result in long-term consequences? Vehicle and human factors. Traffic Injury Prevention 2002;3:89–97.

§ 12:23 Risk factors in whiplash—Female victims

Females generally fare worse in whiplash.

Regarding female victims, see:

Hohl M. Soft-tissue injuries of the neck in automobile accidents. Factors influencing prognosis. J Bone Joint Surg Am. 1974 Dec;56(8):1675–82; Ommaya A, Backaitis S, Fan W, Partyka S. Automotive neck injuries. Ninth Internatl Technical Conference on Experimental Safety Vehicles, US Department of Transportation, National Highway Traffic Safety Administration, Kyoto Japan, Nov 1–4, 1982, pp 274–278; Balla JI. The late whiplash syndrome. Aust N Z J Surg. 1980 Dec;50(6):610–4; Koch, M, Nygren A, Tingvall C. Impairment pattern in passenger car crashes, a follow-up of injuries resulting in long-term consequences. Presented at the 14th International Technical Conference on Enhanced Safety of

Vehicles, Munchen, 1994; Macnab I. Acceleration injuries of the cervical spine. J Bone Joint Surg 46A(8):1797–1799, 1964; Krafft M, Kullgren A, Tingvall C, Bostrom O, Fredriksson R. How crash severity in rear impacts influences short- and long-term consequences to the neck. Accid Anal Prev. 2000 Mar; 32(2):187–95; Richter M, Otte D, Pohlemann T, Krettek C, Blauth M. Whiplash-type neck distortion in restrained car drivers: frequency, causes and long-term results. Eur Spine J. 2000 Apr; 9(2):109–17.

§ 12:24 Risk factors in whiplash—Multiple collisions

Regarding multiple collisions, see:

Richter M, Otte D, Pohlemann T, Krettek C, Blauth M. Whiplash-type neck distortion in restrained car drivers: frequency, causes and long-term results. Eur Spine J. 2000 Apr; 9(2):109–17.

§ 12:25 Risk factors in whiplash—Age of victim

Older occupants are more likely to be injured, middle age and beyond.

Regarding age of victim, see:

Parmar HV, Raymakers R. Neck injuries from rear impact road traffic accidents: prognosis in persons seeking compensation. Injury. 1993 Feb;24(2):75–8; Radanov BP, Di Stefano G, Schnidrig A, Sturzenegger M, Augustiny KF. Cognitive functioning after common whiplash. A controlled follow-up study. Arch Neurol. 1993 Jan; 50(1):87–91; Brison RJ, Hartling L, Pickett W. A prospective study of acceleration-extension injuries following rear-end motor vehicle collisions. J Musculoskeletal Pain 2000; 8:97–113.

§ 12:26 Risk factors in whiplash—Out-of-position occupants (leaning forward/slumped)

Out of position occupants are more likely to be injured.

Foret-Bruno, J., Tarriere, C., & Le-Coz, J.-Y. Risk of cervical lesions in real-world and simulated collisions. Paper presented at the 34th AAAM Conference Proceedings, Scottsdale, AZ; Olsson, I., Bunketorp, O., & Carlsson, G. An in-depth study of neck injuries in rear end collisions. Paper presented at the 1990 September 12–14 International IRCOBI Conference, Bron, Lyon, France; Romilly, D., Thomson, R., Navin, F., & Macnabb, M. Low speed rear impacts and the elastic properties of automobiles. Paper presented at the Proceedings: 12th

International Conference of Experimental Safety Vehicles, 1989, May/June, Gothenburg; Warner, C., Strother, C., & James, M. Occupant protection in rear end collisions: II. the role of seat back deformation in injury reduction. Paper presented at the Proceedings of the 35th Stapp Car Crash Conference 1991, Society of Automotive Engineers, Detroit, MI.

Factors Influencing Whiplash Injury

Sociodemographic and economic status, preinjury health status, and collision-related factors are associated with participants' rating of initial neck pain intensity in Whiplash Associated Disorders. The findings are of importance for interpreting and understanding the underlying factors of pain rating.

Holm LW, Carroll LJ, David Cassidy J, Ahlbom A. Factors Influencing Neck Pain Intensity in Whiplash-associated Disorders in Sweden. Clin J Pain. 2007 Sep;23(7):591–597.

§ 12:27 Litigation & whiplash injury

Factors Predicting outcome after whiplash. One of the many "urban myths" surrounding whiplash is the belief by many defense experts that the existence of litigation itself prolongs symptoms and the need for treatment. Recent research has addressed this issue again. This is the largest and most comprehensive study of this type ever published. Conclusions:

1. "Females fared worse than males, in agreement with all previous studies but one . . ."
2. There is an association between poor outcome and previous whiplash injury.
3. There is a close association between pre-injury back pain and both physical and psychological outcome following whiplash injury.
4. Researchers found a link between increased frequency of visits to a general practitioner pre-accident with poor outcome.
5. There as a "strong association with pre-existing psychological illness demonstrated in this study."
6. There is a "secondary psychological disorder following whiplash injury" which, according to other studies, did not remit within either two years or 15 years.
7. "Front position in the vehicle was one of the principal individual variables associated with poor outcome in this study. This is consistent with other reports and may be due partly to the fact that the majority of rear-seat passengers

were not wearing seatbelts. Wearing a seatbelt increases the risk [4 studies cited] and severity [1 study cited] of whiplash injury."

8. "Early onset of symptoms [7 studies cited], radiating pain and numbness [9 studies cited] and objective neurological signs at the time of examination [6 studies cited] are consistent with a poor prognosis in the overwhelming proportion of the literature examining these variables."

The final conclusions: "A number of variables influence the physical and psychological outcome following whiplash injury and there is considerable overlap between validated physical and psychological outcome measures. **Many of the individual factors that are most strongly associated with poor outcome in this group of patients are present before impact.** This physical and psychological vulnerability may explain some of the variation in response to low violence, indirect neck injury." Lankester BJ, Garneti N, Gargan MF, Bannister GC. Factors predicting outcome after whiplash injury in subjects pursuing litigation. Eur Spine J. 2006 Jun;15(6):902–7.

Logistic regression showed significant association between high physical demand patient occupation and recovery within 6 months from injury (P = 0.036, coefficient 1.5, odds ratio 4.47).

An association between development of **arm pain** (P = 0.01), **upper limb numbness or paraesthesia** (P = 0.03) and **bilateral trapezius pain** (P = 0.04) and persistence of whiplash-related symptoms was also observed. These findings must be taken into account in evaluation and treatment of patients with acute whiplash injuries pursuing litigation.

Karnezis IA, Drosos GI, Kazakos KI. Factors affecting the timing of recovery from whiplash neck injuries: study of a cohort of 134 patients pursuing litigation. Arch Orthop Trauma Surg. 2007 Oct;127(8):633–6.

That litigation status did not predict employment status suggests that secondary gain does not figure prominently in influencing the functionality of these patients. The rather robust effect of litigation status on pain reports is discussed with respect to the potential mediational role of the stress of litigation. Swartzman LC, Teasell RW, Shapiro AP, McDermid AJ. The effect of litigation status on adjustment to whiplash injury. Spine. 1996 Jan 1;21(1):53–8.

These results demonstrate that the potential for secondary gain in patients who have cervical facet ar-

thropathy as a result of a whiplash injury does not influence response to treatment. These data contradict the common notion that litigation promotes malingering. This study also confirms the efficacy of radio frequency medial branch neurotomy in the treatment of traumatic cervical facet arthropathy. Sapir DA, Gorup JM. Radio frequency medial branch neurotomy in litigant and nonlitigant patients with cervical whiplash: a prospective study. Spine. 2001 Jun 15;26(12):E268–73.

All patients who obtained complete pain relief exhibited resolution of their pre-operative psychological distress. In contrast, all but one of the patients whose pain remained unrelieved continued to suffer psychological distress. Because psychological distress resolved following a neurosurgical treatment that completely relieved pain without psychological co-therapy, **it is concluded that the psychological distress exhibited by these patients was a consequence of the chronic somatic pain**. Wallis BJ, Lord SM, Bogduk N. Resolution of psychological distress of whiplash patients following treatment by radiofrequency neurotomy: a randomised, double-blind, placebo-controlled trial. Pain. 1997 Oct;73(1):15–22.

Patients with low back pain or neck pain resulting from a motor vehicle accident showed a statistically significant improvement with treatment despite ongoing litigation. Schofferman J, Wasserman S. Successful treatment of low back pain and neck pain after a motor vehicle accident despite litigation. Spine. 1994 May 1;19(9):1007–10.

Prognostic factors associated with minimal improvement following acute whiplash-associated disorders. A retrospective clinical cohort study was done to identify the prognostic factors associated with a poor response to treatment in the early stages of a whiplash-associated disorder (WAD). Several demographic and clinical factors related to recovery following acute WADs have been identified. However, few longitudinal studies have investigated a multivariable model of recovery that includes socio-demographic, treatment, clinical, and nonclinical factors. In this study a cohort of 2,185 patients with acute or subacute WADs presenting to 48 rehabilitation clinics in six Canadian provinces were investigated for factors associated with failure to demonstrate a minimally important clinical change (10%) in the Canadian Back Institute Questionnaire (CBIQ) score between the initial and discharge rehabilitation visits. The results of multivariable analysis revealed **eight prognostic factors associated with a negative outcome: 1) older age**, 2) **female gender**, 3) **increasing lag**

time between injury date and presentation for treatment, 4) **initial pain location**, 5) province of injury, 6) **higher initial pain intensity**, 7) lawyer involvement, and 8) at work at entry to the clinic. The effect of lawyer involvement was stronger for patients with less intense pain on initial visit (odds ratio = 2.97; 95% confidence interval, 1.77–4.99). Similarly, the effect of work status was stronger for patients with less intense pain on initial visit (odds ratio = 2.02; 95% confidence interval, 1.18–3.46). The conclusions reached are that researchers and clinicians should be aware of the potential for non-injury-related factors to delay recovery, and be aware of the interaction between the initial intensity of a patient's pain and other covariates when confirming these results. Dufton JA, Kopec JA, Wong H, Cassidy JD, Quon J, McIntosh G, Koehoorn M. Prognostic factors associated with minimal improvement following acute whiplash-associated disorders. Spine. 2006 Sep 15;31(20):E759–65; E766.

Chapter 13

Guidelines

Many defense medical examiners or expert witnesses refer to guidelines that allegedly apply to whiplash injuries. They may reference the Quebec Task Force, Mercy Conference, or Federal guidelines. Below is a brief overview of each set of commonly used guidelines.

§ 13:1 Quebec Task Force

In 1995, the Quebec Task Force prepared a study to "redefine" whiplash and its management, with the full text of the article appearing in the April 15, 1995 issue of *Spine.* The study was sponsored by the Quebec Automobile Insurance Agency (Societe de I'Assurance Automobile du Quebec). Spitzer WO, Skovron ML, Salmi LR, Cassidy JD, Duranceau J, Suissa S, Zeiss E. Scientific monograph of the Quebec Task Force on

Whiplash-Associated Disorders: redefining "whiplash" and its management. Spine. 1995 Apr 15;20(8 Suppl):1S–73S.

The Quebec Task Force (QTF) had several objectives, including: (1) creating a tool to assist medical practitioners in diagnosing, classifying and treating patients with whiplash associated disorders (WAD); and (2) to provide guidance in the areas of rehabilitation and treatment of claimants with WAD. The Task Force concluded that, in general, whiplash injuries result in "temporary discomfort," are "usually self-limited," and have a "favorable prognosis." Further, the result of the findings was that pain from whiplash injuries is "not harmful."

The QTF study has been challenged on a number of levels. See e.g. Freeman, Croft & Rossignol, "Whiplash Associated Disorders: Redefining Whiplash and Its Management," Spine 1998; 23 (9) May 1, 1043–1049 ("The validity of the conclusions and recommendations of the Quebec Task Force regarding the natural course and epidemiology of whiplash injuries is questionable."). Note also that current studies indicate pain can affect the immune system, and people with chronic pain have a higher incidence of cancer. Macfarlane GJ, McBeth J, Silman AJ. Widespread body pain and mortality: prospective population-based study. BMJ. 2001 Sep 22;323(7314):662–5).

The QTF study suffers from "selection bias," in that it was followed only to collect data on a return to usual activities or work. No information was collected about whether patients continued to be symptomatic, or if they needed continued care. The cut-off date of studies was 1993. The QTF did not include the work by Australian researchers (Bogduk, Barnsley, Lord, Wallis) on facet injuries from whiplash or some of the most important studies on whiplash, as they were published after the QTF cut-off date.

In the QTF document, only the ICD-9 diagnostic code 847.0 was used as criterion for whiplash injury. Excluded were those who sought treatment, but not compensation; those injured in the course of their employment; those injured who may have sought and received compensation, but were not diagnosed with the ICD-9 code 847.0; those with less than 1 week of time loss; those who were disabled for more than one week, but chose not to seek compensation; those who had no police reports (1743 subjects, 36.6% were excluded); those with delay of onset of symptoms (around 22%).

The QTF study supplied no references to support the claim that WAD is self-limited. There was no mention of ongoing medical treatment or any disability less than total. The QTF did not care if people were in pain or getting medical treatment. They were only concerned about paying total disability claims. If they did not have to pay for total disability, then the patient was considered "recovered."

Further, the literature the QTF relied on (Norris and Watt 1983, Radanov 1993, Hildingsson and Toolanen 1990) indicates that WAD are frequently not self-limited, and that a substantial number of injured individuals have long-term, chronic symptoms as a result of their injuries. Norris and Wat: 66% had neck pain at an average of 2 years after injury; Radanov: 27% were symptomatic at 6 months and, at a follow-up study two-years later, 27% continued to have headaches. Hildingsson and Toolanen: only 42% were asymptomatic and average 2 years after the accident. See Norris SH, Watt I. The prognosis of neck injuries resulting from rear-end vehicle collisions. J Bone Joint Surg Br. 1983 Nov;65(5):608–11; -i—us-Radanov BP, Sturzenegger M, Di Stefano G, Schnidrig A, Aljinovic M. Factors influencing recovery from headache after common whiplash. BMJ. 1993 Sep 11;307(6905):652–5; Hildingsson C, Toolanen G. Outcome after soft-tissue injury of the cervical spine. A prospective study of 93 car-accident victims. Acta Orthop Scand. 1990 Aug;61(4):357–9.

Note that the QTF rejected the very studies they judged reliable. See Norris SH, Watt I. The prognosis of neck injuries resulting from rear-end vehicle collisions. J Bone Joint Surg Br. 1983 Nov;65(5):608–11; Radanov BP, Sturzenegger M, Di Stefano G, Schnidrig A, Aljinovic M. Factors influencing recovery from headache after common whiplash. BMJ. 1993 Sep 11;307(6905):652–5; Hildingsson C, Toolanen G. Outcome after soft-tissue injury of the cervical spine. A prospective study of 93 car-accident victims. Acta Orthop Scand. 1990 Aug;61(4):357–9.). These studies do not support the QTF statement position that only a very small number of individuals will have long-term problems.

§ 13:2 Croft & QTF guidelines—Table I: grades of severity of injury

Grade I	**Minimal:** No limitation of motion; no ligamentous injury; no neurological findings. Lesion is not serious enough to cause muscle spasm.

Grade II	**Slight:** Limitation of motion; no ligamentous injury; no neurological findings. Neck complaint and musculoskeletal signs.
Grade III	**Moderate:** Limitation of motion; ligamentous instability; neurological symptoms. Common symptoms:
	Neck and arm pain
	Cervical herniated disc
	Neck pain with headache
	Cervicoscapulalgia- (pain referred to upper back)
Grade IV	**Moderate to Severe:** Limitation of motion; some ligamentous injury; neurological symptoms; fracture or disc derangement.

§ 13:3 Croft & QTF guidelines—Table II: guidelines for frequency and duration of care in cervical acceleration/deceleration trauma

Daily	3x/wk	2x/wk	1x/wk	1x/mo	T_D	T_N	
Grade I	1 wk	1–2 wk	2–3 wk	<4 wk	—1	<11 wk	<21
Grade II	1 wk	<4 wk	<4 wk	<4 wk	<4 mo	<29 wk	<33
Grade III	1–2 wk	<10 wk	<10 wk	<10 wk	<6 mo	<56 wk	<76
Grade IV	2–3 wk	<16 wk	<12 wk	<20 wk	—2	—2	—2
Grade V	Surgical stabilization necessary—chiropractic care is post-surgical.						

T_D= treatment duration T_N= treatment number.

1 Possible follow-up at 1 month.

2 May require permanent monthly or prn (as needed) treatment.

Regarding the above, see Croft AC. Treatment paradigm for cervical acceleration/deceleration injuries (whiplash). ACA J Chiro 30(1):41–45, 1993; Foreman SM, Croft AC eds. Whiplash injuries: The Cervical Acceleration/Deceleration Syndrome. 3 ed. Philadelphia: Lippincott Williams & Wilkins; 2002.

Chiropractic Treatment in Acute Whiplash Injuries: Grade I & II

Grade I: Mean number of treatments was **20,** mean weeks of treatment was **10.**

Grade II: Mean number of treatments — **34.7,** mean weeks of treatment — **18.2**

Comparison with the Croft Treatment Guidelines:

Davis 2008	**WAD I**	**WAD II**
Mean visits	**19.9**	**34.7**
Minimum	6	15
Maximum	30	66
Weeks Treatment	**10**	**18.2**
Minimum	4	8
Maximum	18	40
Croft — visits	<21	<33
Weeks Treatment	<11	<29

Davis CG. Chiropractic Treatment in Acute Whiplash Injuries: Grades I & II. J. Vertebral Subluxation Res. May 19, 2008.

§ 13:4 Mercy Conference Guidelines

The Mercy Conference Guidelines ("Mercy Guidelines") were created for chiropractic care. They were developed in the early 1990s. The Mercy document makes no comment at all regarding billing codes, CPT codes or EM codes. The insurance industry may subscribe to the Mercy Guidelines, but no chiropractic association in California (ACA, CCA or ICA) endorses the Mercy Guidelines. Furthermore, the Mercy document was based on a literature review that ended in 1991. The literature was mostly on industrial low-back conditions, not on whiplash.

See Guidelines for Chiropractic Quality Assurance and Practice Parameters: Proceedings of the Mercy Center Consensus Conference. Haldelman S, Chapman-Smith D, Petersen DM, eds. Aspen, Gaithersburg, MD, 1993.

§ 13:5 Mercy conference guidelines—Overview of mercy guidelines

Below is a summary of key components of the Mercy Guidelines, which can be found at page 124–125.Acute uncomplicated case (<6 wks symptoms): Up to 5 visits a week for the first 2 weeks, then 3 visits a weeks after that for a maximum of 6–8 weeks (maximum 28 visits) to return to pre-episode status.Subacute case (>6 but less than 16 weeks): average 2 visits a week for 6 to 16 weeks (max 32 visits) to return to pre-episode status.Chronic case: passive care not indicated, unless there has been an acute exacerbation of the chronic condition.Complicated case: exceeds the recommended duration of care, but still fits within the guidelines. Pain >8 days duration before presenting for care may take 1.5x longer to recover. Severe pain may take 2x longer to recover.4 to 7 previous episodes may take 2x longer. Pre-existing conditions, underlying pathologies or anomalies may take 1.5 to 2 times longer. Factors complicating recovery: All may delay recovery and necessitate a need for additional care that may exceed the recommended guidelines for simple, uncomplicated cases.

- biomechanical stress
- psychological stress
- poor compliance
- prolonged static stress
- re-injury exacerbation
- multilevel DJD
- spondylolisthesis

§ 13:6 Mercy conference guidelines

Acute uncomplicated case (<6 wks symptoms): Up to 5 visits a week for the first 2 weeks, then 3 visits a weeks after that for a maximum of 6–8 weeks (maximum 28 visits) to return to pre-episode status.

Subacute case (>6 but less than 16 weeks): average 2 visits a week for 6 to 16 weeks (max 16 visits) to return to pre-episode status.

Chronic case: passive care not indicated unless there has been an acute exacerbation of the chronic condition.

Complicated case: exceeds the recommended duration of care but still fits within the guidelines.

Pain >8 days duration before presenting for care may take 1.5x longer to recover.

Severe pain may take 2x longer to recover.

4 to 7 previous episodes may take 2x longer.

Pre-existing conditions, underlying pathologies or anomalies may take 1.5 to 2 times longer.

Factors complicating recovery:

- biomechanical stress
- psychological stress
- poor compliance
- prolonged static stress
- re-injury exacerbation
- multilevel DJD
- spondylolisthesis

All may delay recovery and necessitate a need for additional care that may exceed the recommended guidelines for simple uncomplicated cases.

Haldeman S, Chapman-Smith S, Peterson SM. Guidelines for Chiropractic Quality Assurance and Practice Parameters: Proceedings of the Mercy Center Consensus Conference. Frederick, Maryland, U.S.A. Aspen Pub. 1992. Chapter 8.

§ 13:7 Articles that report frequency and duration for whiplash victims

Year	Author	Duration	Frequency
1953	Billig	Several Months	3X/day, Then 3X/wk
1958	Seletz	N/A	Start Early, Daily 2–3 wks, Then 3X/wk
1978	Jackson	N/A	Daily 1–2 wks, Then 3X/wk
1986	Ameis	Mild: up to 6 mo Mod: 6mo-3 yrs	Not Reported
1990	Gargan	2 yrs	Not Reported
1992	Mercy Document	Uncomplicated: 16 wks Complicated: 24 –32 wks	Daily for 2 wks, Then 3X/wk for 4 wks, Then 2X/wk for 10 wks = 42 visits 1.5 or 2X the uncomplicated frequency
1994	Schofferman	2 mo — 2 yr 1 mo Mean: 7mo 1 wk	Not Reported

Year	Author	Duration	Frequency
1994	Barnsley	3 mo — 2 yrs	Not Reported
2005	Tomlin-son	3 mo — 2 yrs	Not Reported

Billig H. Traumatic Neck, Head, Eye Syndrome. Journal of the International College of Surgeons 1953; 20(5): 558–61

Seletz E. Whiplash Injuries: Neurophysiological Basis for Pain and Methods Used for Rehabilitation. J Amer Medical Assoc 1958, 1750 – 1755. Jackson R. The Cervical Syndrome; Fourth Edition, Charles C Thomas publisher, 1978: 291.

Ameis A. Cervical Whiplash: Considerations in the Rehabilitation of Cervical Myofascial Injury. Canadian Family Physician 1986;Volume 32.

Gargan MF, Bannister GC. Long-term Prognosis of Soft-Tissue Injuries of the Neck; J Bone Joint Surgery (British) 1990; VOL. 72-B, No. 5.

Haldeman S, Chapman-Smith D, Petersen DM. Guidelines for Chiropractic quality assurance and practice parameters. Proceedings of the Mercy Center Consensus Conference. Gaithersburg, MD: Aspen Publishers, 1993.

Schofferman J, Wasserman S. Successful treatment of low back pain and neck pain after a motor vehicle accident despite litigation; Spine 994;19(9):1007–10.

Barnsley L, Lord S, Bogduk N. Whiplash injury: Clinical Review. Pain 1994; 58:283–307.

Tomlinson PJ, Gargan MF, Bannister GC. The fluctuation in recovery following whiplash injury: 7.5-year prospective review. Injury 2005; 36(6): 758–761.

§ 13:8 Application of guidelines

It is important to note that these guidelines are not intended as recommended treatment plans or prescriptions for care; many patients, particularly those without complicating features, will not require the maximum treatment numbers and duration allowed by these guidelines. Conversely, other patients, due to complicating factors, such as advanced age, prior disease, etc., might require treatment approaches exceeding the guidelines. As always, a clinician's most important management compass is the patient.

Guidelines further allow clinicians to gauge their own clinical efficacy and, in some cases, to suspect that occult lesions may be present. Some patients may require upgrading or downgrading as more clinical or laboratory information becomes available.

See Foreman SM, Croft AC eds. Whiplash injuries: The Cervical Acceleration/Deceleration Syndrome. 3 ed. Philadelphia: Lippincott Williams & Wilkins; 2002.

§ 13:9 A note on the federal guidelines

The "Federal Guidelines" are a referral to the 1994 AHCPR (Guidelines on Acute Low Back Problems in Adults) and do not attempt to define treatment of whiplash injuries.

§ 13:10 Common factors potentially complicating whiplash trauma management

These factors may increase the treatment frequency and/or duration:

- Advanced age
- Metabolic disorders
- Congenital anomalies of the spine
- Developmental anomalies of the spine
- Degenerative disc disease
- Disc protrusion (HNP)
- Spondylosis facet arthrosis
- Rheumatoid arthritis or other arthritides affecting the spine
- Ankylosing spondylitis or other
- Spondylarthropathy
- Scoliosis
- Prior cervical spinal surgery
- Prior lumbar spinal surgery
- Prior vertebral fracture
- Osteoporosis
- Paget's disease or other disease of bone
- Spinal stenosis or foraminal stenosis
- Paraplegia or quadriplegia
- Prior spinal injury

Foreman SM, Croft AC eds. Whiplash injuries: The Cervical Acceleration/Deceleration Syndrome. 3 ed. Philadelphia: Lippincott Williams & Wilkins; 2002.

Chapter 14

Commonly Encountered Defense Studies & Methods

<u>Note:</u> *For a thorough discussion on methods for attacking the weaknesses and flaws in commonly cited defense studies, see*

Finley, Stall, and Fariello, Plaintiffs' Lawyers Guide to Minor Impact Cervical and Lumbar Injuries (Thomson West, 2007-2008).

§ 14:1 Chapter overview

In soft tissue claims, especially those arising from smaller automobile accidents, the handling insurance adjuster may attempt to "educate" the claimant or representing attorney on findings from relevant studies. Similarly, defense expert witnesses routinely cite to such studies as a basis for concluding that a victim could not have been injured, or is exaggerating their injuries. Often, the references are to studies that are considered to be junk science in the legal and scientific communities, and of questionable admissibility in trial courts.

The following sections identify the more commonly cited studies and briefly address the inherent flaws underlying the claimed supporting findings.

§ 14:2 The Allen study—Overview of study

A commonly encountered study that has reached almost mythic proportions in defense circles is the Allen study, in which the authors compare "G" forces from activities of daily living (ADL) and attempt to make comparisons to whiplash trauma. Allen ME, Weir-Jones I, Motiuk DR, Flewin KR, Goring RD, Kobetitch R, Broadhurst A. Acceleration perturbations of daily living. A comparison to 'whiplash'. Spine. 1994 Jun 1;19(11):1285–90.

The authors of the study placed accelerometers (which measure acceleration) on individuals and had them "plop" into chairs, step off curbs, ride a horse, be struck in bumper cars and even hit one researcher in the back of the head with a soft mallet. These findings were published and insurance witnesses began to use this information to "prove" that these were the same forces that the patient experiences in the collisions. The defense uses the study to show that everyday activities generate the same forces as low-speed collisions, and, therefore, nobody can get hurt.

§ 14:3 The Allen study—Problems

There are serious problems with research comparing ADL to whiplash forces and then concluding that soft tissue injury is not possible. The actions tested are not comparable vectors of forces in whiplash injuries. The motions of this testing are not related to those in a rear-end collision. The neck injury criterion of the tests conducted in this study would be close to 0. Attempting to compare simple accelerations of ADL to complex movements such as those that occur in whiplash is biomechanically illogical. The problems with this study are so numerous that at least one appellate court upheld a trial court in not allowing the defense expert to testify, when the opinion was based on Allen. See (*Schultz v. Wells*, 13 P.3d 846 (Colo. Ct. App. 2000).)

§ 14:4 McConnell studies (1993 & 1995)—Overview of study

The 1993 McConnell study reported the results of human volunteer, rear-impact crash testing of four subjects. They determined that, in reference to whiplash injuries resulting from rear impact collisions, the threshold of a "very mild, single event musculoskeletal cervical strain injury" is a delta V (the absolute velocity change of the struck vehicle as opposed to the speed of the striking vehicle at impact) of 4 to 5 miles per hour. See 1993, SAE 930889. McConnell WE, Howard RP, Guzman HU, Bomar JB, Raddin JH, Benedict JV, Smith HL, Hatsell CP. Analysis of Human Test Subject Kinematic Responses to Low Velocity Rear End Impacts: Vehicle and Occupant Kinematics: Simulation and Modeling (SP-975). Society of Automotive Engineers, 930889, Detroit, MI. 1993.

The 1995 McConnell study looked at the movements and acceleration forces sustained by seven human occupant volunteers subjected to repeat rear-end collisions of up to 6.8 mph delta V. They concluded that in a delta V of 5 mph "the likelihood of transient acute neck and shoulder muscle strain injury and possible mild compressive irritation of the posterior neck may increase" for the average vehicle occupant. They also concluded that any injury to the low back is "quite unlikely as a result of a low velocity rear end collision." See 1995, SAE 952724. McConnell WE, Howard RP, Van Poppel J, et al. Human head and neck kinematics after low velocity rear-end impacts—understanding "Whiplash." Society of Automotive Engineers 1995;952724.

See also Castro WH, Schilgen M, Meyer S, Weber M, Peuker C, Wortler K. Do "whiplash injuries" occur in low-speed rear impacts? Eur Spine J. 1997;6(6):366–75.

Typically McConnell and related studies are used to support assertions of claims adjusters or defense experts, such as the following: The impact-related flexion and extension of the cervical spine and thoracic spine in this collision were well within the normal physiological range of movement. Thoracic or cervical sprain, which is injury to the ligaments, was found to be highly unlikely in this type of collision. The mild accident-related motion of the lumbar spine in this collision produces no significant differential forces along the lumbar spine. There is no direct injury mechanism for the lumbar spine, and lumbar strain or sprain is highly unlikely in this accident.

However, the studies are riddled with objectivity problems, as is discussed below, and are of questionable utility or reliability.

§ 14:5 McConnell studies (1993 & 1995)—Problems

The commonly cited studies lack enough objectivity to be useful in whiplash case, as the following points address:

1. The company that McConnell et al. worked for, Biodynamic Research Corp., received over $7.6 million from State Farm from 1990–95. See Superior Court State of Arizona, Maricopa County, Druz v. State Farm, 1997, CV 95-21280. The study was conducted by employees of the company and authors of the article, who testify throughout the country that you can't get hurt.

2. Interestingly, the 1995 McConnell study showed all the participants getting symptoms, suggesting that one can, in fact, get hurt under the best conditions. Whether or not that pain persists for a few hours, a few days, a few weeks, or a few months, depends on the uniqueness of the individual and other aspects of the uniqueness of the collision. This was a "movement of occupant" study and not a study to produce injury.

3. Testimony on studies such as McConnell have been excluded as unreliable in trial courts. See, e.g. *Clemente v. Blumenberg*, 183 Misc. 2d 923, 705 N.Y.S.2d 792 (Sup 1999) *("this court is of the opinion that the literature upon which the expert relies was not independent nor reliable."); Tittsworth v. Robinson*, 252 Va. 151, 475 S.E.2d 261 (1996); *Davis v. Maute*, 770 A.2d 36 (Del. 2001); *see also* Plaintiffs' Lawyers Guide to Minor Impact Cervical & Lumbar Injury (2002, Litigation One) Chapter 13: Overcoming Junk Science Defenses.

§ 14:6 Accident reconstruction damage analysis—Overview of method

In typical soft tissue cases, the defense will likely have sent the matter to a traffic collision reconstructionist and a biomechanist for evaluation. These experts will attempt to utilize formulas or other mathematical equations to "predict" injury, or lack thereof.

§ 14:7 Accident reconstruction damage analysis—Problems

In examining such witnesses, the attorney should have the accident reconstructionist provide the numbers and methodology used to reach his or her conclusions. Often the numbers are based on estimations, or mere guesswork. Determine whether the witness actually collected any measurements, or was merely provided with information from the insurance company or other interested party. The author of *Traffic Accident Reconstruction*, Volume 2, Lynn B. Fricke, said, "You might start to believe your answers are more accurate than they actually are, forgetting that many of the inputs are only slightly better than guesses. Clearly, this is a time to exercise caution and understand the limitation of your analysis." (Id. at 68–27.)

If the reconstructionist used a computer program to reach his or her conclusions, you should know such software assumes collision speeds of 20–50 mph, the ranges of speed of the vehicles that were crashed as stated by the author. Even the creator of one commonly used program, CRASH, states that it should not be used for collisions outside the rage of 10–40 mph Delta-V. Day T. Application and misapplication of computer programs for accident reconstruction. SAE 890738.

In one study, which measured the accuracy of accident reconstructionists, Bartlett et al. found a wide range of variation and uncertainty in measurements on common tasks. This is from trained ACRs doing measurements. See Bartlett W, Wright W, Masory O, Brach R, Baxter A, Schmidt, Navin F, Stanard T. Evaluating the uncertainty in various measurements tasks common to accident reconstruction. In Accident Reconstruction 2002. Warrendale, PA, SAE 2002-01-0546, 57–68, 2002.

Several appellate cases have excluded unreliable accident reconstruction testimony. See, e.g. *Clemente v. Blumenberg*, 183 Misc. 2d 923, 705 N.Y.S.2d 792 (Sup 1999) ("this court is of the opinion that the literature upon which the expert relies was not independent nor reliable."); *Tittsworth v. Robinson*, 252 Va. 151, 475 S.E.2d 261 (1996); *Davis v. Maute*, 770 A.2d 36 (Del. 2001); *see also*Plaintiffs' Lawyers Guide to Minor Impact Cervical & Lumbar Injury (2002, Litigation One) Chapter 13: Overcoming Junk Science Defenses.

Remember too that there is no true relationship of vehicle damage to occupant injury. Robbins, M.C. Lack of Relationship Between Vehicle Damage and Occupant Injury. Society of Automotive Engineers, 1997;970494, Detroit, MI. *See generally, Chapter 5, supra.*

§ 14:8 Accident reconstruction damage analysis—A note on bumper damage

A favorite area of testimony by accident reconstruction experts is to assert that a lack of damage to the vehicle bumper suggests that occupants could not have been injured. Legitimate experts now acknowledge that this testimony is a myth since, subsuent to 1973, bumpers were designed to absorb the impact forces, not to protect occupants.

In Plaintiffs' Lawyers Guide to Minor Impact Cervical & Lumbar Injury (Thomson West, 2007-2008) the author, an accident reconstruction expert, states:

> It is grossly inappropriate to deceive a jury into believing that an ostensibly undamaged bumper reflects the severity of a crash when in fact the design of the bumper is such that its purpose is to survive a substantial crash while exhibiting little residual damage. By law the bumper is supposed to protect the safety systems on the car, but in fact the bumper protects itself by virtue of is energy absorption capability. There is no validity to the argument that a jury should see a bumper photo because it reflects the damage to the car (or lack thereof).

See § 2:1, Chapter 2, The "Undamaged" Bumper Scam.

§ 14:9 Biomechanical injury analysis—Overview of method

The biomechanist will typically present data on the force that is needed to cause failure of a body part. The biomechanist will then state that this was not enough force to cause injury. Most of the testing is done by testing tissues to failure with quasi-static testing methods. This is done by applying a constant force (that is not as fast as the force during the trauma) on a cadaver or cadaver part. It is important to note that most injuries in whiplash are subfailure-not complete failure as in the biomechanic tests.

§ 14:10 Biomechanical injury analysis—Problems with findings

Also important to note in evaluating the biomechanic's findings is that the values cited may be averages for a vehicle. The values for the occupant can be 2 to 3 times that of the vehicle, which is often not mentioned. Peak values that may have a greater influence on injury are usually double that of the average value and also may not be mentioned. The biomechanist will attempt to state that the peak value is only for a few milliseconds and, therefore, doesn't matter. This ignores every value over the average and does not take into account what it may take to fire off the receptors in live humans.

There is a wide variation in human response and tolerance data. This is due to the large biological variations among humans and the effects of aging. Average values are useful in design, but cannot be applied to individuals. *See* King AI. Fundamentals of impact biomechanics: Part I—Biomechanics of the head, neck, and thorax. Annu Rev Biomed Eng. 2000;2:55–81. Additionally, the variables of real-world collisions are great. Some examples include: mass of vehicles, delta-V of target vehicle, make and model of vehicles, head-restraint type and position, crash pulse, mean acceleration and peak acceleration, genetic factors, previous injury, type of impact, head position at time of impact, preparedness for collision, and other factors.

In *Harrison v Smith*, 2008 WL 2673831 (Cal. App. 1st Dist. 2008), the plaintiff attorney had an expert look over the defense experts depositions and reports and write a declaration pointing out the errors. The trial judge then excluded the defense experts.

> A California Court of Appeal demolished a favorite tool used by insurance carriers to defeat low impact auto cases, in an unpublished opinion, reproduced here.
>
> In a personal injury action arising from a rear-end collision, the defendant offered expert testimony that the change in velocity of the plaintiff's vehicle caused by the collision was insufficient to cause the plaintiff's injuries. The trial court excluded the evidence under *People v. Kelly*, 17 Cal. 3d 24, 130 Cal. Rptr. 144, 549 P.2d 1240 (1976). We affirm.
>
> **Background**
>
> On December 10, 2003, Maria Harrison sued Phyllis H. Smith for injuries she allegedly incurred when Smith rear-ended her car while she was stopped at an intersection. Harrison's treating physicians diagnosed her with the following injuries that they said resulted from the accident: a herniated disk in her neck, superimposed on a pre-existing degenerative spine, chronic neck and back pain, and headaches. Smith retained two experts to testify that the accident could not have caused those injuries

because the change in velocity ("delta v") in Harrison's car as a result of the collision was below a minimum threshold for causing such injuries.

Harrison moved to exclude or limit the testimony of the defense experts, Jeffrey Lotz, Ph.D. and Paul Mills, M.D. She argued that the proffered opinions were based on "junk science" that was "taken directly from the 'playbook' followed increasingly by the insurance industry in personal injury litigation across the country." Because the "delta v method" was not generally accepted in the scientific community, the proffered testimony based on that technique was inadmissible under *Kelly, supra*, 17 Cal. 3d at page 30, 130 Cal. Rptr. 144, 549 P.2d 1240. She also argued that Lotz and Mills were not qualified to render the opinions they proffered. Smith opposed the motion.

The trial court ruled that Smith had failed to meet her burden of establishing that the delta v method was generally accepted within the scientific community. The court excluded all expert testimony based on that method.

The case was tried to a jury, which returned special verdicts finding Smith was negligent and her negligence was a substantial factor in causing harm to Harrison. The jury awarded Harrison $79,000 in past economic losses, and $70,000 in past pain and suffering, but nothing for future losses. The court entered judgment March 15, 2006. Smith moved for a new trial on April 7, 2006, based in part on the exclusion of the experts' testimony. The court denied the motion on May 18, 2006. Smith appeals from the judgment and the order denying her motion for a new trial.

DISCUSSION

Expert testimony based on a new scientific technique is admissible if (1) the reliability of the method is established, usually by expert testimony; (2) the expert is qualified to give an opinion on the subject; and (3) correct scientific procedures were used in the particular case. (*People v. Leahy*, 8 Cal. 4th 587, 594, 34 Cal. Rptr.2d 663, 882 P.2d 321 (1994), applying *Kelly*.)The testimony is deemed reliable if the scientific technique on which it is based is "sufficiently established to have gained general acceptance in the particular field in which it belongs.[Citation.]" (*Leahy*, at p. 594, 34 Cal. Rptr.2d 663, 882 P.2d 321.)

The reason for the *Kelly* general acceptance standard is that "[l]ay jurors tend to give considerable weight to 'scientific' evidence when presented by 'experts' with impressive credentials. We have acknowledged the existence of a '... misleading aura of certainty which often envelops a new scientific process, obscuring its currently experimental nature." (*Kelly, supra*, 17 Cal. 3d at pp. 31-32, 130 Cal. Rptr. 144, 549 P.2d 1240.) Although this approach delays the admission of evidence derived from valid new scientific techniques during "an undefined period of testing and study by a community of experts," it assures that judges and juries with little or no scientific background will not attempt to resolve technical questions on which experts cannot even reach a consensus. (*Leahy, supra*, 8 Cal. 4th at pp. 601-603, 34 Cal. Rptr.2d 663, 882 P.2d 321; see also Kelly, at p. 31, 130 Cal. Rptr. 144, 549 P.2d 1240.) The Kelly rule also promotes uniformity of decision. (*Leahy*, at p. 595, 34 Cal. Rptr. 2d 663, 882 P.2d 321.) "[O]nce a trial court has admitted evidence derived from a new technique and the decision is affirmed on appeal in a published opinion, it will become precedent controlling subsequent trials," and each trial court need not confront the issue de novo. (*Leahy* at pp. 595, 603, 34 Cal. Rptr. 2d 663, 882 P.2d 321.)

"Just when a scientific principle or discovery crosses the line between the experimental and demonstrable stages is difficult to define. Somewhere in this twilight zone the evidential force of the principle must be recognized...." (*Kelly*, supra, 17 Cal. 3d at p. 30, 130 Cal. Rptr. 144, 549 P.2d 1240.) The proponent of the evidence bears the burden of establishing general acceptance in the relevant scientific community, not necessarily the scientific reliability of the technique. (*Leahy*, supra, 8 Cal. 4th at p. 611, 34 Cal. Rptr. 2d 663, 882 P.2d 321.) On appeal, general acceptance is a mixed question of law and fact subject to "limited de novo review." (*People v. Reilly*, 196 Cal. App. 3d 1127, 1134, 242 Cal. Rptr. 496 (1987).) Our review is not limited to determining whether a finding of general acceptance is supported by substantial evidence; rather, we undertake "a more searching review-one that is sometimes not confined to the record." (Ibid.) We consider not only the expert testimony that was presented in the trial court, but scientific literature and decisions from other jurisdictions on the question of consensus, "bearing in mind that the needed consensus is that of scientists, not courts." (*People v. Reilly* at pp. 1134-1135, 242 Cal. Rptr. 496.) We must consider both the quality and the quantity of the evidence supporting or opposing the technique. (*Leahy*, at p. 612, 34 Cal. Rptr. 2d 663, 882 P.2d 321.)

I. *The Delta v. Method*

We first set forth the proffered expert testimony. At his deposition, Lotz testified that he planned to express the following opinions at trial:

1. The change in velocity for Harrison's vehicle as a result of the collision was between three and four miles per hour.

2. An accident of that magnitude produces forces on the lumbar spine (low back) that are within the range of those incurred in activities of daily living, do not cause excessive movement or stress on the lumbar spine, and would not be consistent with any acute injury to the lumbar spine.

3. The range of motion of the cervical spine (neck) in a rear-end accident of this magnitude is not exceeded and consequently the risk for hyperextension or injury to the disks of the cervical spine is not exceeded in this accident. The lowest change of velocity that could cause disk herniation to the cervical spine was eight miles per hour.

4. The acceleration forces produced in a rear-end accident of this magnitude are comparable to those of activities of daily living and would not be consistent with a concussion or post-concussive syndrome (head injury).

In summary, it was not likely that Harrison suffered injury other than temporary muscle strain as a result of the accident. "[H]ead, neck and low-back injuries are not likely to occur because of the reasons we have discussed."

Similarly, Dr. Mills averred that he would testify about "the likelihood of injury, for a person of average physiology, resulting from a 3-5 m.p.h. collision. In my opinion, Ms. Harrison suffered no physiologic injury from which she would not be expected to recover with or without treatment in a matter of 3-4 weeks."[1]

Lotz testified that his opinions were based on "studies which relate certain injuries or symptoms to accidents of this magnitude."He specifically cited his own research into the mechanical factors that produce disk injury, biomechanical tests performed on cadavers or animals to help define injury tolerance, studies of human volunteers who experienced rear-end accidents, studies of movements and acceleration forces in the heads of occupants of rear-ended vehicles, and data collected in anthropometric dummies in staged rear-end collisions that focused on head accelerations and low back forces. He explained that based on his review of Harrison's medical records and information he had about her accident, "I don't see anything that creates a reason that she would be different from the literature, or her tolerance for injury would be significantly different. [¶] So I would be comfortable saying that it's more likely than not, from a biomechanical standpoint, that the forces would not have produced an injury in the plaintiff."

We shall refer to the scientific technique described by Lotz as "the delta v method": a method of determining the probability from a low-speed rear-end collision based on the change of velocity in the target vehicle, using data collected in studies of the effects of similar impacts on human volunteers, test dummies, and cadavers.

II. *Applicability of Kelly Test*

For the first time at oral argument, Smith argued that the trial court should not have subjected the delta v method to a *Kelly, supra*, 17 Cal. 3d 24, 130 Cal. Rptr. 144, 549 P.2d 1240, general

[Section 14:10]

[1]Mills testified at his deposition that his opinion was based on his training and experience as an orthopedist, professional meetings, textbooks, and literature regarding the typical course of events after rear-end collisions. The trial court ruled that Mills could not testify about the relationship between delta v and medical causation. He was permitted to testify, and he did testify at trial, regarding his professional opinion as an orthopedist regarding the extent of Harrison's injuries and whether they were caused by trauma.

acceptance test. Smith did not raise this argument in the trial court or in her opening or reply briefs on appeal. The issue is forfeited.[2] (*Ward v. Taggart*, 51 Cal. 2d 736, 742, 336 P.2d 534 (1959); *REO Broadcasting Consultants v. Martin*, 69 Cal. App. 4th 489, 500, 81 Cal. Rptr. 2d 639 (1999).)

In any event, it appears that *Kelly* was the appropriate standard. *Kelly* applies only to new scientific techniques. (*Leahy, supra*, 8 Cal. 4th at p. 605, 34 Cal. Rptr. 2d 663, 882 P.2d 321.) The method is "new" within the meaning of *Kelly* when it "is new to science and, even more so, the law." (Ibid.) The court will look to whether the technique has been the subject of "repeated use, study, testing and *confirmation* by scientists or trained technicians." (Ibid., italics added.) The method is "scientific" because it is based on an experimental process whereby theories are proposed, tested and refined. (See *Whiting v. Coultrip*, 324 Ill. App. 3d 161 (2001) [755 N.E. 2d 494, 498], quoting *Daubert v.*

---

[2]Smith argues that Dr. Lotz's testimony based on his own studies should have been admitted without a showing of general acceptance. She cites cases holding that expert testimony based on personal evaluations of a patient or the subject matter of the expert's testimony are not subject to the *Kelly* test for admissibility. (*Wilson v. Phillips* (1999) 73 Cal. App. 4th 250, 254-256, 86 Cal. Rptr. 2d 204 [psychologist's testimony, based on evaluation of plaintiffs who claimed based on repressed memories that they were sexually molested as children, that plaintiffs' profiles and testimony were consistent with persons who recover repressed memories was not subject to *Kelly* test]; *Arreola v. County of Monterey* (2002) 99 Cal. App. 4th 722, 749-750 & fn. 9, 122 Cal. Rptr.2d 38 [geologist's testimony regarding the likely water flows at the site of a levee that failed during a rainstorm was not subject to *Kelly* test].)

These cases are inapplicable here. Dr. Lotz's personal studies did not involve Harrison or the particular circumstances of Harrison's accident. Rather, they were general studies on "how movement of the spine and forces that are distributed amongst the disks and the facet joints during movement are altered by disk replacement" in order to design devices to replace intervertebral disks; studies of mechanical and other factors influencing disk degeneration based on animal models; studies of how loading influences disk degeneration; studies of compression-induced disk degeneration; a series of studies of tissue properties of the disk relevant to hyperextension or hyperflexion injuries; and studies measuring forces on anthropometric dummies in staged car crashes. The studies are simply part of the body of scientific literature on which the delta v method is based. Smith cites no authority that expert testimony based on the expert's own research into a new scientific technique would be admissible even without a showing of general acceptance. Such a result would contradict the rationale of Kelly, that scientific techniques that are still in a stage of experimentation and scientific debate should not be presented to a jury. (*Leahy, supra*, 8 Cal. 4th at pp. 594-595, 34 Cal. Rptr.2d 663, 882 P.2d 321.)

Further, Smith suggests, without developing the argument, that the court should have allowed Lotz to testify, at least, to the speed of the vehicle. This suggestion was never made in the trial court, nor has Smith established here that this, more-narrow technique passes a *Kelly* analysis.

Merrell Dow Pharmaceuticals, Inc. (1993) 509 U.S. 579, 590, 113 S. Ct. 2786, 125 L. Ed. 2d 469; *Leahy*, at p. 607, 34 Cal. Rptr. 2d 663, 882 P.2d 321.)

Here, the delta v method is relatively new to the law, as we discuss in more detail in section V below. As Lotz testified, the studies on which he relied employed the scientific method. Finally, Lotz's testimony raises the dangers the *Kelly* test is designed to prevent: it is cloaked in scientific terminology such as "delta v" and "g forces" and bolstered by references to scientific studies the jury has no way to evaluate. (See *Leahy*, at pp. 606-607, 34 Cal. Rptr. 2d 663, 882 P.2d 321.)

III. *Smith's Showing in the Trial Court*

Smith did not meet her burden of proof in the trial court of establishing that the delta v method is generally accepted in the relevant scientific community. Indeed, Smith barely presented any argument on the issue.

Harrison challenged both the general acceptance of the delta v method and the qualifications of Smith's experts in her motion to exclude or limit the experts' testimony. In her opposition to the motion, Smith responded only to the argument regarding her experts' qualifications. It is true that in the context of defending Lotz's qualifications Smith argued that "[b]iomechanical causation is not 'junk science.' " However, she never stated that the delta v method was generally accepted in the scientific community; she cited no evidence tending to show general acceptance; and she did not cite the governing legal standard established in *Kelly*. Indeed, she cited no legal authority whatsoever in her opposition to Harrison's motion. At the hearing on the motion, the trial court invited defense counsel to cite legal authority supporting Smith's position, but counsel responded that he could not. The court also asked whether Smith had cited scientific literature showing the delta v method was generally accepted. Defense counsel responded by discussing a single article that had been submitted by Harrison.

Having failed to address the general acceptance argument, discuss any relevant legal authority, or cite expert testimony or scientific literature regarding the general acceptance of the method, Smith cannot reasonably contend that she met her burden of proof. Because she did not meet the argument in the trial court, Smith has forfeited her claim on appeal. Nevertheless, we will review the expert testimony and scientific literature in the record on the general acceptance of the delta v method as well as the state of the case law on the issue. These sources also fail to demonstrate that the method has achieved general acceptance in the scientific community.

IV. *State of the Evidentiary Record*

It appears from the record that many studies have been conducted to measure forces that are created in low-speed rear-end automobile collisions on an occupant of the struck vehicle and to assess what injuries those forces can cause in the human body. However, it does not follow that Lotz's proffered testimony is based on a scientific technique that is generally accepted in the scientific community.[3] First, as discussed in greater detail below, the purpose and focus of most if not all of these studies is to design car seats and head restraints and not to rule out to a high degree of probability whether a particular injury was caused by a particular automobile collision. Second, the studies, insofar as they are described in the record, do not indicate that the scientific community has come to a consensus on the correlation between change in velocity in a target vehicle and the probability of injury to an occupant of that vehicle.

Lotz averred that "[t]here are over 700 articles in the peer-reviewed medical literature that report studies on forces generated within the spine, define the biomechanical strength of spinal tissues, and describe techniques to estimate the body's ability to resist acute musculoskeletal injury." He stated that delta v "is a well accepted standard metric for accident severity." However, he never states that it is generally accepted in the scientific community that these studies provide a reliable foundation on which to assess the probability of injury to an occupant of a vehicle struck in the rear based on the change in velocity of the target vehicle.

Lotz does not provide enough information about the studies to allow us to determine if they establish general acceptance of the delta v method in the scientific community. He does not identify the 700 studies (or a subset of them) or provide copies of them. He acknowledges that many of the studies were generated for different purposes, "such as to develop techniques to prevent and evaluate risk for age-and occupation-related injuries, design medical implants, help surgeons develop treatments for back pain, and help the automotive industry design safer vehicles." At his deposition, Lotz provided a list of 17 studies he claimed supported his opinion, but Smith did not submit copies of those studies to the trial court. His general reference to these studies does not satisfy Smith's burden.

The five published studies that were submitted to the trial court by Harrison also do not demonstrate general acceptance of the delta v method. Instead, the studies, which were conducted for a variety of purposes, suggest that the research into the relationship between change in velocity and injury is in a stage of ongoing experimentation and has not reached a stage of general

[3]In his deposition testimony, Smith said the delta v method was generally accepted in the scientific community because it was based on the scientific method. As explained in Section II above, this fact brings the method within the rule of *Kelly* and does not in itself establish general acceptance.

acceptance. The 1998 Cappon study,[4] for example, discusses the *development* of *testing methods* (primarily a dummy) to assess the protection offered by seat and head restraint systems in rear-end collisions. The paper presents only preliminary findings and specifically states that further study is needed. The 2001 Shimamoto study[5] also discusses the development of a dummy to assess cervical behavior in low-speed rear-end collisions. The conclusion states, "We conclude that the [new model] holds *great promise* as a tool for exposing the mechanism that causes neck injury...." (Italics added.) The 1996 Krafft study[6] states that whiplash "injury as well as the mechanism of the injury are still in many ways unknown. [¶] The purpose of this article is to add different factors that contribute to the knowledge of the origin of this injury." The 1999 Lee study abstract[7] criticizes the " 'one size fits all' " and " 'hard threshold' " approaches often adopted in biomechanical analysis of injury causation and proposes a more comprehensive approach that takes into account "the wide variability in biomechanical data." The 2005 Freeman study[8] compares roller coaster injury data with "*contemporary efforts* to define a lower limit of acceleration below which no significant spinal injury is likely to occur." (Italics added.) The study concludes that "there is no established minimum threshold of significant spine injury. The greatest explanation for injury from traumatic loading of the spine is individual susceptibility to injury, an unpredictable variable."

The scientific literature in the record, therefore, does not demonstrate that there is general acceptance in the scientific community of a particular correlation between change in velocity and probability of human injury. Rather, it appears that the relationship between these factors is currently the subject of experimentation and debate within the scientific community. It may be that the current studies are valid and the correlation will one day gain general acceptance in the community. However, until that occurs, expert testimony based on the experimental data is not admissible at trial.

---

[4]Cappon et al., "A New Test Method for the Assessment of Neck Injuries in Rear-End Collisions," 16th International Technical Conference on the Enhanced Safety of Vehicles (1998) vol. 2, paper # 242.

[5]Shimamoto et al., "Developing Experimental Cervical Dummy Models for Testing Low-Speed Rear-End Collisions," National Highway Traffic Safety Administration RDW, Amsterdam 2001, paper 98-S9-O-10.

[6]Krafft et al., "Whiplash Associated DisorderFactors Influencing the Incidence in Rear-End Collisions," The Fifteenth International Technical Conference on Enhanced Safety of Vehicles (1996) paper 96-S9-O-09.

[7]William E. Lee III, "Biomechanical Analysis and Injury Causation: An Individual-specific and Incident-specific Approach," Association for the Advancement of Automotive Medicine, 43rd Annual Proceedings (1999).

[8]Freeman et al., "Significant Spinal Injury Resulting from Low-Level Accelerations: A case Series of Roller Coaster Injuries," Arch Phys Med Rehab Vol 86 (2005).

V. *State of the Case Law*

Court decisions from other jurisdictions on the admissibility of expert testimony based on the delta v method or similar biomechanical methods fail to demonstrate that the methods have gained general acceptance in the scientific community.[9]

First, all of the decisions that have come to our attention have been published in the last 12 years,[10] which alone suggests that the investigation into a correlation between change of velocity and the possibility of injury is a relatively recent undertaking. Because it takes time for a scientific method to gain general acceptance, the short life of the methodology tends to support a determination that the methodology has not yet achieved general acceptance in the scientific community.

Second, we have reviewed the decisions for discussions of scientific literature on the reliability of the delta v method and have found no indication that the literature reflects general acceptance of the method. Rather, we found commentary to the contrary. A Colorado appellate court, affirming a trial court's finding that scientific studies failed to establish general acceptance of the delta v method, wrote that "there is no agreement, far from it, in the engineering field or in the automobile industry concerning whether there is such a threshold [of injury]." (*Schultz v. Wells* (Colo. Ct. App. 2000) 13 P.3d 846, 852.) A Georgia appellate court wrote, "We find limited evidence in the record that the field of biomechanics includes a technique of determining if specific injuries result from specific accidents, let alone that the technique has reached a scientific stage of verifiable certainty. Simply mentioning that there have been 'cadaver tests' or that volunteers have been filmed in low-speed accidents does not answer the question."(*Cromer v. Mulkey Enterprises, Inc.* (2002) 254 Ga. App. 388 [562 S.E. 2d 783, 787].) A New Jersey court that reviewed 17 studies submitted in support of an expert's testimony wrote: "The record does not establish that experts in the field 'accept the soundness of the methodology, including the reasonableness of relying on this type of underlying data and information.' [Citation.]"[11] (*Hisenaj v. Kuehner* (2006) 387 N.J. Super. 262 [903 A. 2d 1068, 1077] (Hisenaj I), reversed on other

---

[9]There are no published California opinions on this issue. In *People v. Roehler*, the court held that expert testimony based on a biomechanical study (but not the delta v method) was admissible under *Kelly*, but the case is distinguishable because the study was specifically designed and carried out to reflect the actual conditions of the case on trial. (*People v. Roehler* (1985) 167 Cal. App. 3d 353, 387-390, 213 Cal. Rptr. 353.)

[10]The earliest case is *Tittsworth v. Robinson* (1996) 252 Va. 151 [475 S.E. 2d 261] [evidence excluded].

[11]The court in *Hisenaj* also commented that the record "contains no evidence that the seventeen studies are generally recognized and relied upon in the scientific community as authoritative. There is no evidence that they were peer reviewed.... The record is barren of any evidence that the seventeen

grounds by *Hisenaj v. Kuehner* (2008) 194 N.J. 6 [942 A.2d 769] (Hisenaj II); see also Eskin v. Carden (Del. 2004) 842 A. 2d 1222, 1231.)

Other courts that have reviewed studies submitted in support of the method have concluded that the studies were facially unreliable. A New York trial court found that four studies cited by an expert were facially unreliable because they were based on small samples, they involved human volunteers who were associated with the authors or sponsors of the studies, and they inappropriately attempted to "boot-strap" data from other studies using similar but different control variables and methodology in order to overcome the inadequate sample sizes. (*Clemente v. Blumenberg* (1999) 183 Misc.2d 923, 705 N.Y.S. 2d 792, 795 & fn. 2 [183 Misc.2d 923].) A New Jersey court similarly criticized studies that had been described by the expert because they were performed on cadavers or military personnel under controlled conditions dissimilar from an automobile accident and did not support a conclusion that the particular accident in question could not cause the particular plaintiff's particular injuries. (*Suanez v. Egeland* (2002) 353 N.J. Super. 191 [801 A. 2d 1186, 1193]; see also *Hisenaj I, supra*, 903 A. 2d at pp. 1075-1077.)

Third, two of three decisions applying a legal standard comparable to the *Kelly* general acceptance standard[12] deemed expert testimony based on the delta v method inadmissible. (*Clemente v. Blumenberg, supra*, 183 Misc. 2d 923, 705 N.Y.S. 2d 792, 795 & fn. 2; *Whiting v. Coultrip, supra*, 324 Ill. App. 3d 161, 258 Ill. Dec. 111, 755 N.E.2d 494.)[13] We find the third decision, which deemed the testimony admissible, unpersuasive. Although the reviewing court purported to make a general acceptance determination, it actually conducted a review of the expert's qualifications. (*Ma'ele v. Arrington* (Wa. Ct. App. 2002) 111 Wash. App. 557, 45 P. 3d 557, 560.)[14]

Fourth, two decisions from New Jersey extensively examined ev-

---

studies are fairly representative of the prevailing results for these kinds of tests. The record contains no evidence that the size of the data base, 203 subjects over a thirty-four year period, is sufficient to be scientifically and statistically significant."(*Hisenaj v. Kuehner, supra*, 903 A. 2d at pp. 1074-1075.)

[12] Each of these decisions applies the legal standards of *Frye v. United States* (D.C. Cir. 1923) 293 F.1013, on which *Kelly* was based. (*Kelly, supra*, 17 Cal. 3d at p. 30, 130 Cal. Rptr. 144, 549 P.2d 1240; *Leahy, supra*, 8 Cal. 4th at p. 594, 34 Cal. Rptr. 2d 663, 882 P. 2d 321.)

[13] Although *Valentine v. Grossman* also refers to the *Frye* standard, the basis for the trial court's admission of the evidence and the court of appeal's reversal was the relevance of the testimony. (*Valentine v. Grossman* (2001) 283 A.D. 2d 571, 724 N.Y.S. 2d 504, 505-506.) *Valentine* does not rule on the general acceptance of the scientific technique underlying the expert's testimony.

[14] "Tencer has been studying low-speed impacts for five years. His conclusions have been 'pretty much' accepted. [ ] He teaches at the University of

idence produced in support of the delta v method and concluded expert testimony based on the method was inadmissible under a standard similar to the Kelly and Frye standards: "scientific evidence is admissible in a civil case if 'it derives from a reliable methodology supported by some expert consensus.'" (*Suanez v. Egeland, supra*, 801 A. 2d at p. 1189; *Hisenaj I, supra*, 903 A. 2d at p. 1073.) Although *Hisenaj I* was reversed by the New Jersey Supreme Court, the reversal was based on the standard of review. (*Hisenaj II, supra*, 942 A. 2d at pp. 779-780.) The supreme court held that the appellate court erred by augmenting the appellate record with copies of the studies cited by the expert, which had not been admitted into evidence in the trial court, and by not deferring to the trial court's exercise of its discretion. (*Ibid.*) The court specifically stated that it was not disagreeing with the appellate court's assessment of the reliability of the expert testimony or its underlying methodology: "[W]e recognize that the relationship between the studies and literature on which [the expert] relied and [the expert's] opinions in this matter could be attacked as tenuous.... However, we are compelled to restrict ourselves to the record made before the trial court." (*Id.* at pp. 779-780.)

Finally, several other decisions applying standards different from the *Kelly* and *Frye* standards have held that expert testimony based on the delta v method or similar methods was inadmissible because the methods had not been established as a reliable foundation for an expert opinion on whether a particular plaintiff's injuries were caused by a particular accident. (*Tittsworth v. Robinson, supra*, 252 Va. 151 [475 S.E. 2d at p. 263] [general standards for admission of expert testimony]; *Smelser v. Norfolk Southern Ry. Co.* (6th Cir.1997) 105 F. 3d 299, 301, 303, 305 [applying standard of *Daubert, supra*, 509 U.S. 579]; *Davis v. Martel* (La. Ct. App. 2001) 790 So. 2d 767, 771-772 [applying *Daubert* standard]; *Eskin v. Carden, supra*, 842 A. 2d at p. 1231 [applying *Daubert* standard]; see also *Schultz v. Wells, supra*, 13 P. 3d at pp. 851-852 [exclusion was not an abuse of discretion]; *Cromer v. Mulkey Enterprises, Inc., supra*, 254 Ga. App. 393 [562 S.E. 2d 783, 787] [same]; *Martin v. Sally* (2003) 341 Ill. App. 3d 308 [792 N.E. 2d 516, 522-523] [testimony not relevant because it addressed generalities derived from studies, not plaintiff's particular circumstances].) There are also decisions holding such evidence admissible under these different standards, with the courts often commenting that it should be left to the jury to decide how much weight to give the evidence. (*Fussell*

Washington Medical School, he has received a federal grant for his research, and he has written a number of articles about the likelihood of injuries in low-speed accidents. Although [ ], a chiropractor, testified differently about the forces involved in low-speed collisions, other researchers around the world have reached conclusions similar to Tencer. The trial court did not err in ruling that Tencer's work on low-speed collisions is generally accepted in the scientific community."(*Mae'le, supra*, 45 P.3d at p. 560.)

v. Roadrunner Towing and Recovery (La. Ct. App. 2000) 765 So.2d 373, 377 [applying *Daubert* standard; "Any alleged failure... in the analysis or conclusion provides a basis for attack by plaintiffs' cross-examination"]; *Reali v. Mazda Motor of America, Inc.* (D. Me. 2000) 106 F. Supp. 2d 75, 77 [admitted in part under *Daubert*; criticisms "go to credibility, not admissibility"]; *Valentine v. Grossman, supra*, 724 N.Y.S. 2d at pp. 505-506 [relevance]; *Wilson v. Rivers* (2004) 357 S.C. 447 [593 S.E. 2d 603, 605-606 & fn. 5] [applying abuse of discretion standard and clarifying that court had not addressed reliability of expert's methodology].) The California Supreme Court has expressly rejected such an approach. (*Leahy, supra*, 8 Cal. 4th at pp. 601-604, 34 Cal. Rptr.2d 663, 882 P.2d 321.)

DISPOSITION

On the record before us, we find no error in the trial court's refusal to allow appellant to present evidence of the delta v method. The judgment is affirmed. Harrison shall receive her costs on appeal.

Delta-V and Injury

In a whiplash type collision, the dynamic loads generated in the cervical spine are more complex than previously thought. Within the physiological range of cervical motion, considerable shear load was partially produced in the cervical spine, and was able to create micro-injury of soft tissues. This **mechanical model cannot predict the tolerances of the neck structures and injury criteria**.

Matsushita T, Yamazaki N, Sato T, Hirabayashi K. Biomechanical and medical investigations of human neck injury in low-velocity collisions. Neuro-Orthopedics 1997; 21:27–45.

Davis CG. Injury threshold: whiplash-associated disorders. J Manipulative Physiol Ther. 2000 Jul-Aug;23 (6):420.

Note that commentators of these types of tests have pointed out that factors other than selected peak kinematic responses influenced symptom production. **No one parameter was sufficiently strong to successfully predict symptoms.** Extrapolation of the current model outside these test conditions, injury types and injury severities may be inappropriate. The results of this analysis were based on controlled human subjects tests using one vehicle, one seat, and one seated posture. Siegmund GP, Brault JR, Wheeler JB. The relationship between clinical and kinematic responses from human subject testing in rear-end automobile collisions. Accid Anal Prev. 2000 Mar;32(2):207–17.

Studies have shown that one cannot depend on one variable to determine if an injury will occur. **Injury cannot be reliably predicted by knowing the Delta-V**.

Krafft M, Kullgren A, Tin gvall C, Bostrom O, Fredriksson R. How crash severity in rear impacts influences short- and long-term consequences to the neck. Accid Anal Prev. 2000 Mar;32(2):187–95.

The mean acceleration magnitude demonstrated a better correlation with symptom duration, and that the **change of velocity could be misleading predictor of injury**.

Krafft M. When do AIS 1 neck injuries result in long-term consequences? Vehicle and human factors. Traffic Inj. Prev. 2002;3: 89–97.

In a study by of 66 real-life rear-impact crashes were analyzed. They found **no significant correlation** between whiplash associated disorders and crash severity.

Krafft M, Kullgren A, Ydenius A, Tingval, C. Influence of crash pulse characteristics on whiplash associated disorders in rear impacts—crash recording in real life crashes. Traffic Inj. Prev. 2002;3: 141–149.

This notion of **low correlation between grade of whiplash associated disorders and severity of insult** was also found in a study relating hockey injuries to whiplash-associated disorders.

Hynes LM, Dickey JP. Is there a relationship between whiplash associated disorders and concussion in hockey? A preliminary study. Brain Inj. 2006;20:179–188.

Two acceleration levels of the same value can have different jerk values; the rate of change of the acceleration will vary depending on how quickly the peak acceleration is achieved. We show that a peak acceleration of 4.5 g coupled with a jerk of 200 m/s^2 is very different than the resulting head accelerations at a peak acceleration of 4.5 g with a jerk of 400 m/s^2.

Jerk is a parameter that must be evaluated independently of the acceleration level, just like velocity and acceleration. Studies have reported inconsistencies between the two dummies and the human occupant head acceleration responses in the vertical direction at the two different velocities. This lends support to the concept that the kinematic responses of human volunteer subjects are **dependant upon several parameters** and that all pertinent parameters need to be taken into consideration when predicting human responses. As well, caution should be taken when making predictions of injury from extrapolations of data collected at low velocities.

Hynes LM, Dickey JP. The rate of change of acceleration: implications to head kinematics during rear-end impacts. Accid Anal Prev. 2008 May;40(3):1063–8.

Change of velocity (?v), as an estimate of the impact severity, was **not related** to residual problems, neither after frontal (p=0.4), nor rear-end impacts (p=0.5), not even in subjects without any previous neck problems. A "stiff" impact pulse caused residual problems of non-minor grade in 20% of the subjects, without any difference between frontal and rear-end impacts.

The mean delta V of the frontal crashes was 8.1 mph and for the rear impacts is was 5 mph. This is particularly interesting in light of the commonly held belief that the threshold for whiplash injury is a delta V of 5 mph. **The secondary common misconception that is a more or less linear relationship exists between crash speed and injury risk and severity. The authors found a very poor relationship and, in many cases, a reverse relationship**. There also was no correlation between crash speed and time of onset of symptoms.

Bunketorp O, Jakobsson L, Norin H. Comparison of frontal and rear-end impacts for car occupants with whiplash associated disorders: symptoms and clinical findings. IRCOBI Conference — Graz (Austria) September 2004:245–256.

No correlation was found between the impact speed, speed of vehicle struck, with the Neck Disabilty Index.

Crouch R, Whitewick R, Clancy M, Wright P, Thomas P. Whiplash associated disorder: incidence and natural history over the first month for patients presenting to a UK emergency department. Emerg Med J. 2006 Feb;23(2):114–8

Siegmund found that **it is impossible to accurately predict occupant accelerations**, even when the actual accelerations of the vehicle are measured during the test collision.

Peak head accelerations varied widely between the studies, (Severy, Mertz, McConnell, Szabo, Matsushita, Siegmund).

The peak head acceleration at 8–10 km/h (about 5 mph) ranged from 5.0 to 16.6 g.

Siegmund GP, King DJ, Lawrence JM, Wheeler JB, Brault JR, Smith TA. Head/neck kinematic response of human subjects in low-speed rear-end collisions. Society of Automotive Engineers 1997; 973341.

Substantially similar

Where tests are involved, such testimony should be excluded unless there is proof that the conditions existing at the time of the tests and at the time relevant to the facts at issue are substantially similar.

Tarmac Mid-Atlantic, Inc., (1995)250 Va. at 166, 458 S.E.2d at 466;

Runyon v. Geldner, (1989) 237 Va. 460, 463–64, 377 S.E.2d 456, 458–59.

Francis v. Sauve (1963) 222 Cal.App.2d 102, 114–115 [34 Cal.Rptr. 754];

Rudat v. Carithers (1934) 137 Cal.App. 92, 95–97 [30 P.2d 435];

Johnston v. Peairs (1931) 117 Cal.App. 208, 215–216 [3 P.2d 617];

Fishman v. Silva (1931) 116 Cal.App. 1, 8–9 [2 P.2d 473].

Beresford v. Pacific Gas & Elec. Co. (1955) 45 Cal.2d 738 at 749;

Culpepper v. Volkswagen of American, Inc. (1973) 33 Cal. App. 3d 510, at 521.

Different cars have different injury risks. The type of vehicle involve may have an injury risk of 4–5 times higher than another type of vehicle.

Koch M, Kullgren A, Lie A, Nygren A, Tingvall C. Soft tissue injury of the cervical spine in rear-end and frontal car collisions. IRCOBI 1995; 273–83

§ 14:11 Mertz and Patrick (SAE 1967 & 1971)—Overview of studies

The studies by Mertz & Patrick (1967 & 1971) attempted to determine an injury threshold corridor. They based their study on several cadavers and one live volunteer (the author—Patrick). They tested by seeking to find torque at the occipital condyle. With this torque they examined X-rays of the cadaver, noting damage at the C3–4 level. *Mertz HJ Jr, Patrick LM. Investigation of the kinematics and kinetics of whiplash. In Proceedings, 11th Stapp Car Crash Conference, SAE 670919, Detroit MI, Society of Automotive Engineers, 1967; Mertz HJ Jr, Patrick LM. Strength and response of the human neck. In Proceeding 15th Stapp Car Crash Conference, SAE 710855, Warrendale, Pa, 1971.*

They measured the torque at the occipital condyle to tell if there was ligament damage at C3–4. Mertz & Patrick's estimated 42 foot-pounds of torque to ligament damage was for a 50th percentile male, not a women. The cadaver they used sustained ligament damage at C3–C4 at torque of 24.6 foot-pounds. Then they scaled up to measure Patrick based on the greater estimated weight of his head.

To arrive at the 35 foot-pounds of torque as supposedly non-injurious dynamic value, Patrick merely doubled his own static neck strength of 17.5 foot-pounds. Static neck strength means the ability of the neck to resist bending when placed in a fixture containing a pulley mechanism that pulls on the head with increasing force until the neck begins to bend because the neck muscles can no longer resist the force applied to the head.

§ 14:12 Mertz and Patrick (SAE 1967 & 1971)—Problems with studies

Mertz and Patrick also stated in their article that shear forces were not that important to cause injury. It is now known that shear forces are important, and that the muscle activation would occur too late to have any effect on the unaware subject.

In a real life trauma, the joints of the cervical spine undergo maximum deformation during the early part of the whiplash acceleration when the muscle tone activations are minimal or absent. See Deng B, Begeman P, Yang K, et al. Kinematics of human cadaver cervical spine during low speed rear-end impacts. Stapp Car Crash J. 2000;171–88.

It takes some time for the muscle to contact and have enough force to resist movement. Laboratory studies using animals have demonstrated the time to develop muscle forces to be approximately 200 msec. The reaction time of the experimental animal is shorter than that of the human. Tennyson SA, Mital NK, King AI. Electromyographic signals of the spinal musculature during +Gz impact acceleration. Orthop Clin North Am. 1977 Jan;8(1):97–119.

§ 14:13 Mertz and Patrick (SAE 1967 & 1971)—A note on X-rays

Note that in the Mertz and Patrick studies, "X-rays were taken of the cadaver's neck to determine whether a particular sled ride caused any observable neck damage." (Mertz and Patrick, 1971, pg. 234). We now know that X-rays do not detect most lesions. See the following:

In detecting spine lesions, ". . . radiography identified the least number of lesions." Yoganandan N, Cusick JF, Pintar FA, Rao RD. Whiplash injury determination with conventional spine imaging and cryomicrotomy. Spine. 2001 Nov 15;26(22):2443–8.

Most injuries are not seen on plain film X-rays. Only 4 of 245 bone and discoligamentus lesions were detected by X-ray.

Jonsson H Jr, Bring G, Rauschning W, Sahlstedt B. Hidden cervical spine injuries in traffic accident victims with skull fractures. J Spinal Disord. 1991 Sep;4(3):251–63.

§ 14:14 Waddell non-organic signs—Original Waddell study (1980)

Waddell et al evaluated acute work-related low back pain, identifying nonorganic physical signs in 350 North American and British patients. These signs and symptoms are used as screening tools in patients with chronic low back pain for detecting abnormal illness behavior. The signs were associated with other clinical measures of illness behavior and distress. These nonorganic signs are distinguishable from the standard clinical signs of physical pathology and correlate with other psychological data. By helping to separate the physical from the nonorganic, they clarify the assessment of purely physical pathologic conditions. It is suggested also that the nonorganic signs can be used as a simple clinical screen to help identify patients who require more detailed psychological assessment. Waddell G, McCulloch JA, Kummel E, Venner RM. Nonorganic physical signs in low-back pain. Spine. 1980 Mar–Apr;5(2):117–25.

§ 14:15 Waddell non-organic signs—Subsequent studies

Others have attempted to repeat the original study, but none have duplicated it's results.

Because the nonorganic tests are purported to serve as screening tests, cut-off values were selected that minimized false-negative results. Even with optimal cut-off values, <u>none</u> of the nonorganic tests served as effective screening tools. Fritz JM, Wainner RS, Hicks GE. The use of nonorganic signs and symptoms as a screening tool for return-to-work in patients with acute low back pain. Spine. 2000 Aug 1;25(15):1925–31.

In another study, the value of the nonorganic signs in predicting return to activity following an initial episode of low-back pain was determined. One hundred and twenty patients were assessed within 6 months of the onset of their first episode of disabling low-back pain, and again at a mean of 15.3 months following injury. <u>No correlation</u> was found between the presence of nonorganic signs at initial assessment, and either return to activity or resolution of the patient's symptoms. Bradish CF, Lloyd GJ, Aldam CH, Albert J, Dyson P, Doxey NC, Mitson GL. Do nonorganic signs help to predict the return to activity of patients with low-back pain? Spine. 1988 May;13(5):557–60.

§ 14:16 Waddell non-organic signs—Follow-up Waddell study (1998)

In a 1998 "reappraisal," Main and Waddell clarified their findings from the earlier study:

Despite clear caveats about the interpretation of the signs, they have been misinterpreted and misused both clinically and medicolegally. Behavioral responses to examination provide useful clinical information, but need to be interpreted with care and understanding. Isolated signs should not be overinterpreted. Multiple signs suggest that the patient does not have a straightforward physical problem, but that psychological factors also need to be considered. Some patients may require both physical management of their physical pathology and more careful management of the psychosocial and behavioral aspects of their illness. Behavioral signs should be understood as response affected by fear in the context of recovery from injury and the development of chronic incapacity. They offer only a psychological "yellow-flag" and not a complete psychological assessment. Behavioral signs are not on their own a test of credibility or faking. Even Waddel states the signs are only "yellow flag" and not a complete assessment. See Main CJ, Waddell G. Behavioral responses to examination. A reappraisal of the interpretation of "nonorganic signs." Spine. 1998 Nov 1;23(21):2367–71.

§ 14:17 Other studies of note—The Lithuania study

Defense medical experts may attempt to assert that there is no long-term injury in whiplash. The basis for this assertion in the medical literature has its genesis in a famous Lithuania study. Schrader H, Obelieniene D, Bovin G, Surkiene D, Mickeviciene D, Miseviciene, Sand T. Natural evolution of late whiplash syndrome outside the medicolegal context. Lancet 1996;347:1207–11) This study is an attempt to show that there can be acute symptoms, but chronic complaints are no different between the whiplash group and the controls.

In this study, the controls had a high rate of symptoms. Freeman, Croft et al. address the flaws in this study by stating "at least 94% of the acutely injured subjects (29 of 31) in this study would have had to develop chronic symptoms to enable the authors to detect a statistically significant difference between the two groups, an extremely remote possibility. A recalculation of sample size using a meta-analysis-based estimate of effect (expected proportion chronic) of 5% (that is, 33% of the 15% acutely injured subjects) demonstrates that the total study cohort needed to be at least 3000 in order to have sufficient statistical power to discern a significant difference between the two groups." Freeman MD, Croft AC, Rossignol AM, Weaver DS, Reiser M. A review and methodologic critique of the literature refuting whiplash syndrome. Spine. 1999 Jan 1;24(1) :86–96; See also Freeman MD, Croft AC, Rossignol AM. *"Whiplash associated disorders: redefining whiplash and its management" by the Quebec Task Force.*

It should also be noted that many of the defense studies utilized follow-up by mail, with no follow-up medical examination. This included the Lithuania studies. The self reporting of pain/dysfunction may not be the best indicator. At 6 months, 96.6% of patients may self-report as being completely recovered, but upon examination, 73% of the patients were still symptomatic. Costanzo A, Bertolini M. Injuries of the cervical spine caused by road accidents in Italy. J Musculoskletal Pain 2000; 8:1115–122.

§ 14:18 Other studies of note—Canadian government studies

The hypothesis on which the Saskatchewan researchers based their study was taken from the study in Lithuania that showed that there was no chronic whiplash in a country where there was no compensation for injury. This paper is the entire basis for the hypothesis and speculation from the Saskatchewan researchers, who were entirely funded by Saskatchewan Government Insurance. Cassidy JD, Carroll LJ, Cote P, Lemstra M, Berglund A, Nygren A. Effect of eliminating compensation for pain and suffering on the outcome of insurance claims for whiplash injury. N Engl J Med. 2000 Apr 20;342(16):1179–86.

The same authors state the insurance and compensation systems have a large impact on recovery from acute whiplash. Cote P, Cassidy JD, Carroll L, Frank JW, Bombardier C. A systematic review of the prognosis of acute whiplash and a new conceptual framework to synthesize the literature. Spine. 2001 Oct 1;26(19):E445–58.

The government is the only insurer for motor vehicle injuries in Saskatchewan, and everyone's healthcare in Canada is covered under governmental insurance. This paper has become the basis to justify their outcome measure—closure of claims. Cote P, Hogg-Johnson S, Cassidy JD, Carroll L, Frank JW. The association between neck pain intensity, physical functioning, depressive symptomatology and time-to-claim-closure after whiplash. J Clin Epidemiol. 2001 Mar;54(3):275–86.

§ 14:19 Other studies of note—Castro study: no stress-no whiplash?

The desensedefense may use the *Castro* study to state that the psychological elements of the crash—the noise, vehicle damage—is the cause of the patient's condition. This study sought to maximize psychological factors. In all the other crash testing, attempts are made to minimize psychological factors.

In this study, a placebo crash was set up. No actual crash occurred, and the car rolled down a ramp with attending noise. The subjects were then brought back to the rear of the vehicle, and debris was place on the ground. Only 1 of the 51 had what would be a psychological profile to fit this phenomenon of a nocebo response (a placebo response that produces pain) of whiplash injury that we would see for treatment. In the stated, 20% developed acute whiplash syndrome; is this padding the data? One in 50 is 2%. Castro WH, Meyer SJ, Becke ME, Nentwig CG, Hein MF, Ercan BI, Thomann S, Wessels U, Du Chesne AE. No stress—no whiplash? Prevalence of "whiplash" symptoms following exposure to a placebo rear-end collision. Int J Legal Med. 2001;114(6):316–22.

§ 14:20 Other studies of note—Szabo studies: female vehicle occupants

In the Szabo study (1994; SAE 940532), an attempt was made to enhance the epidemiological studies of low speed whiplash with only two female test subjects. Note that the subjects were employess of the testing facility and there were not enough participants to extrapolate to the general population, areas of potential bias.

In the Szabo study (1996; SAE 962432), an interesting note is that the vehicles they used were Volvos. Volvos have been shown to have the lowest neck injury factor (NIF), another possible area of bias. Eichberger A, et al. Comparison of different car seats regarding head-neck kinematics of volunteers during rear end impact. IRCOBI 1996-13-0011.

§ 14:21 Other studies of note—Author's studies

The author of this text has 4 published review papers on the subject of whiplash, which address many of the defense studies cited herein. See Davis C. Chronic pain/dysfunction in whiplash-associated disorders. J Manipulative Physiol Ther. 2001 Jan;24(1):44–51; Davis CG. Injury threshold: whiplash-associated disorders. J Manipulative Physiol Ther. 2000 Jul–

Aug;23(6):420–7; Davis CG. Rear-end impacts: vehicle and occupant response. J Manipulative Physiol Ther. 1998 Nov–Dec;21(9):629–39. Davis CG. Chiropractic Treatment in Acute Whiplash Injuries: Grades I & II. J. Vertebral Subluxation Res. May 19, 2008.

Note that R. Ferrari, M.D. contributes to the defense point of view with opinion articles and letters to the editor relating to my research. Recently, he sent a letter to the editor on my 2001 paper. His letter to the editor and my response are included in Appendix 1 (published in J Manipulative Physiol Ther February 2002).

§ 14:22 Other defense studies of note—Other studies

Schrader H, Obelieniene D, Bovim G, Surkiene D, Mickeviciene D, Miseviciene I, Sand T. Natural evolution of late whiplash syndrome outside the medicolegal context. Lancet. 1996 May 4;347(9010):1207–11. *(Lithuania 1)*

Obelieniene D, Schrader H, Bovim G, Miseviciene I, Sand T. Pain after whiplash: a prospective controlled inception cohort study. J Neurol Neurosurg Psychiatry. 1999 Mar;66(3):279–83. *(Lithuania 2)*

Partheni M, Constantoyannis C, Ferrari R, Nikiforidis G, Voulgaris S, Papadakis N. A prospective cohort study of the outcome of acute whiplash injury in Greece. Clin Exp Rheumatol. 2000 Jan–Feb;18(1):67–70.

Bonk AD, Ferrari R, Giebel GD, Edelmann M, Huser R. Prospective, randomized, controlled study of active versus collar, and the natural history for whiplash injury in Germany. J Musculoskeletal Pain 2000;8:123–32.

§ 14:23 Other whiplash research

Comment:

In recent years, research from Canada addressed the question of whether muscle in jury was a major problem in chronic whiplash. The studies subjected healthy volunteers to impacts ranging from of 4.8 to 15.4 m/s acceleration in controlled crash testing. Surface EMG testing of the sternocleidomastoids, trapezii, and splenii capitis was performed, recorded and compared. The study, cited below, concluded that **"Prolonged symptoms following whiplash injury cannot be explained by biochemically measurable muscle damage."**

Of note, the muscles measured were not segmental stabilizers of the spine, so this commentator finds these studies of questionable significance. Below is an abstract of the study:

Outcome following whiplash injury of the cervical spine is variable, and the pathology of those with prolonged symptoms is uncertain. We undertook a prospective study in 25 patients to identify whether those with prolonged symptoms following whiplash injury exhibit a rise in serum creatine kinase consistent with significant muscle damage at the time of injury. Transient rise in creatine kinase level was seen in only 2 of 25 patients, neither of whom complained of prolonged symptoms. Of the 8 patients who developed chronic symptoms following whiplash injury, none demonstrated a serum creatine kinase rise. **Prolonged symptoms following whiplash injury cannot be explained by biochemically measurable muscle damage**. Scott S, Sanderson PL. Whiplash: a biochemical study of muscle injury. Eur Spine J. 2002 Aug;11(4):389–92.

Another study, Kumar S, Ferrari R, Narayan Y. Electromyographic and kinematic exploration of whiplash-type rear impacts: effect of left offset impact. Spine J. 2004 Nov–Dec;4(6):656–65, has been criticized in published commentary. Coauthor, Ferrari, is a Canadian medical doctor who has asserted that the proper way to explain chronic symptoms from whiplash injury is through a biopsychosocial model. He criticizes other whiplash articles that indicate chronic whiplash is a real entity, but fails to make any criticisms of German and Lithuanian studies he relies upon, which themselves have been seriously questioned.

In the same issue of The Spine Journal *(Nov–Dec 2004), Albert I. King. PhD*, a well-known biomechanical expert, was invited to write a commentary on the Kumar-Ferrari-Narayan study. Below are excerpts from that commentary, followed by key findings in the underlying study that King criticizes:

> "I have been asked to write a commentary on this paper because I felt that the results reported in this paper may be misleading to readers not familiar with the field of impact injury.
>
> There are several different hypotheses on the cause of neck pain resulting from a rear-end impact. The authors did not mention them . . . For researchers in biomechanics, it is our responsibility to ensure not only that our work is supported by good data but that it is also consistent with research in nonbiomechanical areas and with the clinical picture. Looking for a dime under the street light is to be highly discouraged, and making sure that our published results will "do no harm" to the general public is a warning we all need to heed."

Spine J. 2004 Nov-Dec;4(6):656–65; discussion 666–8, Albert I. King, PhD, Detroit, MI.

APPENDICES

APPENDIX 1. AUTHOR'S JMPT ARTICLE AND LETTER TO THE EDITOR

APPENDIX 2. INSURANCE RESEARCH INSTITUTE'S CLAIMS BEHAVIOR STUDY

APPENDIX 1

AUTHOR'S JMPT ARTICLE AND LETTER TO THE EDITOR

When someone publishes an article in a peer-reviewed medical/chiropractic journal, those who read the journal article may submit letters to the editor for criticism on that article. Below is a copy of my article "Chronic pain/dysfunction in whiplash-associated disorders" that was published in the Journal of Manipulative and Physiological Therapeutics (J Manipulative Physiol Ther 2001;24:44–51). *In response to this article, a letter to the editor was sent by Robert Ferrari, M.D., which is also reprinted below. My response to* Dr. Ferrari's letter from the February 2002 issue (Volume 25, Number 2:135 138) *follows.*

§ A1:1 Author's Article: "Chronic pain/dysfunction in whiplash-associated disorders"

Objective: The purposes of this article are (1) to review current knowledge of and recent concepts pertaining to the causes of chronic pain and/or dysfunction following whiplash-type injuries and (2) to acquaint those who treat these types of injuries with possible mechanisms of continued pain and or dysfunction following whiplash.

Data Collection: A review of the literature on mechanisms of injury and neurologic considerations was undertaken. A hand search of relevant medical, neuroscience, chiropractic, and online *Index Medicus* sources and other sources involving mechanisms of nociception, neurotransmitters, and receptors that might evolve from whiplash-type soft tissue injuries was conducted.

Results: Pain is a complex phenomenon that has great variability. Chronic pain appears to involve a deficient descending inhibitory process and/or ongoing excitatory input.

Conclusions: There is a wide variety of reactions by

individuals to any given type of stimulus. Injury may lead to increases in neuronal activity and prolonged changes in the nervous system. Chronic pain may be seen as part of a central disturbance accompanied by disinhibition or sensitization of central pain modulation, mirrored in the immune and endocrine systems. Patients with chronic whiplash syndrome may have a generalized central hyperexcitability from a loss of tonic inhibitory input (disinhibition) and/or ongoing excitatory input contributing to dorsal horn hyperexcitability. Dysfunction of the motor system may also occur, with or without pain. The purpose of treatment should be not only to relieve pain but also to allow for proper proprioception. (J Manipulative Physiol Ther 2001;24:44–51)

Introduction

The types of injury produced in most low-speed motor vehicle collisions are soft tissue injuries involving the spine and nervous system. These injuries are inertial injuries and not crush injuries, which cause a variety of symptoms and syndromes. A human spinal column that is devoid of muscle function is incapable of carrying the loads imposed on it.[1] Without muscles, the spine buckles under very low loads. The average critical buckling load for the osteoligamentous human cervical spine is 10.5 N (SD 3.8). This is approximately one fifth to one fourth of the weight of the average human head.[2] In a low-velocity impact with whiplash, there is complex buckling of the cervical spine. Concomitant flexion and extension occur simultaneously in different regions of the cervical spine, resulting in an S-shaped curvature; motions in the lower cervical levels exceed their physiological motion limits in whiplash-type injuries.[3,4] The soft tissue is seldom torn completely; instead, it is most likely stretched beyond its elastic limit, the result being an incomplete injury.[5] This subfailure injury can significantly alter the tissue's mechanical properties[6]; many subfailure injuries have potential injury consequence.[7] Microscopic collagen fiber failure begins at 3% to 5% strain. Strain greater than 7% to 8% may result in the ligament's undergoing plastic deformation and may cause the load carrying capacity to be lost, even when the ligaments appear macroscopically intact.[8] There is a wide range of variability in (1) ligament strength between individuals, (2) the body positions of occupants in the vehicle, (3) the amount of muscle activation and inhibition, (4) the size of the spinal canals, and (5) the excitability of the nervous system.[9] A whiplash-type injury occurs in deep tissue that may involve the facets, disk, ligaments, or muscles.[10] Deep tissue pain is different from superficial pain: the former lasts longer than the latter[11] and does not follow dermatomal patterns.[12,13] Muscular or deep pain may be driven from both A-β and C fibers.[14] A significantly lower pain threshold has been found in whiplash chronic pain subjects than in normal control subjects.[15]

Discussion

Nociception

The perception of pain involves activation of nociceptors in the periphery, which then activate second-order neurons in the spinal cord. At the cord level, pain signals can be transmitted and modulated. Areas of the brain, thalamus, and brainstem receive the nociceptive information and can originate descending inhibition. Nociceptors are primary afferent neurons that respond to noxious or potentially tissue-damaging stimuli and can be sensitized. Acute pain can induce long-term neuronal remodeling and sensitization.[16] After joint or muscle injury, the spinal cord processes nociceptive information and controls peripheral inflammation. The dorsal horn neurons can be sensitized by peripheral injury with activation of N-methyl-D-aspartate (NMDA), non-NMDA excitatory amino acid, and neurokinin 1 (NK1) receptors.[17] A non-NMDA receptor, α-amino-3-hydroxy-5-methyl-4-isoxazolepropionate (AMPA), appears to set the baseline level of nociception and faithfully transmits the intensity and duration of the stimulus. NMDA receptors enhance noxious information.[18]

After tissue damage, the substances released include potassium (from damaged cells), serotonin (platelets), bradykinin (plasma), histamine (mast cells), prostaglandins (PGE2; damaged cells), leukotrienes (damaged cells), and substance P (SP; primary afferent fibers).[19]

Tetrodotoxin sodium current receptors,[20] nerve growth factor (NGF), NK1 receptors (for SP), δ-μ-κ-opioid receptors, glutamate, NMDA and AMPA receptors, nitric oxide (NO), cyclooxygenase, and other neurotrophic factors and neurotransmitters can also affect nociception.[21] Glutamate is the main excitatory neurotransmitter in the central nervous system and has been implicated in neurodevelopment and synaptogenesis,[22] neurodegenerative disorders, neurotoxicity,[23,24] and synaptic plasticity, as in long-term potentiation (LTP) and long-term depression.[25] Adenosine 5'-triphosphate, which may also evoke nociceptor activation, is known to depolarize sensory neurons and may play a role in nociceptor activation when released from damaged tissue through primary afferent neurotransmission.[26,27]

Presynaptic NMDA receptors found in the afferent terminals in the dorsal horn may control the release of SP and other neuropeptides. Glutamate and SP coexist in primary afferent terminals and are coexpressed and act synergistically in the dorsal horn. The release of SP in the dorsal horn is frequency dependent and appears to be controlled by NMDA receptors in laminae I and II of the spinal cord. Glutamate, an excitatory neurotransmitter in the dorsal horn, has its effects enhanced by SP acting on NK1 receptors.[28] SP is under the control of at least 2 functionally antagonistic glutamate receptors: inhibitory metabotropic receptors (groups I and III) and facilitatory ionotropic receptors (NMDA receptors). The predominance of the mechanisms depends on the pain condition, inasmuch as the pronociceptive function of mGluRs (a type of glutamate receptor) has been found to be mainly associated with inflammation.[29,30] Various intracellular messengers linked to excitatory amino acid receptors (such as NO, arachidonic acid, and protein kinase C) may also play a critical role in the development of persistent nociception after tissue injury.[31–34]

Inflammation

Inflammation increases the sensitivity of the receptors in the periphery and in the central nervous system by altering membrane properties of nociceptors, permitting a higher discharge frequency and contributing to hyperalgesia,[35] and by activating synapses that are usually inactive.[36] Inflammatory pain and the sensitization of peripheral nociceptors can be very rapid and involve non-neuronal cells such as mast cells, neutrophils, fibroblasts, and macrophages.[37] Inflammation increases the sensitivity in the peripheral terminals of A-δ and C fibers (Fig 1).

Inflammation causes A-β fibers, which normally inhibit nociception, to sprout into lamina II in the dorsal horn[38] and express SP as C fibers.[39] Inflammation elevates the neurotrophin NGF,[40] increases levels of PGE2,[41] activates cholecystokinin-B receptors,[42] alters the sensory processing in the substantia gelatinosa,[43] increases nociceptin (also know as *orphanin FQ*),[44] sensitizes tetrodotoxin sodium current receptors[45] that are present in peripheral terminals of primary afferent nociceptors,[46] increases NO that is involved in the maintenance of mechanical allodynia,[47] induces central sensitization in the spinal cord,[48] and increases the number of sensory axons containing ionotropic glutamate receptors that contribute to peripheral sensitization.[49] The medullary dorsal reticular nucleus plays a pronociceptive role in both acute and tonic inflammatory pain, leading to amplification of the nociceptive signal,[50] and it may also underlie the noxious response to the temporomandibular joint.[51]

Cytokines released from an injury may be proinflammatory or anti-inflammatory,[52] Cytokines are small proteins that are essential for healing of connective tissue after injury and play roles in cell-to-cell signaling. The interaction between a cytokine and its receptor is highly specific. The response of a cell to its own cytokine is known as an *autocrine response*; the response of a cell to cytokines produced by adjacent cells is known as a *paracrine response*.[53] Cytokines can also act as endocrine signals. Evidence points to tumor necrosis factor-α (a proinflammatory cytokine) having a role in inducing the hyperalgesic response to inflammation; this is likely to be the consequence of its induction of later-acting intermediaries, particularly interleukin-1-β and NGF.[54] Cytokines may act as a link between the nervous and immune systems.

Mechanisms of chronic pain

Chronic pain can be due to tissue injury, nervous system injury, or both. Pain may be stimulus-dependent or stimulus-independent.[55] In the development of chronic pain, wind-up-type mechanisms and LTP play roles in neuroplasticity to cause hyperalgesia and allodynia. Abnormal processing allows transmission of signals along the central nervous system pathways independent of the degree of nociception that is occurring in the periphery. The term *central sensitization* refers to an increase in spinal cord neuronal excitability and a decrease in threshold. Wind-up, a progressive increase in the magnitude of the C-fiber evoked response, may also produce some characteristics of central sensitization, including expansion of the receptive fields and enhanced responses to C-fiber stimulation.[56] Wind-up differs from LTP in that wind-up requires a very low frequency input and is manifest only during repetitive inputs. LTP requires a brief high-frequency input and is manifest only as a potentiated response to subsequent inputs for very prolonged periods[57]; an ongoing afferent stimulation is not required. LTP can be suppressed by tonically active supraspinal descending systems.[58] Wind-up is not equivalent to central sensitization, but the stimulation that caused wind-up in the dorsal horn may give rise to central sensitization. Both are dependent on NMDA receptors and/or SP acting on neurokinin receptors. The NMDA receptor system in wind-up is changed after inflammation and central sensitization.[59,60]

The NMDA receptor appears to be important for synaptic plasticity, and its function seems to be related to some characteristics of the receptor complex. The NMDA receptor is gated by both ligand binding to the receptor and by the membrane voltage. Activation of the channel can take place only when the membrane of the cell is partially depolarized by activation of other (non-NMDA) receptors. At normal resting membrane potential, the NMDA channel is blocked by magnesium (Mg 2+). Excitatory amino acids acting at non-NMDA receptors may produce a fast excitatory postsynaptic potential, whereas various neuropeptides may induce a slow synaptic potential, generating enough depolarization to remove Mg 2+ from the NMDA receptor channel. Because the NMDA receptor is a high-capacity calcium (Ca 2+) channel, the Ca 2+ ions flow into the cell during NMDA receptor activation. Calcium triggers a number of intracellular biochemical processes that are important for LTP of the particular synapse. These processes include phosphorylation of membrane (receptor) proteins, activation of NO synthase, and activation of immediate early genes coding for factors regulating protein synthesis. The outcome of these biochemical alterations is a potentiation and consolidation of the particular synapse, and this may lead to persistent changes in neuronal excitability. It is assumed that the changes in cellular excitability caused by NMDA receptor-mediated Ca 2+ influx may underlie wind-up.[61]

Chronic pain is characterized by an abnormal sensitivity that may be due to generation of pain in response of low-threshold mechanoreceptive A-β fibers that normally generate innocuous sensations.[62] A decrease in non-nociceptive input may lead to pain by a deafferentation mechanism. The pain in deafferentation is described as "burning, raw, or searing" or as a "tingling, numb sensation."[63] A-β axons may exhibit spontaneous discharges as early as 1 day after injury. A-β fiber modification may cause allodynia by altering the processing of afferent input into the dorsal horn.[64] Because the pathophysiology of chronic pain indicates increased sensitivity to low threshold A-β fiber inputs, low levels of afferent activity are sufficient to maintain a state of central sensitization responsible for sensory changes. Pain and changed somatosensory thresholds may occur after relatively minor axonal damage and nerve sheath inflammation when no axonal damage is present.[65] Repeated low-intensity, non-painful stimulation can result in integration of neural responses and cause severe pain. Sparse nociceptive activity from minor pathologic conditions (minor nerve trauma or tissue inflammation) can become excruciatingly painful as a result of central integration of the neural responses.[66] Generated by tissue injury, persistent small afferent input results in a hyperalgesia at the site of injury and allodynia in areas adjacent to the injury site. Hyperalgesia reflects a sensitization of the peripheral terminal and a central facilitation evoked by the small afferent input, and allodynia reflects a central sensitization.[67] The changes in spinal sensory processing may occur without changes in blood flow[68] or inflammation.[69] Mediated by low-threshold mechanosensitive afferents projecting to sensitized dorsal horn neurons, the nociceptive processes are qualitatively altered in patients with chronic myofascial pain.[70] Patients uffering from chronic whiplash syndrome[71] and patients with fibromyalgia[72] have a generalized central hyperexcitability of the nervous system.

There is also evidence that chronic pain may be seen as part of a central disturbance accompanied by disinhibition or sensitization of central pain modulation, these being mirrored in the immune and endocrine systems.[73] Recent research indicates that pain and immune function mechanisms have mutual features, immunocerebral communication playing an important role in hyperalgesia. Immune parameters have been shown to be related to activity in brain areas involved in pain perception, emotion, and attention.[74] This reflection does not need specific pathways or specific cerebral centers.[75,76]

Dysfunction

Pain is not the only sequela to whiplash. Because the cervical spine is richly supplied with mechanoreceptors and muscle spindles, chronic pain can play a role in locomotor system dysfunction and in its perpetuation[77,78] associated with whiplash trauma.[79] Patterns of normal proprioceptive input are distorted when articular nociception is incurred. This interferes with the precise continuous input necessary for coordinated normal patterns of motion, balance, coordination, and equilibrium.[80] Muscle spindle output from neck muscles is significantly altered when the bradykinin concentration is elevated. This may also induce pain through supraspinal projections and at the same time cause disturbances in motor coordination and proprioception by altering the activity of the γ-muscle spindle system.[81] Hypertonicity of the muscles, autonomic reflexes, and overexcitation of proprioceptors affecting the central nervous system play a preeminent role in the genesis of disequilibrium and chronic postural instability from whiplash-induced injury.[82,83] As a result of disorganized proprioceptive activity, a whiplash injury can cause distortion of the posture control system,[84,85] including oculomotor dysfunction.[86,87]

Some patients who claimed no symptoms after trauma showed oculomotor dysfunction and repositioning dysfunction. Neck pain measured with a cervicobrachial visual analog pain scale did not correlate significantly with oculomotor performance and kinesthetic sensibility. A proprioceptive dysfunction might be one of the most important factors for understanding the morbidity after a noncontact whiplash injury to the neck.[86] Dysfunction related to whiplash trauma may be seen with dysfunction of the smallest muscles (muscles of the eye),[87] which may reveal what otherwise might be overlooked.

Inhibition

Peripheral injury that produces inflammation can result in central sensitization and hyperalgesia. SP and glutamate, acting at the NK-1 and NMDA receptors, are involved in sensitizing spinal neurons inducing hyperalgesia. It is also evident that this is not the only mechanism. A decrease in the effectiveness of inhibitory synaptic transmission leads to increased responsiveness of spinal reflex pathways and pain sensations. In animals, damage to the descending inhibitory systems enhanced wind-up, indicating that wind-up is influenced by supraspinal, descending inhibitory pathways.[88] The inhibition of wind-up-like pain is associated with reduction in the intensity of continuous ongoing pain and with increased pressure-pain thresholds.[61]

Decreases in inhibitory processes—ie, disinhibition and/or an increase in excitatory input—are also involved in central sensitization and hyperalgesia. A disturbed inhibitory mechanism may result in widespread deep hyperalgesia.[89] Attenuated responses of deep dorsal horn neurons are dependent on the previous state of the neuron.[90] Descending inhibitory cortical control is effected by the opioidergic, noradrenergic, and serotonergic systems.[91] Some patients may be genetically predisposed to decreased amounts of opioid receptors,[92] and ischemia can reduce the expression of μ-opioid receptors in the dorsal horn.[93] The greater the quantity of opioid receptors one has, the more likely it is that the result will be less perception of pain.

The midbrain periaqueductal gray (PAG), rostral ventromedial medulla, and spinal cord are components of the endogenous pain modulating pathway[94–96].

These brain stem-descending pathways are involved in modulation of spinal nociceptive neurons in response to transient stimuli and in modulation of spinal nociceptive processes in developing persistent pain. The fine-tuning by descending pathway modulating systems may underlie the variability of perceived pain and hyperalgesia. The imbalance can be a mechanism in acute and chronic pain conditions.[97] The endogenous descending antinociceptive system, including the seratogenic and noradrenergic descending pathways from the medulla and pons into the spinal cord, may be influenced by environmental stimuli. Functions of the PAG include pain, analgesia, anxiety, and cardiovascular control.[98] The descending pathways differentially modulate spinoparabrachial neurons in the superficial and deep dorsal horn in inhibiting nociceptive neurons in the superficial dorsal horn. The descending serotoninergic pathway is more effective in suppressing neuronal hyperexcitability in the deep dorsal horn.[99] PAG μ-opioids activate a descending antinociceptive circuit with a δ-opioid receptor-mediated endogenous opioid link to the rostral ventromedial medulla.[100]

The principal action of serotonin in this process is to limit neuronal excitability. Serotonergic transmission is largely mediated by nonjunctional contacts, which suggests that the actions of seratonin are mediated predominantly by volume rather than by wiring transmission.[101] This release of seratonin may modulate nociceptive transmission in a tonic state-dependent manner.[102] γ-aminobutyric acid (GABA) also reduces nociceptive reflexes, hyperalgesia, and allodynia.[90] In the spinal cord, GABA is concentrated in interneurons of the dorsal horn. Between 24% and 33% of the neurons in laminae I–III are reported to contain GABA.[18] Normal tonic inhibition is partly by means of a GABA-dependent mechanism and, if it is not functioning properly, may play a role in prolonged pathologic states of increased spinal cord excitability.[103] Nociceptive transmission in the dorsal horn is subject to tonic-descending inhibition, and tonic-descending inhibition may prevent plastic changes in nociceptive transmission in the spinal cord.[104]

Activation of NO signal transduction contributes to the sensitization of wide dynamic range spinothalamic tract neurons in the deep dorsal horn, causing simultaneous attenuation in inhibition produced in the PAG.[105] Sensitization of the spinothalamic tract cells is produced in part by disinhibition.[90,105] Tinnitus (an auditory perception not caused by external stimulation) after head injury[106] or whiplash[107] may be due to a type of disinhibition.

Modulation stimulation

Impulses in primary afferent nerve fibers may produce short- or long-lasting modifications in spinal nociception. Afferent stimulation may facilitate or inhibit transmission of nociception information in the spinal dorsal horn. A-fiber stimulation selectively inhibits C-fiber-evoked and noxious stimulus-evoked excitation of dorsal horn neurons. Inhibition may considerably outlast the duration of the stimulus, presynaptic and postsynaptic mechanisms contributing to the inhibition. Somatosensory thalamic stimulation may activate pain modulation circuits. The effective thalamic output from the ventrocaudal nucleus of the thalamus to the cortex is affected by somatosensory input. Stimulation of the ventralposterior lateral nucleus has reduced mechanical alloydynia in experiments.[108] A loss of non-nociceptive input into the thalamus may unmask or strengthen nociception and allow nociceptive neuronal input to be prominent.[109]

Experimental studies suggest that mylinated afferents mediate electrically induced muscle pain and that unmylinated afferents (C fibers) mainly mediate saline-induced muscle pain.[110] Electric nerve stimulation is more effective for immediate relief of myofascial pain, and electric muscle stimulation has a better effect on the immediate release of muscle tightness.[111] The same transcutaneous electric nerve stimulation (TENS) has different degrees of antinociceptive influence on chronic and acute pain.[112] Stimulation frequencies have produced varied results. In one study, low-stimulation frequencies were found to be more effective than high-stimulation frequencies[113]; another study indicated that a high-frequency burst stimulation of A-δfiber strength produced long-term depression of C-fiber-evoked potentials. TENS at high intensities (painful but tolerable) was found to be more effective than stimulation at low intensities. C-fiber synaptic transmission inhibition has been achieved by means of high-frequency stimulation of A-δ fibers.[114] This deep-tissue stimulation on the contralateral side activates inhibitory descending projections from higher centers.[115] The resultant descending inhibition reduces the expression of LTP in dorsal horn cells, and that longterm descending inhibition may override a segmental facilitation.[116] Physical activity can also significantly increase the threshold nociceptive reflex.[117]

Manipulation therapy can also improve pain tolerance. Spinal manipulative treatments show a consistent reflex response of multireceptor origin and may cause clinically observed benefits, including a reduction of pain and a decrease in hypertonicity of muscles.[118-120]

The PAG-mediated descending pain inhibitory system is not the only mechanism associated with manipulative therapy-induced hypoalgesia.[121] The cerebral cortex is involved in pain activity,[122-124] pain facilitation,[125] and pain inhibition.[126] Afferent input evokes changes in the central nervous system and causes changes in the brain, depending on the side being treated (ipsilateral or contralateral).[127] In addition to antinociception, manipulation therapy produces changes in sudomotor, cutaneous vasomotor, respiratory, and cardiac activity. This suggests that activation is through a central control mechanism at a high level of the neuroaxis.[128] β-endorphin levels have also been shown to increase[129] after manipulation.

Conclusion

There is ample evidence that indicates diminished endogenous systems with chronic pain.[130] Injury may lead to increases in neuronal activity that are reflected in gene expression and prolonged changes in the nervous system. The functional result is hyperalgesia and spontaneous pain associated with tissue injury.[131] Pain can be biochemical, with apparently normal structure.[132] Patients suffering from chronic whiplash syndrome may have a generalized central hyperexcitability from a loss of tonic inhibitory input (disinhibition) and/or an increase in excitatory input contributing to dorsal horn hyperexcitability. This may lead to dysfunction of the motor system. The aim of treatment should be not only to relieve pain but also to allow for proper proprioception.[88,133]

References

1. Panjabi MM, Abumi K, Duranceau J, Oxland T. Spinal stability and intersegmental muscle forces: a biomechanical model. Spine 1989;14:194–200.

2. Panjabi MM, Cholewicki J, Nibu K, Grauer J, Babat L, Dvorak J. Critical load of the human cervical spine: an in vitro experimental study. Clin Biomech 1998;13:11–7.

3. Kaneoka K, Ono K, Inami S, Hayashi K. Motion analysis of cervical vertebrae during whiplash loading. Spine 1999;24:763–70.

4. Grauer JN, Panjabi MM, Cholewicki J, Nibu K, Dvorak J. Whiplash produces Shaped curvatures of the neck with hyperextension at lower levels. Spine 1997;22:2489–94.

5. Panjabi MM, Cholewicki J, Nibu K, Babat LB, Dvorak J. Simulation of whiplash trauma using whole cervical spine specimens. Spine 1998;23:17–24.

6. Panjabi MM, Yoldas E, Oxland TR, Crisco JJ. Subfailure injury of the rabbit ACL. J Orthop Res 1996;14:216–22.

7. Herkowitz HN, Rothman RH. Subacute instability of the cervical spine. Spine 1984;9:348–57.

8. Noyes FR, Keller CS, Grood ES, Butler DL. Advances in the understanding of knee ligament injury, repair, and rehabilitation. Med Sci Sports Exerc 1984;16:427–43.

9. Davis CG. Injury threshold: whiplash associated disorders. J Manipulative Physiol Ther 2000;23:420–7.

10. Malanga GA, editor. Cervical flexion-extension/whiplash injuries. Spine: state of the art reviews. Philadelphia: Hanley & Belfus; 1998.

11. Woolf CJ, Wall PD. Relative effectiveness of C primary afferent fibers of different origins in evoking a prolonged facilitation of the flexor reflex in the rat. J Neurosci 1986;6:1433–42.

12. Kellgren JH. On the distribution of pain arising from deep somatic structures with charts of segmental pain areas. Clin Sci 1939;4:35–46.

13. Feinstein B, Langton JNK, Jameson RM, Schiller F. Experiments on pain referred from deep somatic tissues. J Bone Joint Surg Am 1954;36:981–97.

14. Svendsen F, Tjolsen A, Hole K. AMPA and NMDA receptor-dependent spinal LTP after nociceptive tetanic stimulation. Neuroreport 1998;9:1185–90.

15. Olivegren H, Jerkvall N, Hagstrom Y, Carlsson J. The long-term prognosis of whiplash-associated disorders. Eur Spine J 1999;8:366–70.

16. Carr DB, Goudas LC. Acute pain. Lancet 1999;353:2051–8.

17. Sluka KA. Pain mechanisms involved in musculoskeletal disorders. J Orthop Sports Phys Ther 1996;24:240–54.

18. Dickenson AH, Chapman V, Green GM. The pharmacology of excitatory and inhibitory amino acid-mediated events in the transmission and modulation of pain in the spinal cord. Gen Pharmacol 1997;28:633–8.

19. Purves D, Augustine GJ, Fitzptrick D, Katz LC, LaMantia AS, McNamara JO. Neuroscience. Sunderland (MA): Sinauer Associates; 1996. p. 165–77.

20. Cummins TR, Waxman SG. Downregulation of tetrodotoxin-resistant sodium channels and up regulation of a rapidly repriming tetrodotoxin-sensitive sodium current in small spinal sensory neurons after nerve injury. J Neurosci 1997;17:3503–14.

21. Svendsen F, Tjolsen A, Hole K, Doland S, Noland AM. N-methyl D-aspartate induced mechanical allodynia is blocked by nitric oxide synthase and cyclooxygenase-2 inhibitors. Neuroreport 1999;10:449–52.

22. McDonald JW, Johnston MV. Physiological and pathophysiological role of excitatory amino acids during central nervous system development. Brain Res Rev 1990;15:41–70.

23. Meldrum B, Garthwaite J. Excitatory amino acid neurotoxicity and neurodegenerative disease. Trends Pharmacol Sci 1990; 11:378–87.

24. Beal MF. Role of excitotoxicity in human neurological disease. Curr Opin Neurobiol 1992;2:657–62.

25. Baudry M, Massicotte G. Physiological and pharmacological relationships between long-term potentiation and mammalian memory. Concepts in Neuroscience 1992;3:79–98.

26. Chen CC, Akopian AN, Sivllotti L, Colquhoun D, Burnstock G, Wood JN. A P2X purinoceptor expressed by a subset of sensory neurons. Nature 1995;377:428–31.

27. Lewis C, Neidhart S, Holy C, North RA, Buell G, Surprenant A. Coexpression of P2X2 and P2X3 receptor subunits can account for ATP-gated currents in sensory neurons. Nature 1995;377:432–5.

28. Marvizon JC, Martinez V, Grady EF, Bunnett NW, Mayer EA. Neurokinin 1 receptor internalization in spinal cord slices induced by dorsal root stimulation is mediated by NMDA receptors. J Neurosci 1997;17:8219–36.

29. Cuesta MC, Arcya JL, Cano G, Sanchez L, Maixner W, Suarez-Roca H. Opposite modulation of capsaicin-evoked substance P release by glutamate receptors. Neurochem Int 1999;35:471–8.

30. Marvizon JCG, Martinez V, Grady EF, Bunnett KW, Mayer EA. Neurokinin 1 receptor internalization in spinal cord slices induced by dorsal root stimulation is mediated by NMDA receptors. J Neurosci 1997;12:8129–36.

31. Malmberg AB, Yaksh TL. Antinociceptive actions of spinal nonsteroidal anti-inflammatory agents on the formalin test in the rat. J Pharmacol Exp Ther 1992;263:136–46.

32. Yamamoto T, Shimoyama N, Mizuguchi T. Nitric oxide synthase inhibitor blocks spinal sensitization induced by formalin injection into rat paw. Anesth Analg 1993;77:886–90.

33. Coderre TJ, Yashpal K. Intracellular messengers contributing to persistent nociception and hyperalgesia induced by L-glutamate and substance P in the rat formalin pain model. Eur J Neurosci 1994;6:1328–34.

34. Callsen-Cencic P, Hoheisel U, Kaske A, Mense S, Tenschert S. The controversy about spinal neuronal nitric oxide synthase: under which conditions is it up- or downregulated? Cell Tissue Res 1999;295:183–94.

35. Djouhri L, Lawson SN. Changes in somatic action potential shape in guinea-pig nociceptive afferent neurons during inflammation in vivo. J Physiol 1999;520:565–76.

36. Li P, Zhou M. Silent glutamatergic synapses and nociception in the mammalian spinal cord. Nature 1998;393:695.

37. Mendell LM, Albers KM, Davis BM. Neurotrophins, nociceptors, and pain. Microsc Res Tech 1999;45:252–61.

38. Neumann S, Doubell TP, Leslie T, Woolf CJ. Inflammatory pain hypersensitivity mediated by phenotypic switch in myelinated primary sensory neurons. Nature 1996;384;360–4.

39. Ma AP, Woolf CJ. The progressive tactile hyperalgesia induced by peripheral inflammation is nerve growth factor dependent. Neuroreport 1997;8:807–10.

40. Woolf CJ, Shortland P, Coggeshall RE. Peripheral nerve injury triggers central sprouting of myelinated afferents. Nature 1992; 355:75–7.

41. Izumi H, Mori H, Uchiyama T, et al. Sensitization of nociceptive C-fibers in zinc-deficient rats. Am J Physiol 1995;268:1423–8.

42. Schafer M, Zhou L, Stein C. Cholecystokinin inhibits peripheral opioid analgesia in inflamed tissue. Neuroscience 1998; 82:603–11.

43. Baba H, Doubel TP, Woolf CJ. Peripheral inflammation facilitates A-beta fiber-mediated synaptic input to the substantia gelatinosa of the adult rat spinal cord. J Neurosci 1999;19:859–67.

44. Andoh T, Itoh M, Kuraishi Y. Nociceptin gene expression in rat dorsal root ganglia induced by peripheral inflammation. Neuroreport 1997;8:2793–6.

45. Gold MS, Reichling DB, Shuster MJ, Levine JD. Hyperalgesia agents increase a tetrodotoxin-resistant Na+ current in nociceptors. Proc Natl Acad Sci 1996;93:1108–12.

46. Khasar SG, Gold MS, Levine JD. A tetrodotoxin-resistant sodium current mediates inflammatory pain in the rat. Neurosci Lett 1998;256:17–20.

47. Yoon YW, Sung B, Chung JM. Nitric oxide mediates behavior signs of neuropathic pain in an experimental rat model. Neuroreport 1998;9:367–72.

48. Wu J, Lin Q, McAdoo DJ, Willis WD. Nitric oxide contributes to central sensitization following intradermal injection of capsaicin. Neuroreport 1998;9:589–92.

49. Carlton SM, Coggeshall RE. Inflammation-induced changes in peripheral glutamate receptor populations. Brain Res 1999; 820:63–70.

50. Almeida A, Storkson R, Lima D, Hole K, Tjolsen A. The medullary dorsal reticular nucleus facilitates pain behaviour induced by formalin in the rat. Eur J Neurosci 1999;11:110–22.

51. Tsai C. The caudal subnucleus caudalis (medullary dorsal horn) acts as interneuronal relay site in craniofacial nociceptive reflex activity. Brain Res 1999;826:293–7.

52. Cunha FQ, Poole S, Lorenzetti BB, Veiga FH, Ferreira SH. Cytokine-mediated inflammatory hyperalgesia limited by interleukin-4. Br J Pharmacol 1999;126:45–50.

53. Evans CH. Cytokines and the role they play in healing of ligaments and tendons. Sports Med 1999;28:71–6

54. Woolf CJ, Allchorne A, Safieh-Garabedian B, Poole S. Cytokines, nerve growth factor and inflammatory hyperalgesia: the contribution of tumour necrosis factor. Br J Pharmacol 1997;121:417–24.

55. Woolf CJ, Bennett GJ, Doherty M, et al. Towards a mechanism-based classification of pain? Pain 1998;77:227–9.

56. Li J, Simone DA, Larson AA. Windup leads to characteristics of central sensitization. Pain 1999;79:75–82.

57. Woolf CJ. Windup and central sensitization are not equivalent. Pain 1996;66:91–8.

58. Sandkuhler J, Liu X. Induction of long-term potentiation at spinal synapses by noxious stimulation or nerve injury. Eur J Neurosci 1998;10:2476–80

59. Svendsen F, Rygh LJ, Hole K, Tjolsen A. Dorsal horn NMDA receptor function is changed after peripheral inflammation. Pain 1999;83:517–23

60. Carlton CSM, Coggeshall RE. Inflammation-induced changes in peripheral glutamate receptor populations. Brain Res 1999; 820:63–70.

61. Eide PK. Wind-up and the NMDA receptor complex from a clinical perspective. Eur J Pain 2000;4:5–17.

62. Woolf CJ, Doubel TP. The pathophysiology of chronic pain: increased sensitivity to low threshold Ab-fibre inputs. Curr Opin Neurobiol 1994;4:525–34.

63. Tasker RR, Dostrovsky JO. Deafferentation and central pain. In: Wall PD, Melzack R, editors. Textbook of pain. Edinburgh: Churchill Livingstone; 1989. p. 154–80.

64. Shin HC, Oh SJ, Jung SC, Choi YR, Won CK, Leem JW. Activity-dependent conduction latency changes in Ab-fibers in neuropathic rats. Neuroreport 1997;8:2813–6.

65. Greening J, Lynn B. Minor peripheral nerve injuries: an underestimated source of pain? Man Ther 1998;3:187–94.

66. Arendt-Nielsen L, Sonnenborg FA, Andersen OK. Facilitation of the withdrawal reflex by repeated transcutaneous electrical stimulation: an experimental study on central integration in humans. Eur J Appl Physiol 2000;81:165–73.

67. Yaksh TL, Hua XY, Kalcheva I, Nozaki-Taguchi N, Marsala M. The spinal biology in human and animals of pain states generated by persistent small afferent input. Proc Natl Acad Sci 1999;96:7680–6.

68. Andrews K, Baranowski A, Kinnman E. Subthreshold changes without initial pain or alterations in cutaneous blood flow, the area of secondary hyperalgesia caused by topical application of capsaicin in humans. Neurosci Lett 1999; 266:45–8.

69. Alfredson H, Thorsen K, Lorentzon R. In situ microdialysis in tendon tissue: high levels of glutamate, but not prostaglandin E2 in chronic Achilles tendon pain. Knee Surg Sports Traumatol Arthrosc 1999;7:378–81.

70. Bendtsen L, Jensen R, Olesen J. Qualitatively altered nociception in chronic myofascial pain. Pain 1996;65:259–64.

71. Johansen MK, Graven-Nielsen T, Olesen AS, Arendt-Nielsen L. Generalized muscular hyperalgesia in chronic whiplash syndrome. Pain 1999;83:229–34.

72. Sorensen J, Graven-Nielsen T, Henriksson KG, Bengtsson M, Arendt-Nielsen L. Hyperexcitability in fibromyalgia. J Rheumatol 1998;25:152–5.

73. Watkins LR, Maier SF, Goehler LE. Immune activation: the role of pro-inflammatory cytokines inflammation, illness responses and pathological pain states. Pain 1995;63:289–302.

74. Lekander M, Fredrikson M, Wik G. Neuroimmune relations in patients with fibromyalgia: a positron emission tomography study. Neurosci Lett 2000;23:193–6.

75. Jabbur SJ, Saade NE. From electrical wiring to plastic neurons: evolving approaches to the study of pain. Pain 1999;S6:S87–S92.

76. Turrin NP, Plata-Salaman CR. Cytokine-cytokine interactions and the brain. Brain Res Bull 2000;51:3–9.

77. Matre DA, Sinkaer T, Svensson P, Arendt-Nielsen L. Experimental muscle pain increases the human stretch reflex. Pain 1998;75:331–9.

78. Sheather-Reid RB, Cohen ML. Psychophysical evidence for a neuropathic component of chronic neck pain. Pain 1998;75:341–7.

79. Ellis SJ. Tremor and other movement disorders after whiplash-type injuries. J Neurol Neurosurg Psychiatry 1997;63:110–2.

80. Wyke BD. Articular neurology and manipulative therapy. In: Glascow EF, Twomey LT, Scll ER, Idezak RM, editors. Aspects of manipulative therapy. Melbourne: Churchill Livingstone; 1985. p. 72–7.

81. Wenngren BI, Pedersen J, Sjolander P, Bergenheim M, Johannson H. Bradykinin and muscle stretch alter contralateral cat neck muscle spindle output. Neurosci Res 1998;32:119–29.

82. Giacomini P, Magrini A, Sorace F. Changes in posture in whiplash evaluated by static posturography. Acta Otorhino-laryngol Ital 1997;17:409–13.

83. Hinoki M. Vertigo due to whiplash injury: a neurotological approach. Acta Otolaryngol Suppl 1985;419:9–29.

84. Gimse R, Tjell C, Bjorgen IA, Saunte C. Disturbed eye movement after whiplash due to injuries the posture control system. J Clin Exp Neuropsychol 1996;18:178–86.

85. Hinoki M, Hine S, Ushio N, Ishida Y, Koike S. Studies on ataxia of lumbar origin in cases of vertigo due to whiplash injury. Equilibrium Res 1973;3:141–52.

86. Heikklia HV, Wenngren BI. Cervicocephalic kinesthetic sensibility, active range of cervical motion, and oculomotor function in patients with whiplash injury. Arch Phys Med Rehabil 1998;79:1089–94.

87. Mosimann UP, Muri RM, Felblinger J, Radanov BP. Saccadic eye movement disturbances in whiplash patients with persistent complaints. Brain 2000;123:328–50.

88. Gozariu M, Bragard D, Willer JC, Lebars D. Temporal summation of C-fiber afferent input inputs: competition between facilitatory and inhibitory effects on c-fiber reflex in the rat. J Neurophysiol 1997;78:3165–79.

89. Graven-Nielsen T, Babenko V, Svensson P, Arendt-Nielsen L. Experimentally induced muscle pain induces hypoalgesia in heterotopic deep tissues, but not in homotopic deep tissues. Brain Res 1998;787:203–10.

90. Traub RJ. Spinal modulation of the induction of central sensitization. Brain Res 1997;778:34–42.

91. Kharkevich DA, Churukanov VV. Pharmacological regulation of descending cortical control of the nociceptive processing. Eur J Pharmacol 1999;375:121–31.

92. Uhl GR, Sora I, Wang Z. The mu opoiod receptor as a candidate gene for pain: polymorphisms, variations in expression, nociception, and opiate responses. Proc Natl Acad Sci 1999;24:7752–5.

93. Yu W, Hao JX, Xu XJ, Hokfelt T, Elde R, Wiesenfeld-Hallin Z. Spinal cord ischemia reduces µ-opioid receptors in rats: correlation with morphine insensitivity. Neuroreport 1999;10:87–91.

94. Gutstein HB, Mansour A, Watson SJ, Akil H, Fields H. Mu and kappa opioid receptors in periaqueductal gray and rostral ventromedial medulla. Neuroreport 1998;9:1777–81.

95. Hammond DL, Wang H, Nakashima N, Basbaum AI. Differential effects of intrathecally administered delta and mu opioid receptor agonists on formalin-evoked nociception and on the expression of Fos-like immunoreactivity in the spinal cord of the rat. J Pharmacol Exp Ther 1998;284:378–87.

96. Bellgowan PSF, Helmstetter FJ. The role of mu and kappa opioid receptors within the periaqueductal gray in the expression of conditional hypoalgesia. Brain Res 1998;791:83–9.

97. Wei F, Dubner R, Ren K. Nucleus reticularis gigantocellularis and nucleus raphe magnus in the brain stem exert opposite effects on behavioral hyperalgesia and spinal Fos protein expression after peripheral inflammation. Pain 1999;80:127–41.

98. Behbehani NM. Functional characteristics of the midbrain periaqueductal gray. Prog Neurobiol 1995;46:575–605.

99. Wei F, Dubner R, Ren K. Laminar-selective noradrenergic and serotoninergic modulation includes spinoparabrachial cells after inflammation. Neuroreport 1999;10:757–61.

100. Hirakawa N, Tershner SA, Fields HL. Highly & selective antagonists in the RVM attenuate the antinociceptive effect of PAG DAMGO. Neuroreport 1999;10:3125–9.

101. Lovick TA, Parry DM, Stezhka VV, Lumb BM.

Serotonergic transmission in the periaqueductal gray matter in relation to aversive behavior: morphological evidence for direct modulatory effects on identified output neurons. Neuroscience 2000; 95:763–72.

102. Mason P. Central mechanism of pain modulation. Curr Opin Neurobiol 1999;9:436–41.

103. Wall PD, Lidierth M, Hillman P. Brief and prolonged effects Lissauer tract stimulation on dorsal horn cells. Pain 1999;83: 579–89.

104. Gjerstad J, Tjolsen A, Svendsen F, Hole K. Inhibition of C-fibre responses in the dorsal horn after contralateral intramuscular injection of capsaicin activation of descending pathways. Pain 1999;80:413–8.

105. Lin Q, Peng YB, Wu J, Willis WD. Involvement of cGMP in nociceptive processing by and sensitization of spinothalamic neurons in primates. J Neurosci 1997;17:3293–302.

106. Ceranic BJ, Prasher DK, Raglan E, Luxon LM. Tinnitus after head injury: evidence from otoacoustic emissions. J Neurol Neurosurg Psychiatry 1998;65:523–9.

107. Levine RA. Somatic (craniocervical) tinnitus and dorsal cochlear nucleus hypothesis. Am J Otolaryngol 1999;20:351–62.

108. Duncan GH, Kupers RC, Marchand S, Villemure JG, Gybels JM, Bushnell C. Stimulation of human thalamus for pain relief: possible modulatory circuits revealed by positron emission tomography. J Neurophysiol 1998;80:3326–30.

109. Davis KD, Kiss ZHT, Tasker RR, Dostrovsky JO. Thalamic stimulation-evoked sensations in chronic pain patients and nonpain (movement disorders) patients. J Neurophysiol 1996;75:1026–37.

110. Laursen RJ, Graven-Nielsen T, Jensen TS, Arendt-Nielsen L. The effect of differential and complete nerve block on experimental muscle pain in humans. Muscle Nerve 1999;22:1564–70.

111. Hsueh TC, Cheng PT, Kuan TS, Hong CZ. The immediate effectiveness of electrical nerve stimulation and electrical muscle stimulation on myofascial trigger points. Am J Phys Med Rehabil 1997;76:471–6.

112. Cheing GLY, Hui-Chan CWY. Transcutaneous electrical nerve stimulation: nonparallel antinociceptive effects on chronic clinical pain and acute experimental pain. Arch Phys Med Rehabil 1999;80:305–12.

113. Sandkuhler J, Chen JG, Chen G, Randic M. Low-frequency stimulation of afferent A-fibers induces long-term depression at primary afferent synapses with substantia gelatinosa neuron in the rat. J Neurosci 1997;1716:6483–91.

114. Liu XG, Morton CR, Azuke JJ, Zimmerman M, Sandkuhler J. Long-term depression of C-fiber-evoked spinal field potentials by stimulation of primary afferent A-fibers in the adult rat. Eur J Neurosci 1998;10:3069–75.

115. Gjerstad J, Tjolsen A, Svendsen F, Hole K. Inhibition of evoked C-fiber responses in the dorsal horn after contralateral injection of capsaicin involves activation of descending pathways. Pain 1999;80:413–8.

116. Svendsen F, Tjolsen A, Rykkja F, Hole K. Behavioral effects of LTP-inducing sciatic nerve stimulation in the rat. Eur J Pain 1999;3:355–63.

117. Guieu R, Blin O, Pouget J, Serratrice G. Nociceptive threshold and physical activity. Can J Neurol Sci 1992;19:69–71.

118. Herzog W, Scheele D, Conway PJ. Electromyographic responses of back and limb muscles associated with spinal manipulative therapy. Spine 1999;24:146–53.

119. Gillette RG, Kramis RC, Roberts WJ. Suppression of activity in spinal nocireceptive "low back" neurons by paravertebral somatic stimuli in the cat. Neurosci Lett 1998;241:45–8.

120. Terrett ACJ, Vernon H. Activity in nociceptive neurons can be suppressed by somatic stimulation. Am J Phys Med 1984; 63:217–25.

121. Vicenzino B, Cartwright T, Collins D, Wright A. An investigation of stress and pain perception during manual therapy in asymptomatic subjects. Eur J Pain 1999;3:13–8.

122. Bushnell MC, Duncan GH, Hofbauer RK, Ha B, Chen JL, Carrier B. Pain perception: is there a role for primary somatosensory cortex? Proc Natl Acad Sci 1999;96:7705–9.

123. Ploghaus A, Tracey I, Gati JS, Clare S, Menon RS, Matthews PM, et al. Dissociating pain form its anticipation in the human brain. Science 1999;284:1979–81.

124. Coghill RC, Sang CN, Maisog JM, Iadarola MJ. Pain intensity processing within the human brain: a bilateral, distributed mechanism. J Neurophysiol 1999;82:1934–43.

125. Calejesan AA, Kim SJ, Min Zhuo M. Descending facilitatory modulation of a behavioral nociceptive response by stimulation in the adult rat anterior cingulate cortex. Eur J Pain 2000;4:83–96.

126. Kharkevich DA, Churukanov VV. Pharmacological regulation of descending cortical control of the nociceptive processing. Eur J Pharmacol 1999;375:121–31.

127. Carrick R. Changes in brain function after manipulation of the cervical spine. J Manipulative Physiol Ther 1997;20:529–45.

128. Vicenzino B, Collins D, Benson H, Wright A. An investigation of the interrelationship between manipulative therapy-induced hypoalgesia and sympathoexcitation. J Manipulative Physiol Ther 1998;21:448–53.

129. Vernon HT, Dhami MSI, Howley TP, Annett R. Spinal manipulation and beta-endorphin: a controlled study of the effect of a spinal manipulation on plasma beta-endorphin levels in normal males. J Manipulative Physiol Ther 1986;9:115–23.

130. Bruehl S, McCubbin JA, Harden RN. Theoretical review: altered pain regulatory systems in chronic pain. Neurosci Biobehav Rev 1999;23:877–90.

131. Dubner R, Ruda MA. Activity-dependent neuronal plasticity following tissue injury and inflammation. Trends Neurosci 1992;15:96–103.

132. Khan KM, Cook JL, Maffulli N, Kannus P. Where is the pain coming from in tendinopathy? It may be biomechanical, not only structural, in origin. Br J Sports Med 2000;34:81–3.

133. Parkhurst TM, Burnett CN. Injury and proprioception in the lower back. J Orthop Sports Phys Ther 1994;19:282–95.

§ A1:2 Dr. Ferrari's Letter to Editor in Response to Author's Article

To the Editor:

I was initially pleased to read Dr. Davis' theories about the mechanism of chronic pain in patients with whiplash in North America, most particularly his reference to generalized central hyperexcitability from a loss of tonic inhibitory input and/or ongoing excitatory input contributing to dorsal horn hyperexcitability.[1] This phenomenon would perhaps explain the observation that about 35% to 50% of consecutively sampled patients with whiplash in Canadian studies report chronic pain at 6 months after the collision.[2,3] Although I am prepared to explain this theoretical phenomenon to my patients, it occurs to me that it is a wholly unacceptable theory because of its obvious ethnocentrism. The theory is ethnically biased because it excludes most of the whiplash victims in Lithuania, Greece, and Germany who have been studied.

That is, patients with whiplash in prospective studies in Lithuania, Greece, and Germany have been sampled with the same criteria as patients with whiplash in Canadian studies, and they have the very same acute syndrome with the same physical examination findings as identified, for example, in Greece and Germany.[4] Yet after 6 weeks, although many Canadian patients studied are quite willing to developgeneralized central hyperexcitability from a loss of tonic inhibitory input and/or ongoing excitatory input contributing to dorsal horn hyperexcitability, the Lithuanian, Greek, and German patients refused to do so.Indeed, no matter how the patients are collected and studied in North America, there is a sizeable proportion of patients who have chronic pain, and no matter how the patients are selected in Lithuania, Greece, and Germany, they have such a rapid recovery from their injury that they lack the time to developgeneralized centralhyperexcitability from a loss of tonic inhibitory input and/or ongoing excitatory input contributing to dorsal horn hyperexcitability.

I am unclear as to why there should be such an ethnocentric bias to Dr. Davis' approach. Studies have shown, for example, that other chronic pain disorders such as rheumatoid arthritis have the same or worse outcomes in Lithuania as in North America, with a need for extensive therapy and disability programs.[5,6] Lithuanians do not seem to be able to avoid the chronic pain of rheumatoid arthritis (and many other diseases), but they do seem to be able to escape the chronic pain of whiplash to the extent that, if it exists there, it must affect 5% or less according to power analysis. In North America, it affects at least 50% at 6 months. This is a whole order-of-magnitude difference that does not seem to be bridged by dorsal horn hyperexcitability.

The question of how one explains the ethnocentric bias of the theory of hyperexcitability remains; that is, why does it not apply to various cultures? Some have suggested that there are reasons, but this question requires a closer examination of international research.[4]

Finally, there is one other perplexity derived from Dr. Davis' treatise. Do these mechanisms occur in low-velocity collisions? Castro et al,[7] in a recently released publication, have proven that they can produce the acute whiplash syndrome without subjecting the subjects to a collision. That is, they used a placebo collision that fooled the subjects, and acute whiplash syndrome developed in 20% of these previously healthy subjects. If any of them begin to have chronic pain, will it then be correct to assume they have experienced generalized central hyperexcitability from a loss of tonic inhibitory input and/or ongoing excitatory input contributing to dorsal horn hyperexcitability?

-*Dr. Robert Ferrari* 12779-50 Street, Edmonton, Alberta T5A 4L8, Canada

References

1. Davis C. Chronic pain/dysfunction in whiplash-associated disorders. J Manipulative Physiol Ther 2001;24:44–51.

2. Brison RJ, Hartling L, Pickett W. A prospective study of acceleration-extension injuries following rear-end motor vehicle collisions. J Musculoskeletal Pain 2000;8:97–113.

3. Cassidy JD, Caroll L, Cote P, Lemstra M, Berglund A, Nygren A. Effect of eliminating compensation for pain and suffering on the outcome of insurance claims for whiplash injury. N Eng J Med 2000;342:1179–86.

4. Ferrari R, Schrader H. The late whiplash syndrome: A biopsychosocial approach. J Neurol Neurosurg Psychiatry 2001;71:722–6.

5. Dadonlene JH, Uhlig T, Stropuviene S, Venalis A, Boonen A, Kvien TK. Rheumatoid arthritis (RA) patients in Vilnius and Oslo: a comparison regarding disease and health measures. Abstract presented at the 16th EULAR conference. Prague, Czechoslovakia; 2001.

6. Dadonlene JH, Boonen A. Work disability among patients with rheumatoid arthritis in Lithuania. Abstract presented at the 16th EULAR conference. Prague, Czechoslovakia; 2001.

7. Castro WHM, Meyer SJ, Becke MER, Nentwig CG, Hein MF, Ercan BI, et al. No stress—no whiplash? Prevalence of "whiplash" syndromes following exposure to a placebo rear-end collision. Int J Leg Med 2001;114:316–22.

§ A1:3 Author's Response to Dr. Ferrari's Letter

Reprinted from Journal of Manipulative & Physiological

Therapeutics, 25(2):135–138, *Davis, copyright 2002 Mosby, with permission from Elsevier.*

In Response:

A lack of objective data has not prevented Dr. Ferrari from offering an opinion piece.[1] Dr. Ferrari seems to base his opinions on a few flawed studies and arrives at an untestable explanation. He constantly makes comments, writing editorial articles and letters to the editors on almost any study that shows chronic problems after whiplash. In my opinion, his bias is shown by the lack of any critical thinking about the articles on which he relies.

Dr. Ferrari states that the correct model is his proposed biopsychosocial model. That model considers cultural factors, which generate symptom amplification and attribution, as well as the possibility that physical and psychologic causes for symptoms coexist.It negates the concept of chronic injury, which would thus negate the field of neuroscience. This evidently is the basis for his new explanation of ethnocentrism (the concept that the attitudes, beliefs, and customs of one's own group, nation, or people are of central importance and the basis for judging all other groups). Dr. Ferrari's biopsychosocial approach appears to have its genesis in Waddell's nonorganic physical signs in Waddell's low-back pain study.[2] Bradish et al[3] found no correlation between the presence of nonorganic signs at initial assessment and either the return to activity or resolution of the patient's symptoms. These nonorganic signs can be explained by neurologic mechanisms.

Ferrari uses studies that have received considerable criticism. He relies on the Quebec Task Force[4] and studies from Lithuania,[5,6] Greece,[7] and Germany.[8] The problems of the Quebec Task Force findings[9] and studies that reject the notion of chronic problems from whiplash[10] have been addressed. The majority of other studies show that a substantial number of people do have long-term problems with varying degrees of severity. Ferrari now proposes an ethnocentric bias in neuroscience.

From a closer look at the articles he uses for support, it appears that poor studies can and do get published.

The Lithuanian studies recruited subjects from the police station in a former Soviet-controlled country and looked for people who would complain 1 to 3 years after a collision. Eighty-five percent of the participants in these studies were men. Never mind that in many studies there are a greater number of women with chronic complaints. Is this an attempt to eschew real data? In the study in Greece, only 180 people with grade-I and grade-II whiplash who presented to a hospital over a 3-year period were included. Dolinis[11] noted that only 3 out of 254 whiplash subjects had been seen at the emergency room. At this rate, 15,000 subjects did not present to the emergency room. In the study in Germany, a cervical collar was considered a singular therapy. It is evident that the design of the study can influence the outcome.

The ethnocentrism bias Dr. Ferrari proposes is more evidence of the flaws in the Lithuania studies. Do the subjects in Lithuania really escape chronic problems with whiplash? One cannot form a legitimate opinion on the sole basis of these articles. The Lithuanian study was so flawed that the results were not interpretable. The errors in the Lithuanian study that Dr. Ferrari continues to reference are many and fatal, to the point that some who address the shortcomings of the study are asked to become reviewers for that journal.[12]

Merskey[13] has stated that the numbers involved in the Lithuanian study are too few to show a statistical significance. The claim by Schrader et al[5] that late whiplash syndrome "has little validity" is completely unjustified on the basis of their data.

The Lithuanian study by Schrader et al[5] comprised 202 individuals who had been involved in motor vehicle crashes. This cohort was matched for age and sex with a control group of 202 individuals who had no history of a motor vehicle crash. This study was criticized because only a very small proportion of the exposed cohort (15% [31 subjects]) had been injured initially and thus exposed to the putative etiologic agent in late whiplash (an acute whiplash injury). "For the purposes of the current literature critique, a post-hoc sample-size calculation was performed on the data in this study, using an alpha of 0.05 and a beta of 0.20. The smallest detectable difference between the groups was 14.6%. Thus, 94% of the acutely injured subjects (29 of 31) in this study would have had to develop chronic symptoms to enable the authors to detect a statistically significant difference between the 2 groups, an extremely remote possibility. A recalculation of sample size with a meta-analysis-based estimate of effect (expected proportion chronic) of 5% (that is, 33% of the 15% acutely injured subjects) demonstrates that the total study cohort needed to be at least 3000 in order to have sufficient statistical power to discern a significant difference between the two groups."[10] In the second Lithuanian study, the control was slightly worse off than the whiplash group.[6] Is Dr. Ferrari's next proposal that whiplash is therapeutic?

A disconcerting phenomenon is that one poor study is the

genesis of support for another poor study. The hypothesis on which the Saskatchewan researchers based their study was taken from the study in Lithuania, which showed that there was no chronic whiplash in a country where there was no compensation for injury. This study is the entire basis for the hypothesis and speculation from the Saskatchewan researchers, who were entirely funded by Saskatchewan Government Insurance.[14] That article then became the basis to justify their outcome measure, closure of claims.[15] Now these same authors state that the insurance and compensation systems have a large impact on recovery from acute whiplash.[16] Their foundation is as solid as quicksand; however, this is not to say that all insurance-sponsored studies are so biased.

Quality epidemiologic studies are available.[17,18] They contain various cohorts for comparison. These studies show injured subjects have 3 times the rate of problems of noninjured subjects at 7 years.

Dr. Ferrari prefers to use studies that have a 33% to 40% pain level in the control group.[3,4] Perhaps he should use a level of 13% to 14%.[18,19]

Articles should be read along with the abstract presented. A recent article, paid for by an insurance company, stated in the abstract that age over 30, a large amount of damage to the vehicle (half of the vehicle damaged), and admission to the hospital are predictors of long-term treatment for whiplash injury in Japan. One would have to turn the page, however, to find out that the relationship of the degree of vehicle damage to duration of therapy is about the same as that of a vehicle with no damage.[20]

Castro's[21] placebo collision article is another one of those articles. It shows the author's bias,and Dr. Ferrari is grasping at straws in an effort of support. It clearly states in Table 3 that 2 of the 5 subjects did not relate their complaints to the placebo collision. Two others reported symptom duration of 2 days. Only 1 of the 51 had what would be a psychologic profile to fit this phenomenon of a placeboresponse. Is the statement that 20% had whiplash syndrome padding the data?

It is impossible to compare contrived test collisions with real-world collisions. The variables of a real-world situation are too numerous to mention.

Now I am asked to explain the ethnocentric bias of the theory of hyperexcitability and state whether these mechanisms occur in low-velocity collision? In addressing the latter, in complex regional pain syndromes, trivial injury can cause extreme pain. Complex regional pain syndrome can have a mechanism of central nervous system dysfunction,[22] as can chronic whiplash.[23] If the symptoms of a whiplash injury are psychologic and biosocial, physical demands would have no effect on work after injury. However, it has been shown that the greater the physical work demands are, the longer the time off work.[24]

If litigation is such a major factor, why is there no real difference in treatment of litigated and nonlitigated cases?[25,26] The potential for secondary gain does not influence response to treatment. These data contradict the idea that litigation promotes malingering.

Dr. Ferrari also does rheumatologists a disservice by stating that chronic whiplash symptoms do not exist. More studies are showing the importance of the immune system and pain. Immunosuppression is associated with increased pain,[27] and the immune system is involved in the control of inflammatory pain.[28] Hendler et al[29] found that a large number of patients who had been diagnosed with psychogenic pain really had marked pathologic features that were not recognized by the treating physician, because 98% of the patients had an organic origin for their pain complaints.[29]

Pain is only one of the symptoms that should be addressed. There may be nociception without pain. Studies have shown that a decrease in cortical function can lead to a decrease in inhibitory mechanisms.[30,31] Dysfunction may be more important and a better measure than pain, and dysfunction may happen after whiplash without pain.[32–34]

The data once stated that 90% of patients with low back pain would get better in 1 month regardless of treatment. Now we know differently.[35,36] About 75% of patients would relapse. The medical treatment of choice is nonsteroidal anti-inflammatory drugs or that of benign neglect. At best, these treatments might be useful for short-term symptomatic relief.[37] In the end, the patients may seek out treatments they feel are effective.

The flawed basis of certain studies[4-8, 14–16] distorts the reality of the disorder. Dr. Ferrari asserts an ethnocentrism bias by exclusion of the studies from Lithuania, Greece, and Germany. Instead, this is more evidence of the flaws in these studies. The preponderance of the evidence is contrary to Dr. Ferrari's belief. A review of other studies indicates at least a 33% chronic rate after whiplash.[10] There is no rate of chronicity mentioned in the article in question.[38]

Although pain has a subjective component, scientific studies show that different types of nociception serve different functions and give rise to various associated disorders. Victims of motor vehicle collisions with soft-tissue injuries can have both acute pain and chronic pain.

In actuality, people have chronic problems after whiplash. The threshold of such injury can vary widely in terms of the amount of force needed to cause injury and in the symptoms that it produces.[38,39]

-Charles G. Davis, DC 474 S. Citrus, Azusa, CA 91741, USA

References

1. Smythe HA. Rheumatologists and neck pain. Scand J Rheumatol 2000;29:8–12.

2. Waddell G, McCulloch JA, Kummel E, Venner RM. Nonorganic physical signs in low back pain. Spine 1980;5:117–25.

3. Bradish CF, Lloyd GJ, Adam CH, Albert J, Dyson P, Doxey NC, et al. Do nonorganic signs help to predict the return to activity of patients with low back pain? Spine 1988;13:557–60.

4. Spitzer WO, Skovron ML, Salmi RL, Cassidy JD, Duranceau J, Suissa S, et al. Scientific monograph of the Quebec Task Force on whiplash-associated disorders: redefining whiplash and its management. Spine 1995;20(Suppl):S1–73.

5. Schrader H, Obelieniene D, Bovin G, Surkiene D, Mickeviciene D, Miseviciene, et al. Natural evolution of late whiplash syndrome outside the medicolegal context. Lancet 1996;347:1207–11.

6. Obelieniene D, Schrader H, Bovim G, Miseviciene I, Sand T. Pain after whiplash: a prospective controlled inception cohort study. J Neurol Neurosurg Psychiatry 1999;66:279–83.

7. Parthenia M, Constantoyannis C, Ferrari R, Nikifordis G, Voulgaris S, Papadakis N. A prospective cohort study of the outcome of acute whiplash injury in Greece. Clin Exp Rheumatol 2000;18:67–70.

8. Bonk AD, Ferrari R, Giebel GD, Edelmann M, Huser R. Prospective, randomized, controlled study of active versus collar, and the natural history for whiplash injury in Germany. J Musculoskeletal Pain 2000;8:123–32.

9. Freeman MD, Croft AC, Rossignol AM. Whiplash associated disorders: redefining whiplash and its management by the Quebec Task Force. Spine 1998;23:1043–9.

10. Freemn MD, Croft AC, Rossignol AM, Weaver DS,

Reiser M. A review and methodologic critique of the literature refuting whiplash syndrome. Spine 1999;24:86–98.

11. Dolinis J. Risk factors for "whiplash" in drivers: a cohort study of rear-end traffic crashes. Injury 1997;28:173–9.

12. Freeman MD, Croft AC. [Letters]. Lancet 1996;348:125.

13. Merskey H. Whiplash study in Lithuania. Pain Res Manage 1997;2:83.

14. Cassidy JD, Carroll LJ, Cote P, Lemstra M, Berglund A, Nygren A. Effect of eliminating compensation for pain and suffering on the outcome of insurance claims for whiplash injury. N Engl J Med 2000;342:1179–86.

15. Cote P, Hogg-Johnson S, Cassidy JD, Carroll, Frank JW. The association between neck pain intensity, physical functioning, depressive symptomatology and time-to-claim-closure after whiplash. J Clin Epidemiol 2001;54:275–86.

16. Cote P, Cassidy JD, Carroll L, Frank JW, Bombardier C. A systemic review of the progress of acute whiplash and a new conceptual framework to synthesize the literature. Spine 2001;26:E445–58.

17. Berglund A, Alfredsson L, Cassidy JD, Jensen I, Nygren A. The association between exposure to a rear-end collision and future neck or shoulder pain: a cohort study. J Clin Epidemiol 2000;53:1089–94.

18. Berglund A, Alfredsson L, Jenson I, Cassidy JD, Nygren A. The association between exposure to a rear-end collision and future health complaints. J Clin Epidemiol 2001;54:851–6.

19. Ariens GAM, Bongers PM, Hoogendoom WE, Houtman ILD, van der Wal G, van Mechelen W. High quantitative job demands and low coworker support as risk factors for neck pain. Spine 2001;26:1896–903.

20. Hijioka A, Narusawa K, Nakamura T. Risk factors for long-term treatment of whiplash injuries in Japan: analysis of 400 cases. Arch Orthop Trauma Surg 2001;121:490–3.

21. Castro WH, Meyer SJ, Becke ME, Nentwig CG, Hein MF, Ercan BI, et al. No stress—no whiplash? Prevalence of "whiplash" symptoms following exposure to a placebo rear-end collision. Int J Legal Med 2001;114:316–22.

22. Thimineur M, Sood P, Kravitz E, Gudin J, Kitaj M.

Central nervous system abnormalities in complex regional pain syndrome (CRPS): clinical and quantitative evidence of medullary dysfunction. Clin J Pain 1998;14:256–67.

23. Johansen MK, Graven-Nielsen T, Olesen AS, Arendt-Nielsen L. Generalized muscular hyperalgesia in chronic whiplash syndrome. Pain 1999;83:229–34.

24. Gozzard C, Bannister G, Langkamer G, Khan S, Gargan M, Foy C. Factors affecting employment after whiplash injury. J Bone Joint Surg (Br) 2001;83B:506–9.

25. Sapir DA, Gorup JM. Radiofrequency medial branch neurotomy in litigant and nonlitigant patients with cervical whiplash. Spine 2001;26:E268–73.

26. Swartzman LC, Teasell RW, Shapiro AP, McDermid AJ. The effect of litigation status on adjustment to whiplash injury. Spine 1996;21:53–8.

27. Cabot PJ. Immune-derived opioids and peripheral antinociception. Clin Exper Pharm Physiol 2001;28:230–2.

28. Cabot PJ, Carter L, Schafer M, Stein C. Methionine-enkephalin-and dynorphin A-release from immune cells and control of inflammatory pain. Pain 2001;93:207–12.

29. Hendler N, Bergson C, Morrison C. Overlooked physical diagnosis in chronic pain patients involved in litigation, part 2: the addition of MRI, nerve blocks, 3-D CT, and qualitative flow meter. Psychosomatics 1996;37:509–17.

30. Mosimann UP, Muri RM, Felblinger J, Radanov BP. Saccadic eye movement disturbance in whiplash patients with persistent complaints. Brain 2000;123:828–35.

31. Freitag P, Greenlee MW, Wachter K, Ettlin TM, Radue EW. MRI response during visual motion stimulation in patients with late whiplash syndrome. Neurorehabil Neural Repair 2001;15:31–7.

32. Gimse R, Tjell C, Bjorgen IA, Saunte C. Disturbed eye movement due to injuries to the posture control system. J Clin Exp Neuropsychol 1996;18:178–86.

33. Hildingsson C, Weengren BI, Bring G, Toolanen G. Oculomotor problems after cervical spine injury. Acta Orthop Scand 1989;60:513–6.

34. Kessels RPC, Aleman A, Verhagen WIM, Van Luijtelaar ELJM. Cognitive functioning after whiplash injury: a meta anlaysis. J Int Neuropsychol Soc 2000;6:271–8.

35. Croft PR, Macfarlane GJ, Papageorgiou AC, Thomas

E, Silman AJ. Outcome of low back pain in the general practice: a prospective study. BMJ 1998;316:1356–9.

36. van den Hoogen HJ, Koes BW, van Eijk JTM, Bouter LM, Deville W. On the course of low back pain in general practice: a one year follow up study. Ann Rheum Dis 1998;57:13–9.

37. Koes BW, Scholten RJPM, Mens JMA, Bouter LM. Efficacy of non-steroidal anti-inflammatory drugs for low back pain: a systemic review of randomized clinical trials. Ann Rheum Dis 1997;56:214–23.

38. Davis C. Chronic pain/dysfunction in whiplash-associated disorders. J Manipulative Physiol Ther 2001;24:44–51.

39. Davis CG. Injury threshold: whiplash-associated disorders. J Manipulative Physiol Ther 2000;23:420–7.

APPENDIX 2

INSURANCE RESEARCH INSTITUTE'S CLAIMS BEHAVIOR STUDY

With respect to bodily injury claims, the questions of "How much treatment is enough?" and "When did the patient reach MMI (Maximum Medical Improvement)?" are often hotly contested in litigation.

In a recent study of insurance claims by the Insurance Research Council (IRC), *Analysis of Auto Injury Insurance Claims in Four Tort States, the Council* examined auto injury claims behavior in California, Illinois, Texas, and Washington. Comparing auto injury claims from these four tort states, IRC found that California claimants go to chiropractors most often, Illinois claimants are most likely to see an emergency room physician, and Washington claimants are most likely to go to general practitioners, as well as alternative medical providers, such as massage therapists. From 1997 to 2002, per-claimant medical expenses increased the most in Texas, compared with the other three states.

The IRC study examined detailed information from auto injury claims that closed with payment in the four states with similar auto insurance regulations. Key findings from the study revealed the following differences and similarities among bodily injury liability (BI) claims in these four states:

- In each of the four states, neck or back sprains were the most serious injury for at least seven in ten BI claimants and at least three-quarters suffered no disability from the accident.
- In California, 57 percent of BI claimants went to a chiropractor compared with 28 percent in Illinois, 43 percent in Texas, and 46 percent in Washington.
- More than half (53 percent) of California BI claimants' medical fees came from chiropractors, compared with 26 percent in Illinois, and 44 percent in both Texas and Washington.
- From 1997 to 2002, average claimed medical expenses increased by 39 percent in Texas, compared with 25

percent in California, 24 percent in Illinois, and 9 percent in Washington. Over this same time period, medical cost inflation was 22 percent, according to the CPI.

Similar patterns emerged in first-party medical payments (MP) claims in California and Illinois, along with personal injury protection (PIP) claims in Texas and Washington.

In all four states, average BI payments exceeded claimed economic losses, reflecting auto insurance payments for general damages, sometimes referred to as pain and suffering. In 2002, claimed economic losses, mainly consisting of medical expenses, were highest in Illinois and California BI claims, averaging $5,506 and $5,409 respectively. The corresponding average insurance payments to BI claimants were $7,850 in Illinois and $7,830 in California. In comparison with these two states, Texas claimants averaged lower reported economic losses ($4,483) and BI payments ($5,768). Washington BI claimants' economic losses averaged $3,833, the lowest of the four states. However, average BI payments were $7,594 in Washington, near the levels in Illinois and California.

Copies of the complete study are available at $100 each in the U.S. ($115 elsewhere) postpaid from the Insurance Research Council, 718 Providence Rd., Malvern, Pa. 19355-0725. IRC's Web site at www.ircweb.org.

Table of Laws and Rules

CALIFORNIA CODE OF REGULATIONS

Table of Cases

B

Beresford v. Pacific Gas & Elec. Co., 45 Cal. 2d 738, 290 P.2d 498, 54 A.L.R.2d 910 (1955)—14:10

C

Clemente v. Blumenberg, 183 Misc. 2d 923, 705 N.Y.S.2d 792 (Sup 1999)—4:4, 14:5, 14:7

Culpepper v. Volkswagen of America, Inc., 33 Cal. App. 3d 510, 109 Cal. Rptr. 110 (4th Dist. 1973)—14:10

D

Davis v. Maute, 770 A.2d 36 (Del. 2001)—14:5, 14:7

Dunshee v. Douglas, 255 N.W.2d 42 (Minn. 1977)—4:1

F

Fishman v. Silva, 116 Cal. App. 1, 2 P.2d 473 (1st Dist. 1931)—14:10

Francis v. Sauve, 222 Cal. App. 2d 102, 34 Cal. Rptr. 754 (1st Dist. 1963)—14:10

H

Harrison v. Smith, 2008 WL 2673831 (Cal. App. 1st Dist. 2008)—14:10

J

Johnston v. Peairs, 117 Cal. App. 208, 3 P.2d 617 (4th Dist. 1931)—14:10

K

Kling v. City and County of Denver, 138 Colo. 567, 335 P.2d 876 (1959)—4:11

P

People v. Kelly, 17 Cal. 3d 24, 130 Cal. Rptr. 144, 549 P.2d 1240 (1976)—4:4

R

Rudat v. Carithers, 137 Cal. App. 92, 30 P.2d 435 (3d Dist. 1934)—14:10

Runyon v. Geldner, 237 Va. 460, 377 S.E.2d 456 (1989)—14:10

S

Schultz v. Wells, 13 P.3d 846 (Colo. Ct. App. 2000)—14:3

T

Tittsworth v. Robinson, 252 Va. 151, 475 S.E.2d 261 (1996)—14:5, 14:7

Index